EXPERIMENT IN CHANGE

An Interdisciplinary Approach to the
Integration of Psychiatric Content
in Baccalaureate Nursing Education

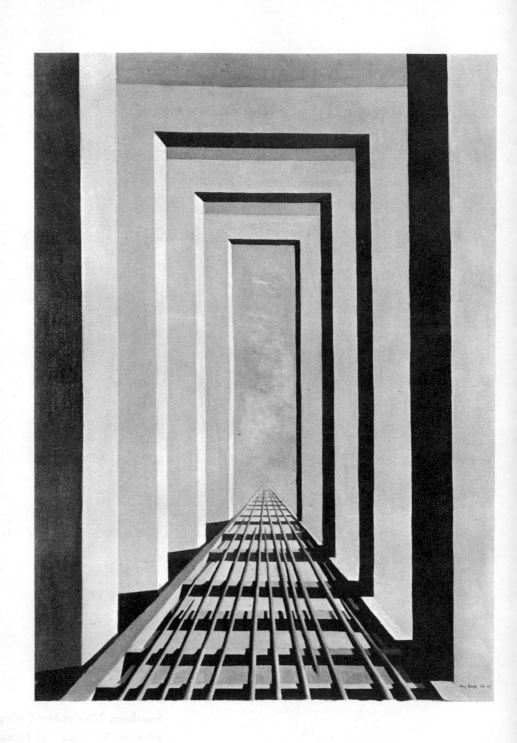

EXPERIMENT IN CHANGE

*An Interdisciplinary Approach
to the Integration
of Psychiatric Content in
Baccalaureate
Nursing Education*

JANE A. SCHMAHL

4757

The Macmillan Company, New York
Collier-Macmillan Limited, London

WY
18
.S348e
1966

FIRST PRINTING

LIBRARY OF CONGRESS CATALOG CARD NUMBER: 66–23792

THE MACMILLAN COMPANY, NEW YORK
COLLIER-MACMILLAN CANADA, LTD., TORONTO, ONTARIO

PRINTED IN THE UNITED STATES OF AMERICA

CREDITS

Appreciation is expressed to Mr. and Mrs. Hugh Chisholm for permission to reproduce as a frontispiece the painting *Detour*, by Kay
Sage, which is from their private collection.

Grateful acknowledgment is made also to the following authors
and publishers who have generously granted me permission to reprint
excerpts from their publications:

Albert & Charles Boni, for an excerpt from *The Woman of Andros* by
Thornton Wilder, copyright, 1930.
Harper & Row, Publishers, Inc., for an excerpt from *Tomorrow and
Tomorrow and Tomorrow* by Aldous Huxley, copyright, 1959.
Alfred A. Knopf, Inc., for an excerpt from *Resistance, Rebellion and
Death* by Albert Camus, copyright, 1960.
Walter Lippmann, for an excerpt from "Leadership and Opinion," in
The Essential Lippmann, published by Random House, copyright,
1962.
Arthur Miller, for an excerpt from *After The Fall*, published by Viking
Press, Inc., copyright, 1964.
National League for Nursing, for excerpts from "The Three Phases of
Psychiatric Integration in Nursing Education," by Jane A. Schmahl
and Montague Ullman, in *Integration of Psychiatric Nursing Concepts
in Baccalaureate Basic Programs*, 1963.
Simon and Schuster, Inc., for an excerpt from *Attorney for the
Damned* by Clarence Darrow, edited by Arthur Weinberg, copyright,
1957; and for an excerpt from *The Open Mind* by J. Robert Oppen-
heimer, copyright, 1955.
Society of Authors, London, for an excerpt from *Man and Superman*
by George Bernard Shaw, published by Dodd, Mead, and Company.

TO AGNES GELINAS,
whose courage made the experiment in change
and this book possible.

But man is a frivolous and incongruous creature, and perhaps, like a chess player, loves the process of the game, not the end of it. And who knows (there is no saying with certainty), perhaps the only goal on earth to which mankind is striving lies in this incessant process of attaining, in other words, in life itself, and not in the thing to be attained, which must always be expressed as a formula, as positive as twice two makes four, and such positiveness is not life, gentlemen, but is the beginning of death.

FYODOR DOSTOYEVSKY, *Notes from Underground.*

FOREWORD

I have read this book with great interest. Anyone who wants to learn about the numerous difficulties and satisfactions of conducting a project in the integration of psychiatric concepts in one basic collegiate program in nursing will find that these difficulties and satisfactions are fully described here. This book is an account of a great human and professional endeavor on the part of a psychiatric nurse and a psychiatrist. Through their efforts, the faculty gained knowledge of psychiatric principles and skill in formulating these principles and applying them to their teaching. The psychiatric team also helped the students to develop the ability to use psychiatric theory in their care of patients.

The integration project was particularly helpful to the faculty and the students in achieving self-understanding. They discovered that knowledge of the self is essential for understanding the problems of others. Some of the faculty members mentioned that it had been difficult if not impossible for them to know their own minds and to assert their rights. They were helped to take stock of themselves, to achieve a realistic perception of their self-worth, and to overcome some of the obstacles to their professional growth.

The faculty members and the students learned a great deal about their attitudes and feelings and those of the patients and families they served. Anger was found to be one of the most commonly experienced feelings in the life of the nurse teacher and nursing student. Another insight that was achieved by the faculty and the students was their recognition of the existence of anxiety in themselves. That every human being, from time to time, is anxious came as a surprise to some.

The work groups in which the participants sought to help one another in the exploration of feelings, attitudes, thoughts, and ideas were one of the most useful experiences in the integration project. Gradually, the members became committed to the idea of examining their professional attitudes and acquired enough courage to share thoughts and feelings that ordinarily are not aired in the presence of others. They were allowed to move at their own pace. There were many rewards of this group experience, but the greatest reward was the spirit of trust, compassion, and comradeship that gradually developed among the faculty and the students.

The straightforward approach and the comprehensiveness of this account should provide other schools of nursing with a picture of psychiatric integration that is in realistic perspective. Although the author has analyzed the process of integrating psychiatric concepts in but one baccalaureate basic program, the mode of problem solving and analysis should be useful to other schools of nursing. In view of the historical importance of this book, the depth and scope of its content, and its vigorous style, one has a first-rate work.

AGNES GELINAS,
Former Chairman,
Skidmore College,
Department of Nursing
New York, New York

PREFACE

This book is an account of the first five years of a study undertaken by the Skidmore College Department of Nursing to investigate and demonstrate the ways in which the various resources at the department's command could be utilized to foster the student's awareness of psychiatric concepts and techniques and to help her apply them in the nursing care of all patients. This study afforded an unusual opportunity for exploring various methods of teaching psychiatric concepts and for collecting data about the processes involved in the incorporation of this teaching in various courses of the curriculum.

The study was supported by a grant from the National Institute of Mental Health (U.S. Department of Health, Education, and Welfare, Grant No. 5–T2–MH–6376). It was carried out under the leadership of a team consisting of myself, as project director, and Montague Ullman, M.D., a psychiatrist.

The project began in February, 1957, when Dr. Ullman and I joined the Skidmore faculty on a part-time basis. The following September, I became a full-time faculty member and continued working on the project as such through July, 1962, when the original grant expired. A second grant permitted the continuation of the project, and I continued to work on the project during the sixth year. It is now in operation under other psychiatric nurse leadership.

This book is based on my experiences and observations during the five-year period from July, 1957, to July, 1962. Like any book, it is also the reflection of the author's total experiences in living. Some of the professionally formative influences that have stamped their imprint on it are the pioneer work of Hildegard E. Peplau, who has clarified the professional nursing role within the context of interpersonal processes—a contribution that has helped to move nursing further toward full professional status; the theoretical formulations of Erich Fromm, Karen Horney, and Harry Stack Sullivan, who have clarified many of the complexities of interpersonal processes within the social context; the contributions of Sigmund Freud, the father of psychoanalysis; the studies of Robert F. Bales, Kurt K. Lewin, Talcott Parsons, and John P. Spiegel, who have made considerable progress in the clarification of the concept of role and group-interaction processes, and the theory of social systems and social change; the communication theory of Jurgen Reusch; the contributions of Nathaniel Cantor, John Dewey, Arthur T. Jersild, Earl C. Kelley and Marie Rasey, and Charlotte Towle, who have studied the role of education in fostering personal change and growth; and the numerous studies in liaison psychiatry by Myer Mendelson and Eugene C. Meyer.

Equally significant are the influences of my psychoanalysis as well as the experiences of study, including supervision of my own psychiatric nursing practice, teaching, and professional relationships with Irene Carn, Gertrude Cherescavich, Mary Carrigan Cronin, Mae Davey, Esther A. Garrison, Sidney S. Goldensohn, Harold Hiatt, Hildegard E. Peplau, Edith Roberts, Daniel Shapiro, Robert E. Switzer, Montague Ullman, William F. Weber, and Charlotte Woehrmann. Finally, I should mention my years as a faculty member at Seton Hall University, School of Nursing; Skidmore College, Department of Nursing; and currently at the William Alanson White Institute of Psychiatry, Psychoanalysis and Psychology, the first psycho-analytic institute to offer courses specifically designed for nurses working in psychiatric settings. My experiences in teaching and clinical practice during these years provided me with an ongoing stream of inspiration from faculty members, students, patients, and clinical personnel.

While writing this book, I quickly became aware that the real meaning of psychiatric integration in nursing can never be precisely or completely ex-pressed in words, because its essence is an experience, a process, a relation-ship, a dynamic force. It is a teaching and learning process and, as such, it is to be understood as living. Psychiatric integration is not what is written in this volume or anywhere else.

What, then, is this book about? In a broad sense, this book is about an educational movement in nursing. It also presents a partial profile of the organizational structure of today's American college and it identifies some of the problems of nursing education when it becomes part of the college social system. More specifically, it is a description of how a study of cur-riculum and teaching functions was transformed into a participant-observa-tional study of intrafaculty, faculty-student, and student-patient interaction. It is an analysis of the process by which Dr. Ullman and I developed into an interdisciplinary team.

In addition, it consists of a series of scenes and emotional experiences so vivid to me that they seem to be happening in the present. It is the story of the satisfactions and the disappointments, the aspirations and the longings, the conflicts and the resistance to change, the joy in achievement, and the frustration and pain of the unfulfillment of needs of a group of faculty members and students who come together in the struggle to improve nursing practice and education. It is a personal account of how their attitudes, reactions, and experiences operate as conjunctive or disjunctive forces in the process of learning to apply psychiatric concepts, and of how these forces are handled.

It is about the faculty member and student who sit in my office and reveal the human emotions of sadness, joy, anger, fear, despair, hope, and love. It is about me as I work to grasp the full meaning of their experience, and about the sense of responsibility, the frustration, and the self-doubt that often accompany my effort to understand and accept them. It is about me as I bump into the wall of loneliness that I erect when I feel lost from my peers. It is about my satisfaction and joy in becoming a dynamic force in the process of professional change and growth.

This book is also about my psychiatrist partner and me as we enter into the complex endeavor of integrating psychiatric concepts in a nursing curriculum. It is about our shared conviction that to deal with psychiatric concepts solely on an intellectual level is a lifeless process, devoid of the meaning and richness of experience and therefore of little worth in changing values and behavior.

It is the story of how we are influenced by the learning experience of which we are a part. It is about us both as we try to teach, supervise, collaborate, confer, administer, only to realize that we can never be the same as we were. It is a running commentary on the steps in our development as a collaborative team and on the ways we handle difficulties that arise.

Lastly, this book represents the accomplishment of what at times has seemed an insurmountable task. In preparing it I have had to face the fact that words are at best a poor counterfeit of the dynamic process which Dr. Ullman and I experienced with our faculty colleagues, with our students, and with each other. More than that, I have had to relive certain experiences which forced me to undergo the anxiety of personal change. Some of these experiences were so painful that they were almost unreportable; for example, at one point I seriously questioned my ability to complete the chapter on interdisciplinary teamwork and was tempted to say, "The devil take the hindmost."

These colleagues and students, who speak through this book, must remain anonymous. Accordingly, fictitious names are used throughout. Some of the faculty members and students, however, may be able to identify themselves and each other. They will need to keep in mind that this book is concerned not with the particular difficulties of individual persons, but with an educational institution and the problems in psychiatric integration.

This account is controversial, as I think it should be. Any effort to conceal difficulties, failures, and value judgments behind laundered words and ambiguous charts and tables would have been unfortunate. Feelings and attitudes should do more than serve as grist for the statistical mill. The department of nursing in which we worked has been a pioneer in baccalaureate education for nursing. From its inception it has been concerned with helping students to grow professionally and personally. In particular, it has put emphasis on helping them to learn to handle effectively the behavior of patients and their families. Its problems to some degree are shared by other collegiate schools of nursing. If they have been accentuated, it is with the conviction that learning more about them, even just facing up to their existence, is the first step toward change. Many of the situations encountered were modified during our association with the project. Perhaps others will be rectified as a consequence of this book.

The reader will also need to keep in mind that in a detailed description of what goes on among faculty and nursing students in the process of psychiatric integration, those aspects which work well tend to be taken for granted and may escape mention. Difficulties, on the other hand, are likely to be more conspicuous than the positive aspects and are easier to write about. It becomes the reader's task to make the necessary adjustments. Many of the findings are also colored by relative subjectivity; other members of the faculty and the student groups might have perceived a particular experience in an entirely different light.

However, to anticipate possible misgivings about the validity of this subjective account for the field of psychiatric integration generally, there is no reason for one psychiatric nurse educator to publish a volume of her own experiences unless it offers something of value to other nurses. It is through the awareness and use of psychiatric concepts and their workability in situations involving other people that these personal experiences become validated. This validation makes it possible for others who are similarly involved to put these experiences to use.

This book, then, has been written for all nurses who are concerned with the broader application of psychiatric concepts. In particular, it should be of interest to teachers and administrators, both in nursing service and in nursing education. It might also be generally helpful to members of the medical and other allied professions and to educators and administrators working in all graduate and undergraduate programs. It should be useful as a tool in in-service education.

It should be emphasized, however, that this book does not provide a stencil of values by which to assess the process of psychiatric integration. Should the reader assume that it is a substitute for experience, it will have failed. And should it provide a magical formula by which dead words are fed to teachers and students of nursing without producing an awareness that these words represent living thoughts that evolved and grew out of actual experiences, it might better not have been written. If, on the other hand, this book functions as a steppingstone to an experience which frees capacity for professional growth, if it excites the curiosity, interest, and imagination of some nurses to delve more deeply into the experience itself—then it will have realized its goal.

JANE A. SCHMAHL
New York, New York

ACKNOWLEDGMENTS

Appreciation is expressed first to the National Institute of Mental Health for having supported the psychiatric integration project with a grant.

Special thanks are due to Skidmore College for the academic freedom that allowed Dr. Ullman and me to test our ideas. I am indebted to Agnes Gelinas, former chairman of the department of nursing, and Val H. Wilson, the late president of Skidmore College, who made it possible for me to take a one-year partial leave, thereby providing the opportunity to begin the preparation of this book. Agnes Gelinas also read the entire manuscript before its publication and she offered many valuable suggestions and generously agreed to write the Foreword. I am grateful to the Danferth Fund which financed the transcription of the tape recordings of faculty and student discussions. My thanks to Shirley B. Knight, registrar of Skidmore College; Edgar R. Sather, formerly chaplain of the college; Frances E. Vernon, director of the vocational office; and Phyllis Hermann Voss, director of admissions, for their interest and cooperation in providing me with much of the data that are used in describing the nursing student population.

My deepest gratitude is expressed to the faculty and students, who, besides participating in the project, gave generously of their time and effort in individual interviews and expressed their willingness to be quoted or paraphrased. It is their voices that are heard in this account, and essentially it is they who have created it.

Much of the project's success can be attributed to my professional colleague, co-pilot, and friend, Montague Ullman, with whom I experienced for the first time the full significance of interdisciplinary collaboration, and who not only reviewed the entire manuscript, but also added an extra dimension to this book by writing Chapter 14.

I wish to express my gratitude to Elizabeth V. Cunningham for her important contribution not only in helping to edit this volume but also for her encouragement and sense of humor during the trying days of revision. The burdensome task of typing successive drafts of the manuscript was performed at various times by Elaine Fox, Joann Kirtland, and Hadley Smith. Thanks to Mrs. Smith, who also transcribed, from tape recordings, numerous faculty and student group protocols.

I wish to acknowledge my indebtedness to Miltiades L. Zaphiropoulos for providing invaluable suggestions about "The Argument" and Chapter 1 of this volume, to Elizabeth Maloney for her useful comments on Chapter 7, and to Esther A. Garrison for providing the information concerning the historical background and development of federal support of psychiatric integration projects in generic baccalaureate nursing programs. I am also indebted to my friend and former psychoanalyst teaching partner in psychiatric nursing at the William Alanson White Institute, William F. Weber, for his scientific critique of the entire manuscript and his valuable suggestions.

From the beginning of the writing of this book, my dear friend and former colleague at Seton Hall University School of Nursing, Mary Carrigan Cronin, generously provided an exacting critique of every aspect of the work. I am grateful for her enduring support and encouragement in the arduous task of bringing this book to its completion.

Although all this expert assistance was invaluable, the responsibilty for the ideas expressed in this book, except where they have been directly quoted, of course, is mine.

CONTENTS

THE ARGUMENT

As psychiatric nurses throughout the country have been exploring and experimenting with methods of integrating psychiatric concepts in nursing education, certain frequently raised issues have become a source of concern and controversy and have created considerable confusion. Some of the questions that have been raised are tangential to psychiatric integration and tend to blur what otherwise might serve as a legitimate focus for investigation. Others, however, are directly relevant and when cast into more precise terms form a basis for discussion that may shed light on psychiatric integration as an educational concept and clarify some problems inherent in its implementation. Before the focus and crucial aspects of the Skidmore project are discussed, consideration of several of these issues is in order.

PRIORITY OF NEEDS

The first issue is, in a manner of speaking, an ethical one for the nurse prepared at the advanced level to teach psychiatric nursing or to function as a clinical expert. The need for such nurses far exceeds the supply, and the question inevitably arises of where she should make her contribution. Catherine M. Norris has declared that psychiatric nurses are supposedly dedicated to improving the care of psychiatric patients, and she questions how such care can be improved "when the energies of so large a number of the leadership group are dissipated in other than psychiatric settings" (6). She has suggested that one of the reasons for the psychiatric nurse's interest in integration may be her feelings of hopelessness about the psychiatric patient and that the psychiatric nurse may be using integration as a respectable way of avoiding the problem.

We cannot limit our definition of those needing psychiatrically oriented nursing care to patients in psychiatric settings. Any psychiatric nurse has but to spend some time on the medical, surgical, obstetric, and pediatric services of a general hospital or in a chronic-disease hospital to recognize the need for such nursing care in these areas. She will recognize, also, that

1

the volume of this need exceeds by many times the amount of care that can be provided by psychiatric nurses—that is, nurses with advanced preparation in psychiatric nursing. How, then, is psychiatric nursing to encompass such a wide area of need?

As early as 1919, Sigmund Freud faced similar problems in the practice of psychoanalysis (2). He pointed out that because of the length of time involved in psychoanalytic treatment, the relatively prohibitive cost of such treatment, and the insufficient number of trained practitioners, psychoanalysts would never be able to treat more than a handful of people. Consequently, the psychoanalyst was faced with the task of adapting his theory and technique to the needs of a greater number of patients and the community at large. Freud said (2),

> It is very probable, too, that the application of our therapy to numbers will compel us to alloy the pure gold of analysis plentifully with the copper of direct suggestion, and even hypnotic influence might find a place in it again, as it has in the treatment of war-neuroses. But whatever form this psychotherapy for the people may take, whatever the elements out of which it is compounded, its most effective and most important ingredients will assuredly remain those borrowed from strict psychoanalysis which serves no ulterior purpose.

In addition to the need to find a way of applying his therapy to numbers, Freud might have mentioned the importance of reaching as many patients as possible during the early stages of their illnesses. At the time he wrote, this problem was enhanced by the fact that psychiatry was treated as the stepchild of medicine. Generally, the psychiatrist was called upon to help only when the patient was thought to be "insane." Early detection of an emotional problem was in most cases impossible because the patient's physician could not recognize it until it had become a hot brick which he could no longer handle.

During World War II, the need to enlist the assistance of all members of the medical profession in dealing with psychiatric problems was recognized, and after the war medical education became engaged in major curriculum revisions designed to incorporate into it both the humanities and psychiatric concepts. Another development aimed at extending the benefits of psychiatric knowledge is what the medical profession identifies as the practice of *liaison psychiatry*. Liaison psychiatry is concerned with the psychological vicissitudes of patients who are admitted to general hospitals primarily because of a medical or surgical condition (4, 5). Not only does it attempt to curtail mental decompensation, but it brings psychiatry into the mainstream of medicine.

Have not these developments in medicine some relevance to nursing? Should not the future professional nurse, like the physician, be prepared and helped to utilize psychiatric knowledge in her nursing practice? If so, it seems overzealous to assume that when psychiatric nurse educators alloy the pure gold of nursing the patients in psychiatric settings with the copper of psychiatric integration, they are foregoing their responsibility to emotionally disturbed patients.

It might also be pointed out that the psychiatric nurse in an integration program may, in actuality, be making a signal contribution to the elimination of what many consider the chief obstacle to the improvement of the psychiatric patient's care—the lack of professional nursing personnel in psychiatric facilities. The adage, "You can attract more flies with honey than with vinegar," has particular relevance for recruiting psychiatric nurses. How does a nurse become interested in working with psychiatric patients? What is the individual nurse's frame of reference? Is it not likely that nurses may become more interested in working with psychiatric patients if such work is presented in its global significance for all nursing?

EDUCATIONAL PLACEMENT

A second issue is raised by those nursing educators who question the educational validity of psychiatric integration projects at the baccalaureate level on the grounds that such projects do not strike at the core of the problem and hence are only patchwork. Norris, for example, has questioned where psychiatric integration programs should be initiated—on the preservice or graduate level of education or in inservice education programs. If psychiatric integration should be undertaken in basic education, she has asked, "How can a faculty member supervise the student in the application of psychiatric concepts in the nursing care of patients if she has not learned them herself?" (6).

Norris has further asked, "If the integrator is going into the clinical situation to supervise students, what does this do to the teacher-student relationship, and how are competitive relationships to be avoided?" If on the other hand, integration is approached through the inservice education of the faculty, she has inquired how faculty members who already are overloaded with professional commitments can have much investment, energy, and interest left for learning to apply and teach psychiatric concepts in patient care.

Her solution is offered in the rhetorical question, "Why don't we teach the nurse teacher *how to teach* nursing in masters programs?" In other words, she has perceived the existence of psychiatric integration programs at the baccalaureate level as the result of inadequate preparation of the nurse teacher and has identified the employment of psychiatric nurse integrators as an admission of this fact.

Most nursing educators would agree that master's education in nursing has a checkered history of successes and failures in adequately preparing nurse teachers. This dilemma, however, is not unique to nursing education.

For years, general education has been harassed by and has struggled with the same problems of teacher preparation. In what can be considered the most revolutionary report ever to have been written on the education of American teachers, James Bryant Conant has delivered a serious blow to the current methods, content, and structure of teacher preparation (1). His recommendations strike at the core of the educational framework, and their implementation requires nothing less than total reconstruction of graduate education.

Whatever our hopes for the future of master's education in nursing, the fact remains that many of today's teachers of nursing have not had the advantage of an education that has prepared them to apply psychiatric content in the practice and teaching of their own clinical area. How are they to get such preparation so that they can teach their students truly professional nursing? This question is, admittedly, a complicated one, and the answer to it is not going to emerge miraculously like Athena with full panoply from Zeus's head. Psychiatric integration projects, however, seem to offer one temporary solution if the psychiatric nurse utilizes the opportunity to share her knowledge and skill with other nurse faculty members. In other words, psychiatric integration should not be considered a substitute for improved master's education in nursing, but rather, a way of handling the effects of inadequate nurse-teacher preparation until much-needed improvements are brought about.

This is not to say that the psychiatric nurse should attempt to help the profession by taking the "total responsibility of trying to upgrade all of nursing" (6). Nurse teachers in other areas must do their part and learn to apply and teach the application of psychiatric concepts in their areas of specialty. If other faculty members consider the psychiatric nurse to be one who pulls their chestnuts out of the fire for them, doing what they should learn to do, then integration programs become a block to any lasting change and growth. The psychiatric nurse should not leave psychiatric patients merely to spoonfeed nurse teachers; she should provide the nutriment of psychiatric knowledge with which they can feed themselves.

THE VALUE OF PSYCHIATRIC INTEGRATION

Many nurses question whether psychiatric integration programs are worth all the time, effort, and money required, including the wear and tear on faculty and the psychiatric nurse teacher. This question is difficult to answer, because psychiatric integration is a learning process that continues over a long period of time. The change it effects is elusive and its validation is difficult in any circumstance and probably impossible within a short period of time.

Nonetheless, the question of yield vis-à-vis expenditure is so important that it should not be entirely sidestepped, even though a complete answer to it is not possible. Those who have invested heavily in psychiatric integration programs have given the subject deep thought, and their conclusions should have some validity. In the case of one such person, the first director of the psychiatric integration project of the Skidmore College Department of Nursing, this analysis has led to a book—this book. In it may be found an account of the costs and benefits which, in the author's opinion, might be charged against or credited to the Skidmore program during the first five years of its existence. It remains for each reader to examine this ledger and come to his own conclusion about whether the Skidmore integration project, during these five years, was worth the price, and possibly to use the findings in evaluating the potential worth of psychiatric integration projects in baccalaureate degree programs in nursing throughout the country.

REFERENCES

1. Conant, James Bryant. *The Education of American Teachers.* New York: McGraw-Hill Book Company, 1963.

2. Freud, Sigmund. "Turnings in the Ways of Psychoanalytic Therapy," *Collected Papers,* Vol. II. London: The Hogarth Press and the Institute of Psychoanalysis, 1924, p. 402.

3. *Integration of Psychiatric Nursing Concepts in Baccalaureate Basic Programs.* New York: National League for Nursing, 1963.

4. Meyer, Eugene. "Disturbed Behavior on Medical and Surgical Wards: A Training and Research Opportunity" in Jules H. Masserman (ed.), *Science and Psychoanalysis: Psychoanalytic Education,* Vol. V. New York: Grune and Stratton, 1962, pp. 181–196.

5. Meyer, Eugene and Myer Mendelson. "Psychiatric Consultations with Patients on Medical and Surgical Wards: Patterns and Processes," *Psychiatry,* **24,** 197–220 (August 1, 1961).

6. Norris, Catherine, M. "The Concept of Integration," *Integration of Psychiatric Nursing Concepts in Baccalaureate Basic Programs.* New York: National League for Nursing, 1963, pp. 18, 20.

PART I

THE
BACKGROUND
OF THE
EXPERIMENT

Chapter One

THE POTENTIAL OF
PROFESSIONAL NURSING

═══════════════════════════

> . . . we must respond to each new challenge, not with our old conditioning, not in the light of conceptual knowledge based on the memory of past and different events . . . but with a consciousness stripped naked and as though newborn. . . . It is our conditioning which develops our consciousness; but in order to make full use of this developed consciousness, we must start by getting rid of the condition which developed it.

> ALDOUS HUXLEY, "Knowledge and Understanding,"
> *Tomorrow and Tomorrow and Tomorrow.*

When, in 1957, the Skidmore College Department of Nursing initiated its psychiatric integration project, it joined the vanguard of a search by many baccalaureate degree programs in nursing for ways in which resources could be more fully utilized in helping their students to learn how to deal with the emotional and social problems of all patients. According to Esther A. Garrison, between 1954, when the first project of this kind was inaugurated, and 1965, the federal government made grants to 119 colleges and universities for such projects, and foundations provided support for an unknown number of others. During this period, the federal grants alone amounted to approximately $11 million (3). If in addition to this sum the foundation donations and the college and university contributions in the form of faculty time are taken into consideration, it is probable that the investment to date in psychiatric integration totals in the neighborhood of $20 million.

These figures challenge those who have been engaged in these projects to explain the need for this comparatively new movement. Has it been brought about by a recently discovered addition to the professional nurse's

9

role—an addition that requires a new kind of preparation? If not, why is it necessary to change or add to the preparation that was provided her in former years? The answers to these questions lie in the evolutionary development of the roles of both physicians and nurses and in the history of psychiatric nursing education.

Developments in the Roles of Physician and Nurse

THE PRESCIENTIFIC ERA

Emotional support for the patient was one of the earliest functions of both medicine and nursing. Until some decades ago there was little the physician could do in the way of treatment because of the few scientifically tested drugs available. As Thomas S. Szasz in his discussion on scientific method and social role has stated, "The treatment which he [the physician] had to offer was to give of himself. He was solicitous, attentive, concerned, devoted, friendly. He gave advice. And finally, he gave medicine which, while of no physiochemical benefit to the organism, served as symbols of magic and hope" (10). This concept of service was personified in the family physician, who was perceived as a combination of magical healer, father confessor, and adviser, whose power and value lay in the physician-patient relationship.

The nurse, historically, was a woman who was responsible for raising and nurturing children. This role was closely tied with mothering, and "caring for" was an inherent part of it. Thus, there emerged the image of the nurse as one who devotedly gives service to the patient through nurturing him and ministering to his needs.

During the era of beginning professional development, then, the role orientation of the physician and the nurse was similar. Both were dedicated to giving of themselves to patients, and the focus of their efforts was the relief of discomfort, emotional as well as physical. However, their psychological ministrations were of an intuitive nature. The field of psychiatry was as yet undeveloped, and other than prescriptions of kindness and firmness, there were no guidelines for dealing with the emotional problems of patients that could be included in the physician's and the nurse's training.

THE ERA OF MEDICAL SCIENCE

The beginning of the twentieth century ushered in the scientific era in medicine. The essential attention to the pathological processes of the various organs of the body was accompanied by increased knowledge of and preoccupation with ways to cure illness by chemical and physical means. With the increasing knowledge of the means by which the body functions, the physician tended to neglect the human aspects of his relationship with the patient. In effect, the patient was impersonalized and meaningful inter-personal communication between him and the physician was hampered. In their discussion of the background and perspectives of medicine, Leo W. Simmons and Harold G. Wolff have spoken clearly on this point (8).

It is easy to understand how medicine, confronted with the amazing achieve-ments of the rapidly striding natural sciences, was compelled to break with its mystical past and adapt a new credo. As a result, from the beginning of the scientific era, the developing methods and viewpoint of the "pure" sciences were turned upon the human body to the neglect of its "spirit." The structure of the body, its functions, and the diseases that plague it, have since then been studied chiefly within the physiochemical or bio-physical frames of reference. Consequently, the distinctive nature of man as a person and the essential one-ness of his psychic and organic life have been largely overlooked.

This change in outlook was reflected in the physician's self-image. As Szasz has stated, "The advent of the era of scientific medicine has meant that the contemporary physician has come to view himself principally as the engineer of the body" (10).

Contributing to the change in the physician-patient relationship was the shift in the locale of medical care. The vast paraphernalia of technology was not transportable in the doctor's bag, but the patient could be transported to the physician's office, the clinic, and the hospital. As a result, instead of a firsthand knowledge of the patient's home environment and family life, the physician now had a card containing a few items of information. The specialization that was occasioned by the tremendous increment in scientific knowledge also played a part in severing the once close relationship; the patient's most critical medical experiences were now often in the hands of a physician whom he had seen only once or twice before.

The patient, too, contributed to the disappearance of the continuing physician-patient relationship. He no longer settled in one place for life, but moved from community to community, changing doctors with each move. As the result of another patient-generated force, the upsurge in demand for health care, the physician was swamped with requests for his services. The most conspicuous change in the physician's behavior was that he was in such a hurry that he became less accessible and less communicative (6).

As the physician and the patient became less and less known to each other, their association took on the quality of a business relationship, characterized by such commercial shibboleths as malpractice suits. In short, the physician had assumed the combined role of scientist, technologist, and business-man (5). It was a role that was not conducive to concern with emotional problems.

The advent of the scientific era also threatened the nurse's traditional role—that of nurturing—but it failed to offer her any compensatory advantage, such as the intellectual stimulation and prestige of scientific inquiry. Technological progress was not in the nurse's hands. Instead, she either borrowed or had thrust upon her a gamut of complicated technical and physical procedures that had formerly been the sole prerogative of the physician. The hallmark of the new nursing was a hard core of technology which included a mass of fastidious details, a variety of rituals, and a facsimile of physical techniques used in medical practice. Instead of concentrating on the development of her unique role, the nurse engaged in the frustrating struggle of trying to become a junior physician, only to end up by feeling that her own role as a nurse was not worthwhile.

The shift from the home to the hospital also interfered with the development of patient-centered and family-centered nursing. Unlike the physician, who was *affiliated* with the hospital and thus retained autonomy, the nurse was *employed* by the hospital and was therefore expected to accomplish assigned tasks. In the interest of "efficiency," her assignment was to a hospital service rather than to patients whom she could accompany from service to service. She was also assigned many new functions in connection with the administration of the clinical unit and, as a result, had less and less time to spend nursing the patient. Moreover, she found that as in many organizations, in the hospital the administrator outranked the doer; the nurse who gave direct nursing care had less prestige than the nurse administrator or teacher. Meaningful involvement with patients held less and less promise for the nurse, and as ancillary personnel were imported into the hospital to assist her, such care was largely turned over to them.

As a result of this behavior, the public's image of the nurse as a devoted, comforting, friendly, compassionate, and caring person began to fade. More and more, the patient began to look upon the professional nurse as a stranger with whom he had little personal and prolonged contact and with whom any contact was likely to be peremptory. Even had the patient been given the time, he was not likely to share his emotional problems with this dehumanized facsimile of a nurse.

However, this public image and the nurse's own view that junior doctorship and administration constituted a successful "nursing" career were overlays on, not substitutes for, the original conception of the essential attributes of a nurse. Underneath them there still persisted the image of the nurse as the nurturer and comforter of the sick. In situations controlled by nurses, such as voluntary public health nursing agencies, this nurturing role continued to be the major one. Leaders in nursing education also continued to make total patient care the dominant theme in the role orientation of their students. After years of struggling to retain the integrity of nursing, these nursing leaders suddenly found support for their efforts from a new development in the medical field—the recognition of the contributions that psychiatry could make to the care of all patients.

THE ERA OF PSYCHIATRY

It was World War II, with its large number of psychiatric casualties, that put the spotlight on the emotional needs of patients and on the responsibility of all health workers for the prevention of personality breakdowns. The acceptance of this challenge by medicine was made tenable by the fact that over the years psychiatry had been slowly accumulating and organizing a body of knowledge about human behavior. Although the large number of variables in man's mental and emotional makeup limited the chances of finding formulas that would predict his emotional reactions to a given stimulus with complete accuracy, enough progress had been made in validating hypotheses concerning human behavior to make psychiatry scientifically respectable. Moreover, in challenging the whole field of medicine to resume its concern with patients' emotional problems, psychiatry had a bonus to offer—teachable content with which to replace the old intuitive operations was now available.

Nonetheless, the challenge of psychiatric integration has not been an easy one for the physician to accept. It requires him to alter his concept of his role and professional self-image and to "recast the moral structure of the traditional therapeutic relationship of physician and patient" (10). Not only must he be tolerant of varying personalities and different value systems, but he must also be cognizant of the implications of these variations on health and illness and their bearing on the degree to which preventive measures and treatment can be effective.

In contrast, psychiatry's challenge has added luster to the nurturing role of the nurse. In a discussion of the concept of nurturing and its role in the therapist-patient relationship, Edwin Kasin has pointed out that nurturing has to do with creating a favorable climate for growth, whereby a person's needs are met as he proceeds through each developmental stage (4). This concept of nurturing has implications for all of nursing. Illness calls forth varying degrees of dependency and thereby accentuates needs that were insufficiently fulfilled in one of the developmental stages. The climate of the nurse's relatedness can and should play a significant part in meeting some of the patient's unfulfilled needs that emerge. The nurse is therefore in a position to help the patient transform his experience with illness into a growth experience.

Thus, the emergence of psychiatry as a force in the health field encouraged the nurse to forsake her excursion down the dead-end path of medical technology and resume identifying and preparing for her unique role. The acceptance of the psychiatric outlook added personal meaning to the nurse's relationship with the patient and re-established nursing as a professional specialty within the health field.

The Contributions of Psychiatry to Nursing Education

To nursing educators psychiatry offers more than a validation of the concept of the nurturing role of the nurse—a concept from which they never departed in theory, although those serving also in nursing service positions may have done so in practice. Psychiatry also offers approaches to problems that have long plagued nursing education.

The first of these problems concerns the development of the student's ability to help the patient to meet his emotional needs. Long a proclaimed objective of educational programs in nursing, this ability was scarcely one that could be taught to students so long as it rested on the flimsy foundation of intuition. Psychiatry provides a substantial amount of teachable material justifying this educational objective. It has established some basic truths about human nature which can serve as a touchstone for judgment. It describes how the individual personality develops and points out how and where miscarriages in such development may occur. It sheds considerable light on the relationship between the intellectual, emotional, and physical aspects of living and has to a certain extent identified relationships between feelings and overt behavior. It has provided a theory of communication which is the core of all interpersonal relationships. It has much to offer concerning the impact of culture on individuals and groups. Finally, psychiatry provides methods and techniques (which may be peculiar to the discipline) for identifying, examining, and solving problems that arise in the environment.

The second problem area relates to the development of the student as a person and a citizen, educational goals that are of considerable concern to collegiate nursing educators. The study of psychiatric concepts can assist the student in her search for personal meaning and can help her to develop her potential for personal involvement and creativity, thereby contributing to her personality growth. Again, by providing a framework for viewing interpersonal and social relations, it contributes to the student's development of social consciousness. An essential characteristic of the professional nurse is that she is more concerned with meeting the needs of others than with self-aggrandizement and practical gain, and her horizon for perceiving these needs must extend beyond her immediate surroundings. As Genevieve Burton has stated, the nursing profession can attain true professionalism only to the extent that it contributes to the long-term solution of international problems, and such attainment depends on the development of emotionally sound, mature individuals (1).

The History of Nursing Education in Psychiatric Concepts

The potential contributions of psychiatry to nursing education were recognized by some nursing educators long before the psychiatric casualties of World War II brought attention to this field. As early as 1914, Effie J. Taylor, a leading nurse educator at the time, advocated that psychiatric nursing experience be considered an imperative for all students, regardless of the setting in which they were planning to practice (11). It was not until 1933, however, that the National League of Nursing Education, the spokesman for nurse educators throughout the country, recognized psychiatric nursing as an area basic to nursing education and recommended that instruction in it be included in all basic nursing curriculums. By 1935, half of the basic programs in the country had made arrangements for their students to have psychiatric nursing experiences, and by 1950, 90 per cent of them had done so.

This period was also marked by considerable progress in the placement of nursing education in institutions of higher learning, and collegiate programs in nursing took the leadership in efforts to develop the nurse as a professional person. Such efforts usually put a sharp emphasis on the liberal arts, particularly the behavioral sciences, which were developing rapidly. The study of the behavioral sciences was considered by nursing educators a second avenue for approaching an understanding of the social and emotional aspects of illness.

The introduction of these instructional units in psychiatric nursing and the behavioral sciences might be regarded as the first attempt at using nursing education to integrate psychiatric concepts into nursing practice. Such phrases as *total patient care*, the *whole person, understanding one's self*, and the *therapeutic use of self*—now nursing clichés but at the time fairly new in the field—were expressive of the hope, if not the belief, that the student was integrating the knowledge gained in these courses into her general nursing knowledge and that her practice would reflect this integration. However, observation of the graduate's performance indicated that this integration seldom materialized to the extent anticipated. As has been pointed out, during this period the nurse tended to detach herself from the patient instead of becoming more concerned with his personal problems. Although this defection could not be attributed wholly to limitations in the nurse's preparation, it did suggest that the courses in the behavioral sciences and psychiatric nursing were not preparing the nurse to work with the emotional problems of all patients.

Upon examination, the limitations of these courses (again with respect to psychiatric integration) became obvious. The behavioral sciences were seldom taught as applied sciences at the undergraduate level but were concerned almost entirely with theoretical formulations, regardless of their applicability to nursing. Even in instances when a fact or principle had relevance for nursing practice, no effort was made to join theory and practice. Nursing educators unrealistically expected that the student could accomplish the integration herself. To the student, however, what she learned in her social science courses constituted one area of knowledge and what she learned in nursing another area.

The hope that the student, unaided, could transfer learning from her psychiatric nursing experiences to her work with other patients also proved to be wishful thinking. At the time the most obvious explanation for the failure was the separation of the personnel who guided the student's learning experiences in psychiatric nursing from the other personnel responsible for the educational program. During this period the collegiate schools of nursing were abandoning the use of hospital nursing-service personnel as teachers of nursing and were employing full-time faculty members whose only responsibility was the education of students. However, the dual-responsibility system persisted in psychiatric nursing because of the shortage of nurses with advanced preparation in this field. The teachers of psychiatric nursing were thus attached to the hospitals in which they worked as supervisors and head nurses, and because these hospitals were usually at a distance from the centers in which the rest of the courses were taught, these teachers were not able to participate fully in such faculty activities as establishing the school's philosophy, determining the curriculum objectives, and planning the curriculum, nor could they serve as consultants to the other faculty members in their area of specialized knowledge. As a result, the psychiatric nursing course tended to be an appendage to the curriculum rather than an integral part of it, and its progress toward a truly college-level orientation was slower than that of the other nursing courses.

As qualified teachers of psychiatric nursing became available and the collegiate schools began to assume the total responsibility for teaching this area of the curriculum, it was hoped that the psychiatric nursing content would be integrated into the rest of the curriculum. However, even with this change in teaching personnel the student gave little evidence of improvement with respect to the application of psychiatric concepts to the care of patients who were not mentally ill. Again accomplishment had not measured up to expectation. A further analysis of the problem was in order.

This analysis revealed how unrealistic it had been to expect that the psychiatric nursing course could adequately prepare the student to deal with the emotional problems of all patients. In the first place, this course was usually placed late in the curriculum after the students had encountered such potentially traumatic experiences as the death of a young child. Secondly, the clinical experiences in psychiatric hospitals were such that the course tended to focus on the psychopathologic aspects of human behavior. Although the differences between the feelings and behavior of mentally ill patients and those of other people are differences in degree rather than in kind, it was difficult for the student to identify the similarities. Her observation of the extreme and often bizarre manifestations of anxiety among psychiatric patients was an inadequate experience for learning how to recognize and deal with the anxiety of the other patients with whom she worked.

But the problem was more than one of curriculum placement and clinical focus—circumstances that might have been rectified by the introduction, early in the program, of a course in psychodynamics in which the clinical units of the general hospital were utilized for clinical teaching. The crux of the problem was the subject matter of psychiatric nursing. The study of feelings and attitudes and how to deal with them is quite different from the study of physical stresses and their alleviation; it involves not only a different body of knowledge but a different approach to learning. In addition to acquiring new knowledge, the student must in many instances change her previous beliefs. This process of re-education requires more than a few months of concentrated study or even periodic study over a span of time; continuing, uninterrupted study is essential.

When the problem was stated in these terms, it was realized that if the student were to utilize psychiatric concepts in all of her nursing activities, the teaching of these concepts and practice in their application could not be relegated to any one course or courses. Use would have to be made of all the opportunities for education and re-education that the entire nursing program had to offer. In other words, to bring about psychiatric integration in professional nursing practice it was necessary to achieve psychiatric integration throughout the educational program in nursing.

Thus the psychiatric integration movement in baccalaureate nursing education came into being. Convinced that it was important for the professional nurse to be prepared to deal with the social and emotional aspects of health and illness in the care of all her patients, the faculties in baccalaureate degree programs in nursing instigated studies aimed at identifying the resources of their programs that could be used and further developed for this purpose. Because this was a new field of faculty inquiry, involving subject matter different from that with which most nurse faculty members were accustomed to deal, the faculties sought persons with expert knowledge about human behavior to guide them in their investigations. The movement spread and, as has been stated, by 1965, at least 119 baccalaureate degree programs in nursing—about 60 per cent of all such programs in the country —had launched what came to be known as psychiatric integration projects.

Deterrents to Psychiatric Integration in Nursing Practice

Justification of the huge outlay for psychiatric integration projects requires the answer to one more series of questions: How is the nursing student's increased knowledge, understanding, and capacity to care for patients going to be used after she graduates? Will the patient's situation be improved because of the nurse's professional knowledge and skill? What of the nurse who has been newly graduated from a baccalaureate degree program? Will she be given the opportunity to use the abilities that she has made such an effort to cultivate? Will she be able to live up to her self-image—the image of a professional nurse—inculcated by her teachers?

The current situation in the hospital makes these questions embarrassing for nursing educators at the present time. The hospital is the environment in which most health care is given and therefore in which most nurses practice, but the forces that since World War II have emphasized the importance of personalized health care have as yet made little impact on it. As far as the hospital is concerned, the era of the technologist is still in full flower. In the hospital setting, individuals and individual events are not significant, and both the patient and the nurse are lost in a fog of anonymity in which every patient is dimly perceived as "the patient" and every nurse as "the nurse," regardless of individual needs and individual abilities.

The atmosphere is made even more hazy by what Harvey L. Smith has termed the "basic duality of hospitals"—the difference between what the formal organizational structure says the workers do and what they actually do (9). An Alice in the wonderland of the modern hospital finds little connection between the terms *nurse* and *nursing*. Much of the nursing of patients is done by unprofessional workers, whereas nurses who have been prepared for this function spend their time working with physicians, administering clinical units, teaching and supervising other personnel, serving as housekeepers and engineers and, during nights and weekends, as hospital administrators, coordinating all these activities. Educated for establishing a therapeutic nurse-patient relationship, the professional nurse is likely to find that after an initial contact with a patient she will never see him again. It is a myth that the nurse is the one professional person who is always available to her patient. There is round-the-clock coverage by the nursing service, but this is by no means synonymous with the patient having his individual nurse and the nurse having her patients.

This contrast between role orientation and role realization cannot help but have a devastating effect on the new nurse. Corwin, Taves, and Haas have found that the impression students have about nursing dissolves, after graduation, into disenchantment—that there is a wide chasm between the nurse's conception of herself as an autonomous, professional person whose primary loyalty is to patient welfare and the reality that, as a staff nurse, she must operate within a large-scale, bureaucratic organization that stresses efficiency, rules, and authority (2).

Nor can the nurse work her way upward to a position where she can practice her profession. Once she leaves the staff level and ascends the ladder of the hospital hierarchy, she is deluged with a profusion of paper work. The opportunities to apply her creativeness—a creativeness which may have been painstakingly developed—become blurred, if not obliterated. Reissman and Rohrer have summed up the dilemma in their description of today's nurse as "having become merely a hub in the complex machinery of the hospital rather than the whole wheel" (7).

The duality of the hospital structure, which is responsible for the nurse's role conflict, stems from two main lines of authority within the hospital. One line extends from the hospital's board of trustees, which consists largely of lay members who supposedly represent the interests of the community served by the hospital, through the ranks of the hospital employees. Heading the other line is the patient's physician, who derives his authority from the fact that he has the final responsibility for the patient's welfare. As Smith has pointed out, "There is almost no administrative routine established in hospitals which cannot be (and frequently is) abrogated or countermanded by a physician claiming a medical emergency . . ." (9). The physician exerts power throughout the hospital—upon nurses, other clinical personnel, and patients.

As a result of the complicated lines of authority, the nurse becomes ensnared in an intricate network of communication. The nurses who are above her, supposedly to help her, frequently do not have the power to make the necessary decisions and institute the changes required for the nurse to be able to take care of patients. Buck-passing, by throwing the responsibility for decisions upward, becomes a way of circumventing feelings of powerlessness. Because the flow of communication continues only when satisfaction outweighs frustration, the nurse, after repeated attempts to communicate problems and suggestions for modifying them, is likely to retreat into passivity and resignation to the status quo. At this juncture she is inclined to consider any attempt at communication as a waste of breath.

Having abdicated her rightful authority and responsibility, she handles her guilt by blaming someone or something for her seemingly insoluble dilemma. Unable to identify her place of appeal in the elaborate power structure and the complicated channels of communication, she vents her anger on the organization as a whole—which she refers to as "they"—on patients, on her peers, and especially on the workers at the level immediately below her in the hierarchy. It is under such fear, individual anonymity, impaired communication, feeling of helplessness, role conflict, and disillusionment with her chosen career that the professional qualities of the nurse, which have been so carefully developed, begin to be replaced by the characteristics of a disgruntled slave.

If this is the result, what price psychiatric integration? In contrast to the old-line goals of nursing education, are baccalaureate students being prepared to be better nurses? If they are being prepared "too well" insofar as they are not permitted to perform the role of the nurse as they have learned it, will they want to do something else, such as function as bargain-basement psychiatrists or junior social workers?

This is not to suggest that nursing educators should give up the ideal image of the nurse. Rather, it is a challenge to them to find some way of dealing with the conflict between the characteristics of the hospital structure and the changing status of the nurse. One possible way to deal with this conflict is to explore how the increasing body of knowledge about the social, cultural, emotional, and physical development of man can be taught in a way that enriches the student's professional equipment and develops a clear conception of the role of the nurse. A second way for nursing educators to reduce the role conflict and undercut the process of professional disillusionment is, as Corwin et al. have suggested, to face up to and explain to their students the reasons for the conflict.

Lastly, nursing educators might well make efforts to search out and work with others who are concerned with providing sick people with effective care. The trend toward integrating psychiatry into medical education cannot help but be reflected in the attitudes of the coming generation of physicians, and these new physicians could prove to be strong allies in helping nurses to resume their rightful role in the hospital. The federal subsidization of psychiatric integration in nursing education indicates the high value that the representatives of the consumers of nursing place on quality nursing care, and it might be assumed that the public will want to get a full return on its investment. A wider interpretation of the aims of nursing to all those who have a stake in the attainment of these aims is one of the most important tasks facing nursing education.

REFERENCES

1. Burton, Genevieve. "Education for Life: Its Place in the Nursing Program," *Nursing Outlook*, 4, 209–212 (April, 1956).

2. Corwin, Ronald G., Marvin J. Taves, and J. Eugene Haas. "Professional Disillusionment," *Nursing Research*, 10, 141–144 (Summer, 1961).

3. Garrison, Esther A., Chief Nursing Section, Training and Manpower Resources, National Institute of Mental Health, U.S. Department of Health, Education and Welfare, from a personal communication.

4. Kasin, Edwin. "The Analyst and the Climate for Growth," unpublished

paper delivered at the meeting of the William Alanson White Psychoanalytic Society of the William Alanson White Institute of Psychiatry, Psychoanalysis and Psychology. New York (January 19, 1961).

5. Lee, Alfred McClung. "The Social Dynamics of the Physician's Status," *Psychiatry*, **7**, 371–377 (November, 1944).

6. Means, John Howard. "Homus Medicus Americanus," *Daedalus*, 712 (Fall, 1963).

7. Reissman, Leonard, and John H. Rohrer. *Change and Dilemma in the Nursing Profession*. New York: G. P. Putnam's Sons, 1957.

8. Simmons, Leo W., and Harold G. Wolff. *Social Science in Medicine*. New York: Russell Sage Foundation, 1954, p. 19.

9. Smith, Harvey L. "Two Lines of Authority: The Hospital's Dilemma," in E. Gartley Jaco (ed.), *Patients, Physicians and Illness*. New York: The Free Press, 1958, pp. 468–469.

10. Szasz, Thomas S. "Psychoanalysis and Medicine," in Morton Levitt (ed.), *Readings in Psychoanalytic Psychology*. New York: Appleton-Century-Crofts, Inc., 1959, pp. 355, 357, 358, 366.

11. Taylor, Effie J. "Mental Hygiene," *Proceedings*. New York: National League of Nursing Education, 1914, pp. 187–190.

Chapter Two

STUDIES IN
PSYCHIATRIC INTEGRATION

Then welcome each rebuff
That turns earth's smoothness rough
Each sting that bids nor sit nor stand, but go!
Strive, and hold cheap the strain;
Learn, nor account the pang; dare, never grudge the throe!

ROBERT BROWNING, "Rabbi Ben Ezra,"
Dramatis Personae.

Because the Skidmore psychiatric integration project did not develop within a professional vacuum, it is important to consider it within the context of all that was happening in the psychiatric integration movement during the five-year period 1957–1962. At the inception of the project, in 1957, the only available literature that pertained to psychiatric integration was a report prepared by Hildegard E. Peplau for the National League for Nursing's regional conferences on graduate education in psychiatric nursing in which some of the therapeutic concepts to be integrated in the undergraduate nursing curriculum were identified (10). Since that time, reports have been published of the psychiatric integration projects conducted in eight baccalaureate degree programs and one master's degree program in basic nursing, namely, the programs at the department of nursing of the Faculty of Medicine, Columbia University (1); the University of North Carolina (3); the University at Pittsburgh (5); the University of California at Los Angeles (6); the Catholic University of America (7); the Cornell University–New York Hospital School of Nursing (8); Yale University (9); the University of Washington (11); and the University of Colorado (13).*

* Eight of these projects were supported by a grant from the National Institute of Mental Health, U.S. Department of Health, Education, and Welfare. The project at the

In addition, three reports of the National League for Nursing conferences on psychiatric integration in baccalaureate nursing education have been made available (2, 4, 12).

In view of the fact that as of 1966, 123 psychiatric projects have been or are being conducted in baccalaureate degree programs in nursing, the picture presented by the available literature is obviously incomplete. Moreover, the information presented in the various reports is not always comparable. As might be expected, the presentations at the national and regional conferences lack the specificity of some of the project reports, particularly with respect to the methods used in the integration process. Moreover, comparable data are not available from all of the nine project reports, the main reason being the fact that they do not all cover the same phases of the integration process. Some of the reports seem to be limited to the exploratory phase, whereas others describe integration in action. Even the reports in this latter group do not always describe the entire project. In particular, the published information about the Columbia University project deals with only one aspect of it—a course taught to first-year students—although there is some indication that the entire project involved all areas of the curriculum.

Three of the reports fall in the first, or groundwork-laying, category— those of the projects conducted at the University of Pittsburgh, Yale University, and the University of California at Los Angeles. Although some of the information in these three reports was of help in placing the Skidmore project in historical perspective, they were not as useful as the other six project reports in the preparation of the summary which follows. This summary will consider types of resources and leadership available to the various projects, the psychiatric concepts that were considered appropriate for integration, the approaches and the methods that were used in the integration processes, and the problems that were identified.

Resources and Leadership

The literature suggests that the kind of leadership and consultation utilized in psychiatric integration projects has a considerable effect on the other variables, such as the concepts identified for integration and the methods used. The consultation and leadership, in turn, seems to be influenced to a large extent by the resources that are available to the school of nursing. Four factors, in particular, seem to play an important part in charting the future direction of the project.

The first factor is the geographical distance between the facilities used for teaching nursing and those used for instruction in other subjects. When

Cornell University–New York Hospital School of Nursing was supported by the Russell Sage Foundation.

the instructors in nursing and the instructors in liberal arts education are close to one another, collaboration is possible, because the project director is able to work with the faculty in the total educational program. In the instance of Skidmore College, the instruction in nursing is provided two hundred miles from the college campus. In these circumstances consultation with members of other disciplines and departments was exceedingly difficult and real collaboration with them was impossible.

A second factor is the presence or absence of a full-time faculty member who has the responsibility for planning and teaching the course in psychiatric nursing. It was not possible to determine from the literature how many of the eight schools were totally responsible for all instruction in psychiatric nursing, although there was some indication that in all of them there were psychiatric nurses on the faculty in addition to the one who worked in the integration project. During the 1957–1962 period of the integration project at Skidmore College, the psychiatric nursing course was taught at a cooperating agency to whose personnel the faculty of the department of nursing had delegated the responsibility for teaching and supervising the students. The project director, therefore, was the only psychiatric nurse on the faculty during the period covered in this book.

The third factor concerns the levels of instruction in psychiatric nursing offered at the institution. It is only recently that psychiatric nursing has begun to be considered other than a stepchild among the clinical nursing specialties, and unless there is a graduate program, its importance still is not given full recognition. When there is a graduate program, the faculty gets caught up in the excitement that comes from the research which is part of such a program but which is missing in a baccalaureate program. With the existence of a graduate program there is, therefore, greater faculty acceptance of psychiatric nursing and stimulation of the psychiatric nurse who works in integration. With the exception of Cornell University–New York Hospital School of Nursing and the department of nursing at Columbia University, the seven other schools offered graduate curriculums in psychiatric nursing during the entire period or part of the period in which the integration project was in progress. At the time of the integration project, Skidmore College did not offer graduate programs in any of its departments. The department of nursing, however, provided some learning experiences for students enrolled in graduate programs in nursing at other universities. During the integration project, two students in graduate programs in psychiatric nursing had learning experiences in relation to this project.

The fourth factor relates to the existence or nonexistence of a department of psychiatry in the medical school of the educational institution and of psychiatric services under the auspices of the university. With the exception of the Catholic University of America, the literature indicated that all of the eight universities have medical schools with departments of psychiatry.

It was not possible, however, to ascertain the number or kind of psychiatric services that are under the jurisdiction of the universities.

Through contractual agreement, the base hospital of the Skidmore College Department of Nursing is the New York University Hospital, New York. During the period of the project, this hospital did not have a psychiatric inpatient service, and although consultants in psychiatry from the New York University department of psychiatry were appointed to the hospital, a highly developed and systematic psychiatric consultation service was not in progress. Without the psychiatrist on the integration team, the nature of the curriculum pattern in the department of nursing and the limited inter-disciplinary resources available within the organizational structure would have completely separated the discipline of psychiatry from the non-psychiatric part of nursing.

In regard to the responsibility for the leadership and direction of psychiatric integration projects, six of the nine projects were directed by a nurse, and in four cases—the Catholic University of America, the University of Colorado, the University of Pittsburgh, and the University of Washington—the project director was a psychiatric nurse. In the other two instances—Yale University and Columbia University—a public health, mental-health nurse consultant directed the project. The other three projects were directed by social scientists, of whom two were sociologists (the Cornell University–New York Hospital School of Nursing and the University of North Carolina) and the third an anthropologist (the University of California at Los Angeles).

Despite the lip service that the nursing profession generally (and psychiatric nursing specifically) pays to the value and importance of interdisciplinary teamwork, as far as can be determined from the literature, the University of North Carolina and the Columbia University schools were the only ones that utilized an interdisciplinary team approach during most of the project. In these two schools, members from three disciplines—nursing, psychiatry, and sociology—were involved on more than a consultative basis. The reports of these projects, which were prepared by members from each of these disciplines, are a further demonstration of interdisciplinary collaboration.

The literature reveals that two other projects availed themselves of some kind of interdisciplinary consultation (which, of course, is not synonymous with collaborative teamwork). At the University of Colorado a consultant group composed of three psychiatrists, two psychologists, one sociologist, a professor of education, and two psychiatric nurses, all of whom were outside of the school of nursing, gave assistance to the project through three annual meetings. In the project at the Cornell University–New York Hospital School of Nursing, psychiatric consultation from the psychiatric division of the medical center was used to help nursing service personnel to handle the behavioral problems of patients, and guest lecturers from the faculty of the medical college contributed to the course on social science concepts.

With the exception of the article about the Columbia University project, in which students were taught the psychosocial aspects of patient care by teaching teams, each of which consisted of a nursing instructor, a nursing service supervisor, a psychiatrist, and a sociologist, the literature is vague about the way in which psychiatrists participated in the integration projects. Moreover, the role of the psychiatric nurses does not come through very clearly. In the Skidmore project, although a psychiatric nurse was the project director, a psychiatrist and the psychiatric nurse functioned as an interdisciplinary team for the duration of the five-year project. In 1962, when for the first time those with the major responsibility for leadership in the integration projects in baccalaureate degree programs came together at the National League for Nursing work conference in Chicago, the psychiatrist member of the Skidmore integration team was the only participant from a discipline other than nursing.

It should be pointed out, however, that the values of a multidisciplinary approach were recognized at other conferences sponsored by the National League for Nursing. At the five regional conferences in 1958, papers on psychiatric integration were presented by nursing administrators, nurses who represented every clinical area of teaching, psychiatric nurses who were teaching in integration programs, psychiatrists, psychologists, and sociologists (2). Again, at the 1959 National League for Nursing conference in Boulder, Colorado, the invited participants included nurse educators, psychologists, psychiatrists, and sociologists and a philosopher and anthropologist (12). This group engaged in provocative discussions of problems related to a wide range of subjects that had a bearing on psychiatric integration—the nursing profession's perspective regarding the upgrading of the profession, the definition of illness and health, the relative value of self-awareness and understanding, the inevitable dialectic between the individual and the group, the essence of professional nursing, the use of verbal communication and interpretation by the nurse, the identification of concepts versus their translation into action, and the differing perceptions of psychiatry with particular reference to the controversy over a dynamic versus a technological position. Some of the participants' remarks implied severe criticism of the psychiatric nurses' points of view. Analysis of the report of this conference reveals that one of its major contributions was its demonstration of some of the difficulties in communication that frequently occur among members of different professions.

Four of the educational programs (those in the Catholic University of America, the University of Colorado, the University of North Carolina, and the University of Washington) indicate that steering and advisory committees were organized for the purpose of administering the projects. These committees generally were composed of the administrative head of the educational unit in nursing and representatives from other departments in the college or university.

During the initial phase of the Skidmore project a subcommittee composed of the chairman of the department of nursing, instructors in medical-surgical, pediatric, and public-health nursing, and the project director was organized for the purpose of giving direction to the integration program. Because of the relatively small number of full-time faculty members in the department of nursing, however, communication with the total group proved more advantageous in this situation than working through the subcommittee, and to avoid duplication of activities the subcommittee was abolished.

Identification of Psychiatric Concepts to Be Integrated

The reports of the nine integration projects vary considerably with respect to their discussion of the psychiatric content taught. Some of them make no mention of the specific content; for example, the article about the Columbia University project describes the methods used in teaching psychosocial concepts but does not indicate what the concepts were. Other reports describe the content with considerable detail but do not indicate how it was identified. Still others describe structured studies designed to identify the concepts which the professional nurse needs to know and be able to apply. The literature also indicates that the selection of the concepts to be integrated was strongly influenced by the discipline of which the project director was a member.

In the Cornell University—New York Hospital School of Nursing project, which was directed by a sociologist, the content taught to the nursing students covered concepts which were identified as (1) culture, subculture, and social class; (2) authority; (3) value judgments; (4) psychosocial aspects of physical disability and rehabilitation—fear, body image, depression, and anxiety.

In contrast, the concepts selected for integration at the University of North Carolina and the discussion of these concepts in the report of this project bear the imprint of the special knowledge and skill of the three participating disciplines—sociology, psychiatric nursing, and psychiatry. This report discusses in some detail the concepts of regression, denial of illness, unconscious motivation, and stress. It also mentions a partial list of concepts found to be useful in nursing care—role behavior, self-concept, nonverbal communication, adaptation, homeostasis, sensory deprivation, cultural isolation, ego defense, denial, and perception. In addition, a second major area of content, "life and illness experience" and "behavior in illness," was taught to sophomore and junior students in small group seminars that were jointly conducted by the psychiatrist, sociologist, and nurse project coordinator.

The report of the integration project conducted by a psychiatric nurse at the University of Pittsburgh consists primarily of a tabulation of the psychological principles that were being taught in the nursing curriculum. The distribution, duplication, and depth of content were investigated, but no attempt was made to identify the specific principles or concepts that should be integrated in the curriculum.

At the Catholic University of America the psychiatric nurse project director studied course offerings and course outlines and had individual interviews with the faculty members for the purpose of identifying what "human relations content" was currently being taught in the total curriculum. The content which the faculty considered helpful to nursing students in their professional relationships was categorized under the following headings: (1) human growth and development—principles of normal growth and development, psychodynamics of individual and group behavior; (2) understanding of behavior, one's own and that of others—unconscious motivation, the concept of culture, the interplay between physiology and the emotions, the concepts of anxiety, dependency and independency, guilt, resentment, rejection and hostility, and defense operations; (3) interpersonal relations—the concepts of role and communication; (4) psychosomatic aspects of nursing care —the meaning to the patient of illness, hospitalization, surgery, terminal illness and dying, and rehabilitation.

At the University of Colorado and the University of Washington, where the integration projects were directed by psychiatric nurses, systematic studies were made for the purpose of identifying those psychiatric concepts that the nurse needs to know and to apply in her work with patients. Although the methodology of these studies was similar, there were distinguishing points of emphasis. At the University of Colorado, in the interaction between the nursing student and her patient, the emphasis was on the student's role as a participant observer. For example, the student was asked to record the emotional problems she had identified in the patient, what she and the patient did and said during the interpersonal transaction, her feelings in the situation, and her speculations about the patient's feelings. In the University of Washington study, the student was also asked to record what both she and the patient said and did; however, the principal focus was on the student. She was asked, for example, to record a situation with a patient in which she felt some discomfort and to speculate about the ideas or reasons for her feelings.

In these two studies, analysis and classification of the problem situations also represent two different points of view. Although the University of Colorado study focused on the patient in the collection of the data, the data were analyzed and classified according to student problem categories—for example, "blocks exploration of the problem by reassurance" and "asks personal questions and cannot deal with the answers." Conversely, although the student was the principal focus in the collection of the data in the University of Washington study, the reasons for the student's discomfort were classified according to the patient's behavior—for example, "The patient directly blocks or interferes with the student's attempts to provide physical nursing care, by hesitating to accept it, refusing it, undoing it, or running away"; "the patient's verbal or nonverbal behavior is perceived by the student as having sexual connotations." Despite the fact that the project directors proceeded from two different vantage points, they ended up with similar data— both identified patient and student problems in nurse-patient relationships, but they did so in different sequence.

In the University of Colorado study, the following concepts, which were extracted from the students' written process recordings, were considered fundamental to examining any interpersonal relationship: (1) awareness of self precedes awareness of others; (2) it is through communication that one's view of one's self, other people, or a situation becomes confirmed, modified, or changed; (3) comparative freedom from self-blame for events in which one participates is a requisite to examining one's participation in the event and to trying out new skills in a situation; and (4) the problem-solving process can be applied to the nurse-patient interpersonal relationship. One of the most fascinating and useful parts of the report is the discussion of the "teacher's guide for introducing mental health concepts," in which the concept of helplessness was developed.

In the University of Washington study, the broad concepts of anxiety, role behavior, verbal and nonverbal behavior, and basic human needs were identified as threads that continue throughout the nursing program. The University of Washington study also went one step beyond the University of Colorado study by identifying four major categories of behavior that are possible in a nurse-patient relationship—(1) aggressive behavior; (2) withdrawal behavior; (3) compliant behavior; (4) therapeutic behavior; and (5) problem-solving behavior.

In addition to the reports of the integration projects, the literature derived from various National League for Nursing conferences contains material relative to the psychiatric concepts that should be included in a baccalaureate nursing program. Peplau's presentation at the regional conferences on graduate psychiatric nursing education contains a precise study of the dynamic interaction between the patient and the nurse, a formulation of the concepts relating to the functions of the nurse, and a beginning, although extensive, checklist of socio-psychiatric curriculum content (10). This report represents one of the first attempts at a systematic identification of those psychiatric concepts that should be integrated throughout the undergraduate nursing curriculum.

The National League for Nursing's five regional conferences in 1958 focused primarily on a description of the methods and experiences that had been utilized in psychiatric integration. Although these descriptions were punctuated by beginning attempts to identify some of the principles and dynamics underlying psychiatric integration and to provide a conceptual framework for integration as a process, the formulation of specific principles and concepts remained a task for the future.

The report of the proceedings of the 1959 work conference at Boulder, Colorado, represented another step toward identifying and formulating the major components in nursing which serve as the basis for integrating psychiatric concepts in the undergraduate nursing curriculum. The following four areas were studied—(1) the philosophy underlying the integration of psychiatric concepts; (2) the identification of components in a therapeutic nurse-patient relationship; (3) the supervisory process in teaching psychiatric concepts; and (4) the identification of psychiatric concepts to be integrated (12). The following ten concepts were considered to be among the most important for psychiatric integration.

1. All behavior is meaningful, is purposeful, and can be understood.

2. Some degree of anxiety is basic to the growth and learning process.

3. An understanding of one's self may lead to an understanding of others.

4. The individual's body of knowledge plays an important role in his perceptions and decisions.

5. Mastery of action depends on conscious awareness and the ability to make a decision, to take a risk, and to accept the consequences.

6. There is a basic potential in man that seeks actualization under the proper conditions.

7. Man functions and experiences both as an indivdual and as a member of a social group.

8. Personality and behavior are influenced by man's interaction with his environment.

9. Love is the force that helps to liberate the capacity to love one's self and to love others.

10. Man's sense of reality arises from his continuous struggle with the forces about him.

The first two concepts were further developed and discussed in some detail.

As for the Skidmore project, the members of the psychiatric team agreed that in the process of identifying the psychiatric concepts to be integrated, a good deal of time and effort would be expended. Because their long and broad teaching experiences in university settings and their close contacts with patients, nurses, physicians, and nursing and medical students had given them a fairly clear picture of the psychiatric concepts that are most useful in patient care, they decided to limit their work to selecting the particular concepts to be taught and to exploring the sequence and manner in which these might best be presented.

Approaches to Integration

The reports of the various projects reveal that integration personnel can use a variety of approaches in fulfilling their responsibility to provide the students with opportunities to learn about psychiatric concepts and how to utilize them. Besides the avenue between project personnel and students, there are the less direct routes that utilize the curriculum, or the instructional personnel, or those whom the student observes in the clinical situation. From these reports it would seem that the selection of the approach or approaches used in a project, besides being dependent on the available resources, is likely to be governed by several other factors.

The first factor is the philosophy and the goals of the educational program in which the project is being conducted. The second is the discipline to which the project director is oriented. The psychiatric nurse educator, for example, because of her orientation toward helping patients and students to change and grow, may be inclined to value change in the current situation over scientific investigation as an end in itself. The social scientist, on the other hand, is oriented toward and dedicated to the pursuit of scientific knowledge through the identification and analysis of problems—a goal which may not include attempts to resolve the problems.

The third factor in the selection of an approach is the degree of theoretical knowledge the faculty members have of psychiatric concepts and their ability to apply this knowledge in the teaching-learning process. The fourth factor is the nature of the organizational structure of the educational and clinical settings, particularly as these pertain to the constellation of power and its effect on methods of decision making and the process of communication. The last, but by no means the least, determinant is the willingness and the capacity of the faculty members and the project director to change.

As has been pointed out, the reports of three of the projects—those conducted at the University of Pittsburgh, Yale University, and the University of California at Los Angeles—do not describe the actual process of integration, so that the approaches that were envisioned when the reports were prepared are more or less a matter of surmise. From the preliminary work outlined in the University of Pittsburgh report, it might be assumed that the approach anticipated was via the curriculum. The report of the Yale University project shows that in identifying the principles that guide nursing practice, which apparently was the goal of this project, the project director worked with students and nursing personnel in the clinical situation, and it may be that this approach was the one envisioned for the future.

In the preliminary report of the project at the University of California at Los Angeles, four interlocking aspects of curriculum and teaching were analyzed—(1) the patients with whom the students work, who were studied to see if emotional problems exist in all areas of patient care; (2) the nursing staff in instructional situations, whose functions were investigated to see how they handled these problems in patient care; (3) the structure of the school of nursing; and (4) the content of psychiatric concepts. This analysis suggests that the process of integration would require helping the faculty members in the selection of patients for study, as well as in curriculum development and teaching, and working with the nursing service personnel in the clinical learning field.

Although the preliminary viewpoints revealed in these three reports are of interest, those who have engaged in the actual process of integration will probably agree that such viewpoints may well change as a project develops. When a blueprint that calls for concepts to be introduced in the content of such-and-such courses reaches the point of implementation, it may be discovered that the instructors of the courses need considerable help before they are competent to teach the concepts. Again, consideration must be given to the vast array of learning situations to which the students are exposed. The project director who anticipates carrying the whole burden of student instruction in psychiatric concepts may find, when the project begins, that her efforts are negated, even though unintentionally, by the teaching of other, less knowledgeable, instructors. Lastly, there is the question of priorities. Although in theory it may be desirable to utilize to the maximum every route to the students, in practice the project personnel may find it necessary to direct their major efforts along the more important channels and to bypass or skim over the other ones.

In short, in the case of the three integration projects for which only preliminary reports are available, one can only surmise the anticipated approach to the integration process. Furthermore, even assuming that the surmises are correct, a discrepancy between the planned and the actual approaches is highly possible. For these reasons, the summary of information about approaches to psychiatric integration is based on the information supplied in the reports of the other six projects.

All of these six projects utilized a dual approach—a direct one, in which the psychiatric project personnel worked with students, and an indirect one, in which they attempted to improve the student program through working with the faculty members. In each instance, moreover, it would appear that the project personnel helped the faculty members improve their competence in teaching psychiatric concepts. In five of the schools the faculty members were also helped to identify the places in the curriculum where psychiatric concepts might well be emphasized. Whether this assistance was given in the sixth program (at Columbia University) is not indicated in the article on its project.

This focus on faculty as well as students is in line with the consensus among nursing educators and social scientists that the success of psychiatric integration is dependent on the ability of the faculty group as a whole to apply psychiatric concepts in the work with patients, students, nursing personnel, and co-workers. The importance of the psychiatric integrator's work with faculty was further acknowledged when this aspect of the psychiatric integration process received major attention at the 1962 National League for Nursing conference in Chicago. The report of the Skidmore project in particular emphasized this point (14).

Besides focusing on the faculty and the students, the Cornell University–New York Hospital School of Nursing put a major emphasis on the nursing service personnel. The sociologist who directed this project points out that because nurse faculty members have dual positions in this school, part of their responsibility being to the school and part to the hospital's nursing service, much of the integration process had to occur within the clinical situation. The University of Colorado made a course in interpersonal relations in nursing available to the associated nursing service personnel. In the Columbia University project some nursing service supervisors in medical and surgical services were members of the multidisciplinary teaching teams and, as such, participated in the post-seminar discussions of these teams.

Like the other integration projects that are fully reported in the literature, the Skidmore project utilized the double-focus approach of working with the faculty members and students. One essential difference in the work with the faculty, however, was the psychiatric team's emphasis on the recognition, identification, and resolution of those issues in intrafaculty relations that were impeding the teaching-learning process. The psychiatric nurse project director also held a series of seminars for the nursing service personnel of the base hospital of the department of nursing.

Methods of Psychiatric Integration and the Role of the Project Director

In identifying the methods of psychiatric integration that were employed and the various roles that were taken by the project directors, the relationship between the goals of the integration project, the nature of the subject matter, the methods of integration, and the role of the project director can hardly be overestimated or overemphasized. Even though a diversity of methods are presented in the literature—a diversity which functions as a safeguard against the formulation of a blueprint for psychiatric integration

—some direction in which psychiatric integration is moving is clearly discernible.

The project personnel worked with the faculty in a group in various ways. At the Catholic University of America, this work was primarily done in curriculum meetings in which the content that was to be included in all the nursing courses was discussed. There is no indication in this report, however, that the faculty members took the role of learners. At the Cornell University–New York Hospital School of Nursing a committee of members was utilized for the purpose of previewing the content that was to be included in the social science course for students. In the Columbia University project, the senior psychiatrist or an equivalent staff member held weekly conferences with the nursing instructors who were members of the teams teaching psychosocial aspects of patient care. However, these discussions apparently centered on methodological concerns—techniques of group leadership and methods of integrating resource people into the teaching team— rather than on psychiatric content per se.

In three of the projects—the University of Colorado, the University of North Carolina, and the University of Washington—besides participating in the various meetings devoted to curriculum development, the project director worked with the total faculty as a group on a systematic and scheduled basis for the specific purpose of helping the faculty members to increase their knowledge of psychiatric concepts and their skill in applying them. At the University of Colorado and the University of North Carolina, one-year lecture-discussion courses were provided for the faculty members, and at the University of Colorado the course was repeated each year for new faculty members. Apparently the project at the University of Washington was the only one in which group work with the faculty was carried on consistently over a sustained period of time (four years). In all three projects the faculty's attendance at the courses and group discussions was on a voluntary basis. It was not possible to ascertain the frequency of faculty group discussions devoted to the integration project in the other settings.

In the three described situations the content for discussion included theoretical concepts. In the lecture-discussions at the University of Colorado and the less formal faculty seminars at the University of Washington, interpersonal relationships in clinical practice served as the framework for the discussion of theory. Both situations made extensive use of the faculty members' process recordings.

Interestingly enough, despite the orientation of social scientists and psychiatric nurses to group dynamics and interactional processes, the University of Washington report was the only one that indicated a focus on the interactional processes between the faculty members and the two psychiatric nurse project directors during the faculty group discussions. Ventilation of attitudes toward the integration project and the two psychiatric nurses was encouraged. The identification of some of the phases of inter-action through which the faculty members and the project directors passed constituted an important part of the report.

As for the work with individual faculty members, each of the Columbia University teaching teams, following their sessions with students, held con-ferences during which the psychiatrist and sociologist members of the team helped the nursing instructor to become conscious of her behavior during the session so that she might become more secure in her role. The other five projects reported that individual conferences between faculty mem-bers and the project director were utilized and that these constituted a valuable tool in the integration process. Another method of working with the individual faculty member that was used in these five projects consisted of the psychiatric nurse on the project staff alternating between doing col-laborative teaching and participating as a resource person in the instructor's clinical conferences and seminars with students.

In the project at the Cornell University–New York Hospital School of Nursing, the individual faculty members, who had dual positions in educa-tion and service, were worked with in clinical conferences in the clinical setting. In the University of North Carolina project, the psychiatric nurse member of the project staff observed lecture-discussion classes for the pur-pose of identifying the psychiatric concepts that were currently included in the curriculum and noting the teaching-learning process between the nurse teacher and the student in the clinical area.

The broad spectrum of methods used with the faculty members indicates that the project director took at least one of several roles with them—teacher, consultant, resource person, counselor, and peer. Frequent combinations of these seemed to be (1) teacher and resource person; (2) teacher, resource person, and counselor; and (3) resource person and peer. In the article on one phase of the Columbia University project, the role of the project director is not specified. In the other five projects, the role of consultant seemed to be the project director's least frequent role with the faculty members, the exception being the Cornell University–New York Hospital School of Nurs-ing, where the social scientist project director assumed this role.

In the Skidmore project the psychiatric team members employed the con-cept of interactional process in their work with the faculty group and pre-sented psychiatric concepts from within the experiential framework of intrafaculty relationships as well as teacher-student-patient relationships. In contrast to the other projects, attendance at the faculty discussions was not on a volunary basis. The team members worked with individual faculty members in clinical conferences with students; as in the Columbia Uni-versity project the instructor took the roles of learner, in relation to the team, and teacher, in relation to the students. The general use of individual conferences with faculty members may have occurred at a later date in the

Skidmore project than in other projects. The content of the individual conferences with the faculty members consisted primarily of student problems,
how to counsel students, and difficulties in intrafaculty relationships.

Concerning the methods of psychiatric integration with students, the
project personnel in four schools (the Cornell University–New York Hospital
School of Nursing, the University of Colorado, the University of North Carolina, and Columbia University) organized and participated in courses in
social science and psychiatric concepts for students. In one situation, a
thirty-hour course was offered to students in their first clinical year (8). In
the other two settings, a two quarter-hour course and a fifteen-hour course
were offered to junior students, the latter course being expanded to include
an experimental group of sophomore students (3, 13). At Columbia University, the twenty-week course for first-year students consisted of seminars
that were based on interviews with patients presented at the seminars.

In the other five projects the project directors participated in informal
seminars and clinical conferences with students. In the project at the University of North Carolina the clinical learning experiences of the students
in communicable-disease and long-term-illness nursing, medical-surgical,
pediatric, obstetric, and psychiatric nursing, plus the nursing care of Negro
patients with medical-surgical conditions, were observed by the psychiatric
nurse who worked on the integration project. The majority of the projects
appeared also to utilize the method of individual conferences with students.

In regard to the project director's role with students, as far as it can be
determined from the literature, none of the project personnel in any of the
settings had any responsibility for the supervision or evaluation of students.
The project director's roles with students, as with the faculty members, were
those of teacher, resource person, and counselor.

During the first year of the Skidmore project, the psychiatric nurse, who
functioned as a full-time instructor in medical nursing, was responsible for
the supervision and evaluation of students, which included the assignment
of grades. From that point on, however, the students participated in an integration program and were no longer evaluated by the psychiatric nurse.
Beginning in the second year, the psychiatrist taught a twenty-hour course
in social science concepts and the psychiatric nurse taught a thirty-hour
course in interpersonal relations in nursing. One or both members of the
project team participated in conferences in every clinical area except obstetric nursing. Individual conferences with students also became one of
the team members' most important functions.

As for evaluating the results of the psychiatric integration projects, no
built-in evaluation methods as part of a project design or approach were
reported in the literature, nor as far as it can be determined, was any valid
instrument developed for measuring precisely what occurred. This is of
especial interest in view of the fact that three of the projects were directed

by social scientists, who are oriented toward the construction of evaluation tools.

The University of Colorado utilized four sources of information in the attempt to measure changes—the scores on the National League for Nursing Achievement Test in Psychiatric Nursing, the Professional Examination Service's Student Public Health Nursing Test, and the State Board Examination Pool test in psychiatric nursing, and the process records of student-patient interactions.

The Catholic University of America designed an objective-type questionnaire which included two projective-type drawings of nurse-patient situations. Rating scales were used by the instructors to estimate the student's understanding of the principles and processes that pertain to dealing with patients' emotional problems.

All the schools utilized direct observation in evaluating the growth of the students and the faculty members. In at least two situations the students were asked for written, subjective evaluations of the impact of the project on themselves (8, 11). In one situation the project director interviewed each faculty member individually as a way of appraising the results of the project (11). The literature gives no evidence as to whether, in any of the projects, the project personnel's own change and growth were considered in the evaluation process.

In the Skidmore project no objective tool for evaluation was developed. The psychiatric nurse used the methods of ongoing participant observation and individual interviews with all the faculty members, selected students, selected members of the nursing service personnel, and the educational director of the cooperating agency where the course in psychiatric nursing was taught.

Emergent Problems

The literature reveals that the most frequent, complicated, and serious problems emerging in the integration projects were those that arose between the faculty and the project director, and that the majority of these problems related to the faculty members' ambivalent attitudes toward change. The defenses against anxiety that were aroused in response to change varied considerably. Some faculty members were openly hostile to the proposed change and the project director; some completely withdrew from participation with the project director; and some expressed verbal acceptance and attempted to ingratiate themselves. Difficulties were also created by authority and status differences between the faculty members, who took the role of learners, and the project director, whose central role was that of teacher and therefore rational authority. Again, the use of a different language and different theoretical orientations created difficulties in communication.

The second problem identified in the literature concerned the faculty members' insufficient theoretical knowledge of psychiatric concepts. Perhaps an even more important problem was their inability to transfer theoretical knowledge to the working problems of nursing and nursing education.

The third problem pertained to the faculty members' expectations that the project director would share information about the problems the students had confided to her and about the project director's conflict between concealing confidential information and sharing pertinent aspects with the faculty.

In the Skidmore project two other problems with serious implications for the integration process emerged. The first concerned the difficulties associated with the synthesis of the psychiatrist and the psychiatric nurse as an interdisciplinary team. Just as difficulties arose in regard to the work of the project director with the faculty in other projects, the differences in the disciplines of the psychiatrist and the psychiatric nurse and the issue of status relations between them presented numerous hurdles. The second problem pertained to the tendency of the faculty members and the students to fragment the emotional-social and the physical components of patient care.

Unraised Issues

Although the literature places heavy emphasis on the problems arising from the project director's work with the faculty, the report of the University of Washington is the only one that deals with the step-by-step integration process of the project director with the faculty and that identifies some of the difficulties that occurred in the integration process. As far as can be gleaned, none of the literature spells out the steps of how the project director, be he social scientist or psychiatric nurse, became integrated with other members of the project staff. For the most part, the literature focuses on the anatomy of integration—structure and content. Although the story of the Skidmore project is also concerned with structure, its primary focus will be on the process—the physiology of integration.

REFERENCES

1. Betz, Lorraine, Bernard Schoenberg, and Jay Schulman. "Multidisciplinary Teaching of Patient Care in a Group Setting," *Nursing Forum* 1 (4), 41–59 (Fall, 1962).

2. *Concepts of the Behavioral Sciences in Basic Nursing Education*, Proceedings of the 1958 Regional Conferences on Psychiatric Nursing Education. New York: National League for Nursing, 1958.

3. Gifford, Alice J. (ed.). *Unity of Nursing Care: A Report of a Project to Study the Integration of Social Science and Psychiatric Concepts in Nursing.* Chapel Hill: University of North Carolina, School of Nursing, 1960.

4. *Integration of Psychiatric Nursing Concepts in Baccalaureate Basic Programs.* New York: National League for Nursing, 1963.

5. Jahraus, Agnes. *Psychological Content in a Nursing Curriculum.* Pittsburgh: University of Pittsburgh, School of Nursing, 1960.

6. Kaufman, Lorraine. "The Integration of Psychiatric and Mental Health Concepts in a Generic Baccalaureate Program," *Nursing Research,* **6,** 75–76 (October, 1957).

7. Kupka, Mary Ellen. *The Teaching of Psychiatric-Mental Health Nursing in the Basic Professional Nursing Program.* Washington, D.C.: The Catholic University of America, 1962.

8. Macgregor, Frances Cooke. *Social Science in Nursing.* New York: Russell Sage Foundation, 1960.

9. Orlando, Ida Jean. *The Dynamic Nurse-Patient Relationship: Function, Process and Principles.* New York: G. P. Putnam's Sons, 1961.

10. Peplau, Hildegard E. "Therapeutic Concepts," *Aspects of Psychiatric Nursing.* New York: National League for Nursing, 1957.

11. Pesznecker, Betty L., and Helon E. Hewitt. *Psychiatric Content in the Nursing Curriculum—A Study of Integration Process.* Seattle: University of Washington Press, 1963.

12. *Psychiatric Nursing Concepts and Basic Nursing Education.* New York: National League for Nursing, 1960.

13. *Report of the University of Colorado School of Nursing Experience in the Integration of Mental Hygiene Concepts in the Basic Collegiate Program.* Denver: Bureau of Nursing Research and Studies, University of Colorado School of Nursing, 1960.

14. Schmahl, Jane A., and Montague Ullman. "The Three Phases of Psychiatric Integration in Nursing Education: A Conceptual Framework," *Integration of Psychiatric Nursing Concepts in Baccalaureate Basic Programs.* New York: National League for Nursing, 1963, pp. 4–13.

Chapter Three

A CONCEPTUAL FRAMEWORK FOR PSYCHIATRIC INTEGRATION

The very process of interaction with that which was previously unknown produces new content, new stuff, new realities, new things to understand and to love, as well as new instruments of observation, new ways of knowing, new modes of esthetic apprehension. These, too, will change the nature of man . . . by broadening the doorway through which he passes, so that he may see more of the vista he approaches and may as he does so become always a larger man.

GARDNER MURPHY, *Human Potentialities*

The differences in the approaches to psychiatric integration in baccalaureate degree nursing education that have been recorded in the literature indicate the possibility that there may be differences in the philosophies that underlie these approaches. Accordingly, it would seem incumbent upon anyone who attempts to render a full account of a psychiatric integration project to state his position on issues relevant to the development of the project. This chapter represents a statement of the beliefs held by the psychiatric nurse who directed the psychiatric integration project at Skidmore College.

The Goals of Nursing Education

The goals and methods of psychiatric integration are inextricably tied to the goals of collegiate nursing education. The choice of the methods utilized in a psychiatric integration project therefore hinges on what those who are guiding the project perceive as the short- and long-term goals of nursing education and what they believe are the appropriate avenues for approaching these goals.

The methods chosen for the Skidmore project were influenced by the belief that the broad objective of collegiate nursing education is to prepare the student to find rational solutions to professional nursing problems through the process of giving comprehensive nursing care by ministering to the physical, emotional, and social needs of patients and their families in whatever setting she finds them. This is not to say that the undergraduate nursing program can prepare its students to function as clinical specialists. The graduate of a baccalaureate degree program in nursing should be prepared to collect the data about a patient's problem, to analyze these data, and to identify the nursing problems. She should be able to understand behavior so that she can respond appropriately to nursing problems at the time of their occurrence and not be traumatized by them. She also should be able to recognize when a particular problem is beyond her depth and know the resources to use for help. She should not, however, be expected to initiate and implement nursing interventions which require her consciously to set up situations in which the patient's problems come into the open and then are dealt with. This task is the responsibility of the clinical specialist prepared in a graduate program in psychiatric nursing.

It is further believed that a predominant characteristic of collegiate nursing education should be a learning structure in which the student not only acquires the necessary knowledge and skills but also develops the feelings, attitudes, and appreciations that make it possible for her to think and behave in a way that is appropriate to the practice of professional nursing. Assistance in the development of such a structure is the main purpose of a psychiatric integration project.

The Meaning of Psychiatric Integration

A second important factor in determining the approaches and methods used in a psychiatric integration project is the meaning accorded the term *psychiatric integration*. Because of the various interpretations that are put on the words *psychiatric* and *integration*, this term is subject to a considerable number of connotations. Insofar as the word *psychiatric* is concerned, the confusion and conflict about its use in connection with integration projects has stemmed from a debate over whether such other terms as *mental health, mental hygiene, human relations, social science,* and *behavioral science* would be more appropriate.

The choice of *psychiatric* for use in the Skidmore project was based on the concept of psychiatry as a scientific discipline that is concerned not only with psychopathology and the care and treatment of patients with serious emotional disorders, but with all the psychological and social aspects of human experience and with the fostering of personality growth and the prevention of developmental misfortunes. According to this concept, the same principles govern the entire range of behavior from the so-called normal to the grossly abnormal. Within this context psychiatric nursing is both a specialty and an aspect of all professional nursing practice.

This continuum is denied by those who equate psychiatry with only its psychopathologic aspects and who use *mental health* or *mental hygiene* in connection with efforts to prevent mental illness and to promote positive health. Also, as Peplau has pointed out, these terms connote a static concept of health by implying that there is an artificial split between the mind and the body so that the mind can be sick or healthy apart from the body (18).*

As for the use of *behavioral science* and *social science* in connection with integration efforts, it is true that the social sciences, and more specifically those that are designated as behavioral sciences, provide a body of facts which the health professions can use. It remains for the health professions, however, to select the facts relevant to their practice and place them within appropriate value systems by identifying their relationship to the processes involved in the achievement of health goals and the development of such professional qualities as compassion. This translation of the theoretical concepts of the behavioral sciences into terms that reflect their applicability to health and professional conduct involves more than a reformulation; a substantive change also takes place. Just as the concepts of such sciences as anatomy, physiology, and physics acquire new meaning when they are adapted for use in orthopedics, so the behavioral science concepts acquire a new dimension when adapted to psychiatry.

In other words, the use of *psychiatric* in connection with projects directed toward helping students of nursing learn to deal with the emotional aspects of health and illness is more than a matter of semantic hair-splitting. It indicates a viewpoint with respect to both the dynamics of human behavior and the frame of reference for teaching them.

Integration is also a term that may be variously interpreted when used in connection with psychiatric integration projects. A number of meanings have been attached to it and the acceptance or nonacceptance of some of these meanings as relevant to the educational process is likely to affect the goals not only of a psychiatric integration project but of an entire educational program in nursing.

Probably most nurse educators would agree that *integration* refers to a process by which a student unifies the various items of knowledge that she

---

* The terms *mental health* and *mental hygiene* came into wide use in connection with the movement that developed in the early 1900's to improve the care of the "insane," to initiate programs for the prevention of "insanity," and to educate the public regarding psychopathologic behavior. In this movement the currently available knowledge about behavior was utilized (2), but no efforts were directed toward gaining any new knowledge of behavior. This latter task has remained within the province of psychiatry.

needs in order to provide a patient with total or comprehensive nursing care—care that takes into account all his nursing needs, physical, psychological, and social. It also refers to the end point of this process—the student achievement of integration through the process of integration.

The term *integration* is also used to denote the curriculum arrangements through which a student is helped to unify this knowledge. Instead of compartmentalizing in a single course or group of courses content that applies to many nursing situations, the content is woven through all appropriate areas of the curriculum and is presented in such a way that the student can perceive its relevance to each area. For example, when certain psychiatric concepts are identified as applicable to the care of patients ill for reasons other than those labeled "psychiatric," such as medical-surgical patients, these concepts are integrated into the course in medical-surgical nursing. Such integration involves teaching the concepts in the various learning experiences in this course in such a way that a student learns about the nursing care that a patient requires. She will also learn how to identify and take into account the patient's and his family's emotional response to his illness and rehabilitation and the impact of cultural and social factors on these responses. Such integration is not synonymous with teaching psychiatric nursing and medical nursing; rather, it represents teaching medical-surgical nursing in a comprehensive and unified course. However, it does contribute to the student's preparation for nursing psychiatric patients through laying a groundwork for or reinforcing her learning experiences in the psychiatric nursing course.

As has been stated, these interpretations of the word *integration* with respect to both the student's integration of knowledge and the integration of curriculum content in an educational program would be accepted by most educators. In all probability the majority of educators would also acknowledge the existence of a further meaning of this term, that is, the "unification of a person's knowledge, feelings, and attitudes into a harmonious whole." However, some nursing educators question whether helping the student to achieve this latter type of integration is a proper objective for an educational program. Rather, they believe that the goals of an educational institution should be limited to helping the student to acquire scientific knowledge and to develop intellectual discipline. The development of a unified approach to life, because it requires the student to change her existing attitudes as well as to acquire new knowledge, they regard as solely within the province of psychotherapy. In other words, re-education is not included in their concept of education.

The team that guided the Skidmore psychiatric integration project accepted integration according to its broadest definition—the one that includes both the process by which knowledge is synthesized and the process by which the student grows toward a wholeness of personality—as an essential goal of professional education for nursing. They also considered it the responsibility of the psychiatric integration project to contribute toward the attainment of this goal. This viewpoint stemmed from their belief concerning the limitation of professional performance that is based solely on the possession of scientific knowledge and their conviction that fundamental changes in behavior can be brought about by educational, as opposed to psychotherapeutic, means.

The Goal of Change and Growth

This discussion of the direction in which the student should be helped to grow in a baccalaureate degree program in nursing and in a psychiatric integration project associated with such a program will be limited to the attitudes and appreciations required for the fulfillment of the nurse's professional role. It should be emphasized, however, that this limitation in no way reflects the belief that these are the only objectives of collegiate nursing education, nor is it implied that the student's professional growth can be considered apart from her growth as a person and a member of society. Rather, it is believed that there is considerable overlapping in the qualities that make for maximum self-fulfillment in these three aspects of a nurse's life.

The argument for accepting change in a student's approach to life as an essential goal of baccalaureate education in nursing is based on an analysis of the requisites of the practice of professional nursing. Knowledge about the nursing needs of patients and the ways in which a nurse can help patients to meet these needs is certainly an essential for such practice, but the possession of such knowledge does not necessarily result in its application. The nurse is a human being, not a data-processing machine, and the knowledge with which she has been "programmed" is not the only determinant of her behavior in a situation. Her feelings, attitudes, and appreciations affect the degree to which she applies her knowledge, and in fact may decide whether or not she applies the knowledge at all. Thus, her preparation for assuming the role of a professional nurse is incomplete unless it fosters her growth toward appropriate attitudes, especially her attitudes toward the subject matter under study and the teaching-learning process. Specifically, two areas of growth would seem to be important—the development of a willingness to become personally involved in one's professional activities and the realization of one's potentials for creativeness.

PERSONAL INVOLVEMENT

As the emotional aspects of nursing care have moved from an intuitive level to one that permits the conscious application of scientific principles, nursing educators have begun to consider the disquieting reality that something has been lost thereby—the personal meaning of nursing to the student. Often the objectivity required for the scientific observation of a nursing problem and response to this problem has been equated with emotional detachment and the maintenance of Spartan self-control. When this line of reasoning is carried to an extreme degree, it distorts the learning of nursing into a quest for theoretical knowledge and the acquisition of a blueprint for the manipulation of one's environment. Such an outlook can lead only to professional hollowness—to the "sense of emptiness" which Arthur T. Jersild has identified as a recurrent problem among teachers (8). Its result is student lack of interest in the subject matter of nursing—the patient—and thus, eventually, the extermination of any motivation to acquire knowledge and any inclination to participate in the life of the classroom.* A feeling of personal involvement in what she is doing and learning is essential if the nurse or the student of nursing is to derive any real meaning from the practice of her chosen profession.

True, such a feeling should not be allowed to interfere with the nurse's performance of measures that are required for the patient's well-being or recovery. To this extent the nurse must remain objective; nor is personal involvement synonymous with a movement from a professional to a social relationship in which the nurse uses the patient to satisfy her own needs and ends.† The personal involvement referred to here is the type of involvement in which a nurse truly cares about what happens to a patient and, in a broader sense, is one in which she is willing and able to invest herself in what she believes in and hopes for in the practice of her profession. Such investment requires her to have reasonable awareness of her own feelings and their effect on her interpersonal relationships; for example, she is not content with self-assurances that she means to be kind, but undertakes to learn how she can implement her intentions. Thus, her search for a personal meaning in nursing results in an insatiable hunger for understanding and discovery rather than for material gain.

The search for meaning in nursing is unmistakably a personal search. Nonetheless, it is one toward which an educational program can stimulate a student by penetrating her illusion of detachment and helping her to discover, formulate, and refine meaning in the practice of nursing in whatever context it occurs. This task is one which collegiate programs must undertake

---

* William F. Weber, in an unpublished paper describing a clinical seminar for psychiatric nurses in which he and I collaborated at the William Alanson White Institute of Psychiatry, Psychoanalysis and Psychology, has identified the psychiatric nurse's fear of becoming involved and inability to become involved—to allow herself to feel for patients and to permit such feelings to come into awareness—as one of her chief problems (26).

† Norris has identified five differences between a social and professional relationship. She discusses these within a psychodynamic framework which includes principles of goal getting, expectations, communication, participant observation, and steps in problem solving (17).

if nursing is to survive as a profession, or develop into one. To be valid, nursing's claim for professionalism must be based on concern for the patient as well as on a scientific approach to the patient's problems. Unless nurses reach a clear understanding of the meaning of personal involvement and, in so doing, cease to carve the image of the professional nurse out of the quicksand of myth and conformity, the nursing profession can expect only increasing distress and eventually professional death.

CREATIVENESS

A nurse's ability to remain personally involved in the practice of nursing is contingent upon her capacity to be creative and her opportunity to exercise her creativeness. Unless she can view each nursing situation as a challenge to her creative ability, her sense of personal involvement will disappear and be replaced by a preoccupation with prescribed procedures and routines.

In a penetrating analysis of the nature and processes of creativeness, Gardner Murphy has pointed out that creating is much more than sheer combining, which consists principally of associating or connecting things together, and has identified *emergence* as being the central principle underlying creativeness (16). In emergence, new methods and tools of conceptualization are required of the individual at each level of integration. According to Murphy (16),

> Emergence defines the process by which co-working factors result in a *new form of organization*. It is the appearance of a new total arising from a series of interdependent changes, no one of which has any specific predictive power for a new system of functions.

Creativity in nursing requires the individual nurse to integrate "much that is in our sensory world, in our cognitive world, in our affective and impulsive world—a single, unified representation of what we make out of the universe itself" (16). For the student of nursing, the integrative task is a joy or a burden, depending on the concomitant feelings that are aroused in her. Her integrative capacity is dependent on positive past experiences, a strong self-concept, and some achievement of success and satisfaction in effecting constructive innovations.

It therefore becomes the task of nursing education to encourage the student to take a fresh look at problems and practices and attempt innovations that hold some promise of bettering the existing routine. Such a task is admittedly difficult in a learning situation that deals with people rather than with things or ideas that can be tested without endangering human welfare. The nursing student's (and the nurse's) freedom to make innovations is to some extent limited by her responsibility to the individuals entrusted to her care. The proposed innovation, if given a trial, may prove to be more effective than the old method, but is it safe to try it? The old method may be cumbersome or even useless, but after all it is "tried and true."

The fact that nursing education takes place in a setting that exists primarily for service rather than educational purposes also is a barrier to the development of creativity. As has been pointed out, the bureaucratic structure of the hospital frequently requires the nurse to conform by eliminating such superfluous qualities as a spirit of inquiry and a desire to innovate.

Despite these handicaps it is essential that educational programs that purport to prepare professional nurses fan the flame of creativity in their students. Otherwise, instead of being a profession which, through the contributions of each generation of its members, is kept abreast of scientific and social progress, nursing will be, at best, a skilled occupation whose members continue to use the hand-me-down practices of their grandparents.

Education versus Psychotherapy

The process of fostering personal involvement and creativity is considerably different from that involved in helping the student to acquire knowledge. Although in previous experiences the student may have acquired some erroneous "facts" relevant to nursing, such information is usually minimal and easily abandoned. The student's growth in knowledge is therefore largely a matter of acquiring new knowledge. In contrast, the student enters her program in nursing with a whole system of values and definite patterns of emotional responses that are deeply embedded and are by no means so readily relinquished as is her factual information. Her development of appropriate professional attitudes and feelings, therefore, often involves *change.*

Because the area in which this change takes place involves the subject matter of psychiatry—emotions, attitudes, and appreciations—the goal of change is one to which a psychiatric integration project might be expected to contribute. Such was the thinking that led to the inclusion of the student's change and growth in the direction of appropriate professional attitudes as one of the aims of the Skidmore College psychiatric integration project.

In determining the approach to this goal, however, the members of the psychiatric team were careful to bear in mind the differences between education and psychotherapy, so that the activities of the integration project would stay within the bounds of those that are legitimately characterized as educational. Such clarification is particularly important in any nursing education venture because of the concern on the part of many nurse educators that nursing education, in its endeavor to incorporate psychiatric concepts in its curriculum content, has moved too far in the direction of psychotherapy.

This confusion between educational and psychotherapeutic endeavors is understandable in view of the historic influence that the development of psychoanalysis has had on American education and its efforts to incorporate the personal growth of students among its goals. The similarity of goals has also been a factor. For both education and psychotherapy the ultimate purpose is the fullest possible development of the individual (25). As John Walker Powell has stated, "Education and therapy are complementary phases of a single process—the learning process as directed to the achievement of effective maturity" (20). Although it is not unusual for two quite separate disciplines to share the same ultimate goal (for example, medicine and nursing), the existence of a common purpose can obscure, in the minds of some people, the differentiating characteristics.

The confusion about the boundaries between education and psychotherapy has been compounded, in the case of nursing educators, by the fact that in the process of adapting psychoanalytic theories for use in nursing education and nursing practice, certain misunderstandings and misinterpretations have occurred. Among these misunderstandings are those occasioned by the reckless use of the word *therapy*; many people, including psychiatrists and educators, have tended to use this word in connection with any activity that is carried out in groups or that deals with feelings (21). As a result, whenever the goal of an educational endeavor in nursing includes professional growth and change, and particularly when the teaching method emphasizes the learner's subjective responses to the curriculum content, the question is likely to arise, "Is this education or psychotherapy?" The issue is practically certain to evoke concern when, as in the case of some psychiatric integration projects, a faculty or some other group not formally designated as "students" is the focus of teaching.

For these reasons, the psychiatric nurse director of the Skidmore College integration project believed it important for her to define the differences between education and psychotherapy, particularly those differences that would be observed in the utilization of a purely educational approach to psychiatric integration, the psychiatric nurse noted the following:

1. The goal of education is further growth of the individual. Its attainment, therefore, involves change for something better. The emphasis is on the achievement of competence and awareness. Its sphere of work is the external world and social reality as it is composed of mental, physical, and aesthetic activities (24). It teaches the individual how to examine what he thinks about what he feels (20). Education does not aim at personality reorganization, although personality change may be a by-product. The teacher is concerned with the handling of judgments and the student's impulse to generalize beyond legitimate implication (20).

The goal of psychotherapy, on the other hand, is the acceptance of one's self, including one's limitations. Psychotherapy is primarily a *corrective* experience. It is concerned specifically with correcting distortions in perception and communication. It pays more attention, therefore, to feelings than to the verbal content of communications. Its focus is on widening the knowledge of a person's internal world. Through self-awareness one is able to relinquish distortions that impede effective living. The psychotherapist is concerned with the patient's faulty handling of his emotions.

2. In education there is a program, a curriculum, and a definite body of knowledge that has to be learned (25). The problems and issues that are explored are limited to those arising in connection with the particular field of study or professional activity. The teacher accepts the content and tries to help the student to distinguish among the various ideas contained in it. In clarifying the function of education, Nathaniel Cantor has stated, "The teacher's function is to deal with a student's difficulty only insofar as his work in the course is concerned" (4). Psychotherapy covers a much broader field which includes problems and issues arising in all interpersonal relationships.

3. Education is concerned primarily with motivational factors in terms of *conscious* desires and wishes. It does not pass these boundaries into the unconscious. Understanding unconscious motivation, however, can increase one's sensitivity to conscious attitudes and reactions. The emphasis of education is on the present condition. Psychotherapy focuses on the individual's genetic and unconscious motivational factors and therefore utilizes past experiences with significant persons.

4. Education achieves enhancement of the self-concept by enlarging social activities, stimulating interests, and redirecting anxiety (24). Through focusing on anxiety and its resolution, psychotherapy frees, but does not stimulate, interest.

5. Education directs change through the use of evaluation, approval, and disapproval. Not only does the teacher impart information and guide the student in the formation of new skills, but she takes a stand. In this way, the teacher is a rational authority (25). In psychotherapy, change evolves. The task is not to influence or control directly. The psychotherapist avoids giving approval, disapproval, praise, and so on, and hence does not engage in evaluation as such (25).

6. The teacher works primarily with positive attitudes and channels the negative reactions (25). The psychotherapist has the task of uncovering negative attitudes, although he does not stimulate them. He must handle the patient's transferential reactions without reacting with countertransference.

7. Education is an acculturation process. Therefore, not only is the teacher a helper of individuals, but she also is a carrier of the culture, in that she is an implementor of the social group's standards. The psychotherapist is primarily a helper of individuals.

As the nursing profession becomes more aware that nursing education can be a means of achieving personal growth, more learning problems which

involve aspects of the personality will be faced, worked through, and resolved. In learning how to help students in this manner, nursing educators
must be careful to observe the boundary lines between education and psychotherapy, so that they can give the students the benefits of what they, as
educators, have to offer without infringing on the domain that properly
belongs to the psychiatrist.

The Methods of Psychiatric Integration

TEACHING PSYCHIATRIC CONCEPTS

Emphasis on the educational program's responsibility for stimulating the
student to undertake a search for personal meaning in nursing and for
helping her to develop her capacity for creativity does not depreciate the
importance of providing her with the knowledge that is essential for professional use. If nurses are to utilize a scientific approach in dealing with
the emotional aspects of nursing problems, nursing education must make
available to students of nursing the relevant facts and theory from the
growing body of knowledge about human behavior.

Imparting this essential knowledge, however, is only the first step in the
process by which the teacher helps the student to learn psychiatric concepts.
If this knowledge is to be useful, the student must translate it into her
behavior, and such translation does not follow automatically from the
acquisition of the knowledge. The student must be helped to establish a
bridge between the theoretical content relating to human behavior and the
application of this content in the care of patients.

It might seem strange that this type of teaching cannot be taken for
granted, because traditionally nursing has been taught as an applied science,
and work with patients has constituted the major share of the learning
experiences. However, in the case of the emotional aspects of nursing care,
nursing educators have sometimes tended to confuse the content of nursing
education—essential knowledge—and the desired result of this education—
the ability to translate this knowledge into nursing practice. If a student is
able to describe the stages of growth and development, the various forms
of interpersonal interactions, and so on, it is often assumed that she will be
able to apply her knowledge in the care that she gives to patients.

Possibly this assumption is a matter of historical development. The introduction of instruction in the behavioral sciences into the nursing curriculum
coincided with other attempts to "professionalize" nursing education
through the addition of courses in the liberal arts. It is possible, therefore,
that knowledge about human behavior is sometimes regarded as "horizon-
broadening" knowledge which, by the very fact of its possession, will make
the nurse a more "educated" person and therefore a better nurse. Whatever

the reasons, the fact remains that nursing instructors have felt far less responsible for helping the student to bridge the gap between behavioral science knowledge and its application to the care of patients than they have in the case of the knowledge derived from such sciences as physiology, microbiology, and chemistry.

This method of dealing, or not dealing, with content relating to human behavior raises several questions. In the process of professionalization, has nursing education become entangled in the speciously logical pattern of equating the possession of knowledge with understanding? In their professional self-consciousness, have nursing educators been caught up in impatience for professionalization to the point where they are operating on the delusion that the mere possession of more knowledge will automatically raise nursing to a status equal to that of other professions? Does increased knowledge necessarily enhance the role of the nurse? Have nursing educators become overly concerned with knowing instead of thinking?

When knowledge is perceived in this light, it freezes rather than kindles the student's imagination. It narcotizes instead of awakening thought. If nursing educators and students are inclined to perceive knowledge as primarily information accumulated by scholars of the past, there will be little connection between these tombstones to dead experience and what we call "education for living"; the faculty and the students become passive voyeurs of life but can know very little about living. If nursing is to develop its potential for helping patients with their emotional problems, the psychosocial aspects of illness, like the physiological aspects, must be taught as laboratory subjects.

This is not to say that the methods utilized in teaching the physical aspects of care are sufficient for teaching psychiatric concepts. To be able to deal with physiologically induced problems, the student does not have to have suffered from the condition herself. To deal with emotionally generated problems, however, requires more than an intellectual grasp of the content. For example, to know the definition of anxiety and even to be able to identify its manifestations in a person is not the same as to understand what anxiety means to a person to the extent that one can interact with him in a way that is helpful to him. The development of this kind of understanding comes from a study of one's own experience with anxiety.

Thus, the teaching of psychiatric concepts involves experiential teaching —the method by which the teacher helps the student to recognize, describe, analyze, validate, and synthesize the meaning of her experiences. In an experiential teaching-learning situation, therefore, the learner is as much the subject of study as the patient or other person whom she is studying. The threat of exposure involved in such study makes experiential teaching one of the most difficult of all teaching methods.

EFFECTING CHANGE

The Group Approach. The methods for helping nursing students grow in the direction of the attitudes and appreciations that are consistent with the professional practice of nursing are far more complex than the methods involved in teaching psychiatric concepts. Much of this complexity is derived from the influence that the group has on the individual's attitudes. As Kurt K. Lewin has pointed out, as long as the values of the group remain the same, the individuals in the group will hold on to them tenaciously (13). On the other hand, group decision has the power of changing the standards, values, and atmosphere of the group, thereby facilitating growth in the individual.

Therefore, the most potent method of bringing about behavioral change in nursing students is to involve them in a group. As Lewin and Grabbe have stated (14),

> Re-education is a process in which changes of knowledge and beliefs, changes of values and standards, changes of emotional attachments and needs, and changes of every day, do not occur piecemeal and independently of each other, but within the framework of the individual's total life in the group.

In his study of the resolution of social conflicts, Lewin has further pointed out that changes of this kind require a change in group atmosphere rather than in single items (13).

Jacques Eliott has identified several strengths in group interaction as a method of facilitating real change that have relevance in the education of nursing students (7).

1. Group interaction offers an opportunity for the students to meet the anxiety that the total educational experience arouses in them.

2. It fosters mutual support among the students by universalizing their feeling experiences and providing a practical milieu in which to ask questions and raise issues.

3. It helps the students to transform the large body of diverse course material, life experiences, and lecture material into the gestalt of nursing.

4. It provides a dynamic medium for learning through experiences that are shared emotionally as well as intellectually.

The Process. Motivation alone does not lead to change; action is the link between the desire to change and the achievement of change (12). Lewin has identified three steps in the process.

The first step is to unfreeze the present level of values of the group. Because no change can occur in a group until the individual members are no longer hostile toward a new set of values, beliefs, and attitudes—at least to the point of maintaining a neutral open-mindedness—a crucial aspect of

Ganong Joan + Warren

Nursing Management

'76

:ine is in good taste? _____

in poor taste please note it k

_____

_____

sections of the magazine that

d   4. Let's

se Times   5. Adven

                           6. This

ng that might be done to add t

Thank you very much.
This will help us ha
THESE TIMES, EDITORI

the unfreezing process is catharsis (1). Catharsis involves a deliberate emotional shake-up by which complacency and self-righteousness are penetrated, thus helping to eliminate prejudice. The ventilation of negative reactions is the prelude to change.

The second step in working toward change is to move to the new level of values. Verbal expression of the new values indicates progress in this direction, but it is not the equivalent of actual change. The third step is to freeze the group on the new level, or, as Ronald Lippitt has put it, to generalize and stabilize the change (15). Through such freezing the new value system is made relatively secure against change.

Impediments to Change. Those who attempt re-education of this kind must take into account the obstacles to change within a group. One of these obstacles is the resistance to change on the part of the group members, for despite the influence that group values have on a group member, in the final analysis the individual members determine whether the group values will change. As P. W. Bridgman has stated (3),

> One of the most important things to remember if we hope to understand the functioning of society is that no particular situation can come to pass, no matter how desirable on general principles nor how universally acceptable, unless there is some specific mechanism by which the succession of detailed steps necessary for its realization can occur. In society the detailed steps are the actions of the individuals who compose the society.

Lippitt has identified four reactions on the part of individuals within the group that operate against change in the group (15). These reactions are (1) reluctance to admit weaknesses; (2) fear of failure or awkwardness in trying to initiate a new practice or behavior pattern; (3) a fatalistic expectation of failure instilled by previous unsuccessful attempts to change; and (4) fear of losing some current satisfaction, such as power over and dependency on others. Generally, group equilibrium takes on a value of its own, and in going against the group standard, an individual risks being banished from the group.

A second major force that impedes goal-directed change is a hierarchal structure in the group. Regardless of the type of social system that exists, change is always imminent, but in a hierarchy, effort is directed toward keeping change consistent with orthodox ideas. A primary behavior pattern in a hierarchal structure is that of dominance and submission, which destroys the free flow of communication. Thus, any genuine change in the nursing student group is dependent on a change in the traditional power constellation in faculty-student relationships.

Techniques. Those who are attempting to bring about change must take into consideration both the steps that must be accomplished—unfreezing (by catharsis), movement, and freezing—and the forces that tend to obstruct change. These considerations obviously rule out teaching techniques by which knowledge is transmitted without a prior determination of the emotional set of the group members, especially the lecture method with its hierarchal implications. The method that holds most promise is face-to-face discussion in which the members of the group can clarify and work through the concrete issues they are facing at the time that these issues arise.

The first requirement of the group discussion method is that there be enough continuity for the individuals to coalesce into a group. Therefore, arrangements are made for the students to meet at regular intervals.

In line with the need for a democratic rather than a hierarchal structure, there is no dominant leader; the teacher is a member of the group, not outside it, and like the other members voices her reactions to issues. Nor is there any fixed agenda; the issues to be discussed emerge during the meeting. The atmosphere is an unhurried one. Silences occur frequently. Irrelevant topics are raised as a means of escape from affect-laden material. Therefore, enough time is allowed at each meeting for the discussion to be continued until some sort of resolution is reached.

The depth of the professional problems raised is related to (1) the ability of the teacher to involve the total group and to help the students to identify and clarify issues, (2) the degree of mutual trust and confidence that is established among them, and (3) the degree to which some constructive action is possible. Besides creating a matrix for the resolution of conflicts at the level of action, this method of teaching creates a laboratory in learning participant observation and problem solving and in developing creativeness. One of the chief functions of the teacher is to combat the students' feelings of hopelessness about the possibilities for change, including resignation to a perpetuation of the status quo.

The Role of the Nurse Teacher

HELPING THE STUDENTS TO LEARN PSYCHIATRIC CONCEPTS

The nursing educator is the moral watchdog for the nursing profession. As a nurse she is responsible for assuring safe and effective nursing care. Within this context the patient is the principal concern. Hence, the nurse teacher is obligated to help the nursing student to achieve clinical competence and must focus on what the student needs to develop this competence.

The nurse teacher is a resource person, and as such she is both a primary source of knowledge and a guide to further sources of knowledge. She plans and guides the students in experiences in which they can discover knowledge or acquire skill in applying their knowledge, and she helps them to integrate what they learn in these experiences. Sometimes she makes arrangements for another expert to present material.

At first glance it might appear that this method of securing the cooperation of an expert might be used for instruction in psychiatric concepts. On
second thought, however, it is obvious that the method of teaching those
concepts—experiential teaching—involves more than the sprinkling of psychiatric content throughout the curriculum according to prearranged schedule;
the student must be helped to examine and reflect on her experiences with
other people as they occur. Accordingly, the experiential teaching of psychiatric concepts is best accomplished by the instructor who guides the student's
clinical learning experiences in the course in which the concepts are being
integrated.

This instructor has an opportunity to know the total nursing situation in
which the student's experience occurred—the patient's physical condition,
his relationships with his family, his behavioral tendencies, the student's
characteristic reactions to situations of this kind, and so on—and is therefore
in a position to help the student explore all aspects of the situation, possibly
including some of which the student is unaware. Moreover, in assigning a
student to a patient, the instructor can, to a certain extent, observe the
educational principle of from-the-simple-to-the-complex with respect to the
patient's emotional as well as physical nursing needs. For example, the
nursing problems of a patient who has undergone a prostatectomy might be
regarded as fairly simple insofar as the physical aspects are concerned, but
the emotional aspects might make the care of such a patient an extremely
complex nursing situation.

The integration of psychiatric concepts throughout the nursing curriculum, then, can occur only to the degree that every instructor on the nursing
faculty is able to teach psychiatric concepts, principles, and processes along
with the physical aspects of nursing care. It is therefore important that every
nurse instructor not only have a "book knowledge" of psychiatric concepts
but be able to use these concepts in whatever she does professionally. As
Norris has pointed out, one cannot expect students to synthesize psychiatric
concepts into their nursing care if their instructors have not done so
(17).

It is therefore crucial for the nurse teacher to find ways to strengthen her
knowledge of psychiatric concepts and her skill in teaching these concepts
to students. To do so may make a demand upon her to become a learner.
The learner role in this instance is much more difficult than any she may
assume with respect to other clinical areas. If, for example, a pediatric
nursing instructor needs to acquire additional knowledge or skill in medical-
surgical nursing, she will be able to do so and to incorporate this knowledge
in the content that she teaches without changing her behavior in any way.
If she is not skilled in teaching psychiatric concepts, however, she will not
only have to learn a new method of teaching but will have to undergo a
behavioral change. In response to the expectation of change, she is bound

to experience varying degrees of anxiety. Anxiety, however, can be a spear-head to learning and growth.

Helping the Students to Change and Grow

Interpersonal Relations in the Classroom. In meeting the student's edu-cational needs, the nurse teacher encounters and must work with the stu-dent's emotional responses to illness and death, the authority-dependency conflict, the complexities related to an organizational structure, and the difficulties arising from the communication process. She has to deal primarily with the ingredients of perception, for it is these that make meaningful experience possible.

The way the student achieves the goals of nursing education is through her relationships with the teacher and her compeers. It is almost impossible to exaggerate the influence that any teacher exerts, either knowingly or otherwise, on a student's attitudes toward what she is teaching. In a dis-cussion of the relationship of the teacher's personality and the quality of the interpersonal relations in the classroom to what is learned by the student, Joseph Katz has stated, "academic subject matter can be recognized to assume many additional forms. It can be sentimental, pragmatic, polemical, censorious, ego-syntonic, ego-alien, subjective, objective, phantasy-oriented, reality-oriented, expressive, constructive, collectinglike, abstract-schizoid, and so on" (9).

Inherent in the student-teacher relationship is the concept of the teacher as a model. Through the transference phenomenon (which classically refers to a process in psychoanalysis in which the patient reacts to the psycho-analyst as though he were an important figure in the patient's past life), the student consciously and unconsciously identifies with the teacher. Because of this transference phenomenon, the teacher, in her relationships with students, may take on some aspects of various roles, such as those of mother or older sister, boss, chum, or colleague. Because the quality of the teacher-student interactions plays an essential part in influencing the degree of professional and personal growth that is realized, the transference phenom-enon can be an aid or an obstacle to learning.

Leadership Responsibilities. Directly or indirectly, the nurse educator is a powerful force in molding society. Because of the nature of her relation-ships with students, parents, patients, nursing service personnel, members of other disciplines, and professional colleagues in her own and other insti-tutions, every nurse educator holds a leadership position. The degree of goal-directed and permanent change that occurs within a group of nursing students is dependent on the quality of the faculty members' leadership and the distribution of leadership among them.

As a leader in nursing education, the nurse teacher plays the role of change-agent. In this role she presents opposing points of view, and so modifies previous attitudes and creates the possibility for change and growth (10). She also is confronted by and creates situations in which some individual or group value is challenged or is perceived as being neglected or violated.

Because such situations inevitably arouse anxiety, it is incumbent upon the nursing leader to recognize anxiety, to be able to tolerate it, and to utilize the appropriate principles and processes in resolving it. Peplau has stated that all leadership positions carry a threefold responsibility with respect to stress—(1) to recognize the cues of stress in students and co-workers; (2) to intervene constructively; and (3) to take preventive actions toward reducing stress and minimizing the possibilities of its occurrence (19).

If the nurse educator is to effect lasting change by initiating constructive intervention in affect-laden situations, she must understand the relationship between the presence of anxiety, frustration, aggression, and conflict as well as such principles that pertain to group functioning as group composition and contagion, special and spontaneous group processes like the formation of cliques, and group psychological phenomena such as the development of scapegoats (6). Other knowledge necessary for utilizing the group process in effecting change includes the concepts of psychological force and tension, learning theory, and such principles of psychoanalysis as those pertaining to unconscious motivation, defense patterns against anxiety, communication theory, free association, transference, and countertransference.

Constructive intervention represents the core of leadership. The essence of intervention is the willingness and the ability to investigate situations that disturb the equilibrium and to explore the needs, expectations, and goals of those persons with whom one works. In this exploration the leader assiduously searches for and collects the pertinent data, which include such subjective material as the attitudes, feelings, thoughts, reactions, modes of communication, and patterns of behavior of the other person or persons, and analyzes these data by consciously formulating meanings and then consensually validating the interpretations with those who are directly concerned.

In constructive intervention, the nursing leader, whom Peplau has colorfully referred to as the "pacemaker," is concerned with changing the social system as contrasted with the "peacemaker," who is primarily concerned with perpetuating it (19). The nursing leader openly challenges destructive practices, even if in so doing she risks the disapproval and blame of her colleagues. Instead of working toward maintaining "peace at any price" by pretending that interpersonal conflicts do not exist (in the hope that merely wishing will make it so), the leader directly confronts individuals and the group in the effort to uncover the differences and to harmonize them.

Obstacles to Role Performance

For the nurse teacher to help the student develop personally and professionally, she too must have the opportunity to change and grow. In a collegiate setting there are many elements conducive to such growth—the resources for continued study and self-development, the stimulation of students and faculty colleagues, and the atmosphere of excitement about the future of professional nursing that pervades the settings in which this future is being planned. There are also obstacles to the nurse teacher's development, particularly with respect to the qualities she needs for her pacemaker role. Perhaps the greatest of these is the hierarchal structure in which she must operate.

The nursing profession has developed within a hierarchal social structure in which the concept of high status and low status is a hallmark. Moreover, nursing education has not rid itself of this structure as it has moved into institutions of higher learning. Thus, to her surprise and sometimes to her disenchantment, the nurse teacher finds herself confronted by problems of status, power, authority, communication, and decision making corresponding to those in the hospital and a similar aggregate of rules and regulations (although they may not be explicitly stated) promulgated to preserve the status quo and to enforce individual conformity. She must face the fact that she has exchanged the hospital hierarchy for the ladder of rank and authority of the collegiate setting.

CHARACTERISTICS OF THE COLLEGE HIERARCHAL STRUCTURE

Upon reflection, it is obvious that a hierarchal structure is a characteristic that one would expect to find in the American college. Every college and university is a subculture which, although it has its own idiosyncratic values and concerns, reflects the politics and the economies of the larger society to which it belongs. Like the rest of our society and its other institutions, it is organized on neither purely democratic nor strictly authoritarian lines.

As a corporate enterprise, much of its activity must be devoted to surviving, expanding, and maintaining a strong position in relation to other institutions (22). For such a large-scale organization to carry out a complex program, decisions must be made and men must be induced to carry them out (5). A great deal of power (the ability to influence behavior) must be exercised.

It is particularly difficult for professionals to function within a hierarchal group structure, because it is sustained not by a recognition of differences in skill and contributions of those who work together, but by the predomination of special distinctions and privileges accorded to the individual teacher. Although the individual faculty member knows he is being evaluated and that he is competing with his colleagues for a high-status position, he frequently is confused about the ground rules of the competition (27).

These interpersonal tensions and rivalries lead to the formation of factions or cliques that are organized on the basis of the individual faculty member's vested interests, needs, goals, roles, and real or perceived position within the educational hierarchy. Caplow and McGee have said, "There are factions in all faculties, and at least some of the factions are the same everywhere" (5).

Because the college and university faculties are organized into an hierarchal structure, deliberate and concerted change of any kind is extremely difficult. Speaking to this point, Nevitt Sanford has said (22).

> In order to resist the pressures from the outside as well as to further their most immediate interests, faculties have fostered an ingroup spirit, built up traditions of faculty prerogatives, installed the machinery of campus democracy. They are the very things that now make change very difficult, even when the impulse to change arises largely from the faculty itself. Measures contrived for one purpose tend to be put in the service of other purposes as well, until they become autonomous.

As far as the achievement of the goals of psychiatric integration is concerned, the most detrimental effects of the hierarchal structure in the college or university result from the obstacles it puts in the way of intrafaculty communications, decision making, and the individual faculty member's feeling of freedom to function creatively.

EFFECT ON COMMUNICATION

Because of the way power is distributed in the American college, communication problems rank at the top of the list of those conditions that prevent educational reform. Caplow and McGee have recognized, for example, that a low-status faculty member generally will complain to the chairman or dean only when the problem seems to be out of the latter's control, for to complain about matters within his control would be to challenge his authority. "Thus, complaints about the chairman will be made to peers, one of whom will carry the tale to the chairman. In this way the status of the peer is enhanced, because the act of making the complaint to him implies that he can do something about it. The peer in turn is able to confront the chairman because the complaint is not his own. As an intermediary, he is not challenging the chairman's authority and will not fear retaliation" (5).

EFFECT ON DECISION MAKING

The adverse effects of the hierarchal structure on the making of decisions is to a certain extent related to the conflicts and pressures that are built into the role of the departmental chairman. A comparison of the chairman's role with the foreman's role in a factory, as described by Caplow and McGee, helps to clarify some of these pressures. As the foreman represents management to the workers and the workers to management, so the chairman represents those persons who are above in the vertical axis of power, such as the dean and the president, to those lower-status persons, the teachers. He also represents his faculty to the dean and the president. Because of his professional identification with the faculty group, he is closer to it than to the higher-status group. Since, however, the higher-status persons appointed him to his job and, through the budget allocation and the degree of freedom they permit him, influence his ability to do his job effectively, he must be close to them also.

The chairman's relationship with the upper-status persons is largely in the decision-making area, and many of the decisions involve confidential information, such as those pertaining to budget matters, the promotion of faculty members, and the granting or the withholding of certain rights and privileges. Therefore, the chairman must conceal from his professional colleagues much of the content of his communication with higher authorities. His possession of secret information tends to arouse distrust in him and repeatedly leads to a breakdown in communication between him and his colleagues (23).

One result of this frequently untenable position is that the chairman may be inclined to "pass the buck" by throwing upward the responsibility for all the decisions—especially the invidious budget decisions—that wreak hardship on the individual faculty member. Conversely, he may lay claim to those decisions which result in pleasant outcomes (5).

This vagueness about who is actually responsible for what decisions tends to cloud the whole decision-making area. Uncertain of the types of decisions in which the departmental chairman has a voice, the faculty tends to be unsure of its prerogatives and responsibilities for making recommendations about matters that require action by administrative authorities and even, at times, about its obligation to make decisions that fall within its own sphere. Thus, it can happen that even when the need for change is felt, it does not come about because of the haziness about the machinery necessary for engineering it.

EFFECT ON INDIVIDUAL CREATIVENESS

In a hierarchal structure there are strong pressures on the individual to remain in his assigned place and do his assigned job—but no more. As Harold H. Kelley discovered in his study of experimentally created hierarchies, conditions of low status which are also nonmobile toward a higher one and those of high status which have the potential for further upward mobility are more detrimental to total group cohesiveness than any other

status-mobility combinations investigated. Hostility results from the perception of persons at the other level either as threats to one's own desirable
position or as occupants of a coveted but unattainable position (11). Much
of the antagonism that is frequently directed toward the faculty member who
functions as a consultant, for example, generally arises from the fear of the
high-status persons that in some way he will usurp their position in the
hierarchy or from the desire of the low-status persons to have his position
for themselves.

It is this interplay of statuses that makes it extremely difficult to assimilate
the nonconformist within the college department. The nonconformist is
likely to be perceived as dangerous because he is a threat to the status quo.
Yet to be creative one must be a nonconformist in the sense that one must
abandon the worship of tradition and be willing to challenge orthodoxy.

As frequently occurs in the hospital setting, the nurse teacher in a collegiate setting may use the problems associated with the authority-
dependency conflict, which is an inherent aspect of the college hierarchy,
defensively. When she is afraid or unwilling to use initiative, to take responsibility and leadership, to explore alternatives, to compromise, to set limits,
she may be inclined to blame those persons who are on the next level above
and below her in the hierarchy. The ability to innovate may be lost. Like
the nurse who practices in the hospital, she may unwittingly become an
actress playing numerous roles, thereby failing to discover and develop her
own.

Implications for Psychiatric Integration Project

To summarize, then, in formulating the conceptual framework for the
Skidmore psychiatric integration project, the psychiatric nurse project director incorporated the belief that the goals of professional nursing education
include the student's personal and professional growth as well as accumula-
tion of knowledge and development of skills. A large contribution to the
achievement of these goals can be made by the integration of psychiatric
content and the utilization of educational methods based on psychodynamic
principles. These methods must take into account the extent to which the
success of any efforts to bring about goal-directed and permanent change is
dependent on the group and the atmosphere in which the group operates.

The nursing student is the ultimate reason for the educational activities
directed toward psychiatric integration. However, because the nurse teacher
has a pivotal position in these activities, she too must be helped to strengthen
her knowledge of psychiatric concepts and her skill in teaching these concepts. She must also be encouraged to develop further the qualities of
leadership that are implicit in her teaching role. As is the case with students,
the importance of the group and its organization must be taken into con-

sideration in helping the faculty member. Thus, a psychiatric integration project involves an appraisal of all elements of the educational program in nursing—the students, the faculty, the curriculum, and the policies and organization of the nursing unit and the institution in which it functions— to determine the assets that can be capitalized on and the places where further strengthening is desirable and feasible. The personnel responsible for guiding the integration project should, of course, be included in this evaluation.

This is not to say that all the problems that are identified can be resolved by psychiatric integration. Psychiatric integration is not a panacea; it cannot, for example, change the hierarchal structure of the American college. The particular structure of the individual college and the available resources, including the amount of money and time that are available for integration activities and personnel, have to be considered, and these will determine the depth to which various aspects of the total situation are approached. The differences in approach to psychiatric integration in the long run, therefore, provide a mirror of each college's unique characteristics.

REFERENCES

1. Allport, Gordon W. "Catharsis and the Reduction of Prejudice," *Journal of Social Issues*, 3–10 (August, 1945).

2. Beers, Clifford. *The Mind That Found Itself*. Garden City: Doubleday, Doran and Company, Inc., 1929.

3. Bridgman, P. W. *The Way Things Are*. New York: The Viking Press, Inc., 1961, p. 253.

4. Cantor, Nathaniel. *Dynamics of Learning*. Buffalo, N.Y.: Foster and Stewart, 1946.

5. Caplow, Theodore and Reece J. McGee. *The Academic Marketplace*. New York: Basic Books, Inc., 1958, p. 206.

6. Dollard, John, et al. *Frustration and Aggression*. New Haven, Conn.: Yale University Press, 1939.

7. Eliott, Jacques. "Interpretive Group Discussion as a Method of Facilitating Social Change," *Human Relations*, 1, 533–549 (1948).

8. Jersild, Arthur T. *When Teachers Face Themselves*. New York: Bureau of Publications, Teachers College, Columbia University, 1955, p. 169.

9. Katz, Joseph. "Personality and Interpersonal Relations in the College Classroom," in Nevitt Sanford (ed.), *The American College*. New York: John Wiley and Sons, Inc., Chap. 9, p. 389.

10. Kelley, Earl C. *Education for What Is Real*. New York: Harper and Row, 1947, p. 114.

11. Kelley, Harold H. "Communication in Experimentally Created Hierarchies," *Human Relations*, 39–56 (April, 1951).

12. Lewin, Kurt K. "Frontiers in Group Dynamics," *Human Relations*, 1, 5–41 (1947–48).

13. Lewin, Kurt K. *Resolving Social Conflicts.* New York: Harper and Row, 1948, pp. 49, 50.

14. Lewin, Kurt K., and Paul Grabbe. "Conduct, Knowledge and Acceptance of New Values," *Journal of Social Issues,* 53–64 (August, 1945).

15. Lippitt, Ronald. *The Dynamics of Planned Change.* New York: Harcourt Brace and Company, 1958, pp. 180, 181.

16. Murphy, Gardner, *Human Potentialities.* New York: Basic Books, Inc., 1958, pp. 134, 140, 258.

17. Norris, Catherine M. "What Insights Can Psychiatric Nurses Contribute to the Development of Curriculums in Basic Professional Nursing?" *Concepts of the Behavioral Sciences in Basic Nursing Education.* New York: National League for Nursing, 1958, pp. 264–270.

18. Peplau, Hildegard E. "Integration of Mental Hygiene: Psychiatry in the Basic Professional Nursing Program," unpublished paper, delivered at the Work Conference on Curriculum, New Jersey State League of Nursing Education, Newark, N.J., Dec. 1, 1950, pp. 24–37.

19. Peplau, Hildegard E. "Leadership Responsibility in Toleration of Stress: The Leader's Role in Helping Staff to Tolerate Stress," unpublished paper, prepared for Conference on Preparation For Leadership in Psychiatric Nursing Service, Department of Nursing Education, Teachers College, Columbia University, June 7–8, 1963.

20. Powell, John Walker, et al. "Group Reading and Group Therapy: A Concurrent Test," *Psychiatry,* 15, 33–51 (February, 1952).

21. Redl, Fritz. "Resistance in Therapy Groups," *Human Relations,* 1, 307–313 (1947–48).

22. Sanford, Nevitt. "Higher Education as a Social Problem," in Nevitt Sanford (ed.), *The American College.* New York: John Wiley and Sons, Inc., 1962, pp. 10–30.

23. Schutz, William C. "What Make Groups Productive?" *Human Relations,* 8, 429–465.

24. Searle, M. V. "Some Contrasted Aspects of Psychoanalysis and Education," *British Journal of Educational Psychology,* 276–296 (February, 1932).

25. Symonds, Percival A. "Education and Psychotherapy," *Journal of Educational Psychology,* 40, 1–32 (1949).

26. Weber, William F. "An Educational Experience for Psychiatric Nurses in the Use of Self and the Awareness of Interpersonal Processes," unpublished paper, 1964.

27. Wilson, Logan. *The Academic Man: Sociology of a Profession.* London: Oxford University Press, 1942, p. 62.

Chapter Four

NURSING DEPARTMENT PROFILE

This is the true joy in life, the being used for a purpose recognized by yourself as a mighty one. The being thoroughly worn out before you are thrown on the scrap heap; the being a force of Nature instead of a feverish selfish little clod of ailments and grievances complaining that the world will not devote itself to making you happy.

GEORGE BERNARD SHAW, "Epistle Dedicatory,"
Man and Superman

The fashioning of any psychiatric integration program, as has been pointed out, should take into account the educational environment in which it is to be conducted and the people who will be involved in its operation. For this reason a summarization of the general characteristics of the program and personnel of the Skidmore College Department of Nursing appears to be a suitable starting point for describing the process of psychiatric integration in this educational program during the years 1957–1962.

General Characteristics of the Department of Nursing

Skidmore College is a four-year college for women, located in the town of Saratoga Springs, New York. It was granted a charter in 1911 and was incorporated in 1922. One of its purposes is to provide its students with the opportunity for both liberal arts education and concentration in areas of special ability or professional interest. At the time of the integration project, the average enrollment was 1,200 students.

The educational unit in nursing, which was established in 1922, is organized as a department of the college, headed by a chairman who is directly responsible to the dean of the faculty. It offers a curriculum of eight semesters plus two summer sessions, leading to the degree of Bachelor of Science. Students enter the program directly from high school and, upon graduation, are qualified for beginning positions in all fields of nursing practice. At the time of the project, 141 credits were required for graduation, of which 60 were earned in general education courses and 81 in nursing courses.

The philosophy of the Department of Nursing, as formulated by the total faculty, has been stated as follows (2).

> The faculty believes that the basic professional program in nursing should be based on the needs of the students and the nursing needs of our society. In meeting these needs, we also believe that nursing has purposes and functions that are distinct, unique, but interdependent with other professions.
>
> We believe that nursing education needs to concern itself with health and social values of the community, the way people grow and develop, and the way culture hinders and facilitates growth. It is also concerned with the way people learn, and the way this learning is affected by the nature of significant relationships such as teacher-student and nurse-patient.
>
> Because we believe the nurse is responsible for nursing diagnosis and treatment, we believe we have the responsibility to help the student develop an inquiring mind, and to become a self-governing citizen able to exert her own self discipline.
>
> Since the nurse can best achieve her goals through collaboration, as a colleague, with all other members of the health team, we believe the faculty has the responsibility to help the student further develop as an individual so that she can function in a significant way in any of her roles as a woman, such as nurse, wife, mother, teacher and citizen.
>
> We believe that, to the degree she realizes her fullest potentialities and capacities, she will be able to meaningfully influence others—her patients and their families, members of the health team, and the community.

The need for the department of nursing to expand its clinical resources led it, in 1942, to move to New York City, 200 miles from Saratoga Springs, where it continues to maintain its headquarters at the New York University Medical Center. All the clinical nursing courses are taught in New York City; the general education courses in the curriculum are the regular courses provided for all Skidmore students at the Saratoga Springs campus.

In 1944, retroactive to 1942, the nursing program was accredited by the National League of Nursing Education, and it was the first basic collegiate program in the country to be accredited for preparing students for public health nursing practice.

During the five years of the integration project, the average enrollment in the nursing program was between 140 and 150, and the enrollment in the sophomore and junior classes amounted to about twenty-seven students each. Instruction in the nursing curriculum was provided by the twelve full-time faculty members (including the psychiatric nurse project director), the psychiatrist, and numerous other personnel who taught varying aspects of pharmacology and the medical sciences on a part-time basis and the personnel in three affiliating agencies.

The Students

The Skidmore student is usually between seventeen and eighteen years old when she enters college. At the time of the integration project about 82 per cent of the approximately 1,200 students enrolled in the college were from the Eastern seaboard, 10 per cent from the Midwest, 4 per cent from the South, 1 per cent from the West, and 3 per cent from other countries. The communities from which most of the students came had a population of 10,000 or less.

For the most part the students' parents were in the upper middle socio-economic group. The girl's father generally had completed college and was practicing a profession. Contrary to the stereotype of the student in a woman's college, the majority of students had been graduated from second-ary public schools, although some had been educated in private schools where they had lived away from home. Frequently the student had grown up with the unquestioning idea of completing college. She majored in liberal arts, in fine arts, or in a professional area, such as elementary or physical education, business, or nursing.

The admissions policy of the college regarding religion was clarified by Phyllis Hermann Voss, director of admissions, in a letter to the editor of *Skidmore News*. She stated (3),

> The first time a student is asked to declare her religious affiliation is in June, *after* she has been accepted and paid her deposit. At that time she is asked to complete a card which goes to the chaplain's office and is available for the local church of that faith so the student may be welcomed in the fall by the minister.

Only a small number of Negro students were enrolled in the college. Concerning this fact, the director of admissions has stated (3),

> As for Negro students, the small number we have on campus is a reflection of the number of applicants we have had. Intensive recruitment has produced eight applicants in 1960, and all eight have met our standards academically and personally. All eight have been accepted.

Julius K. Robinson, director of school-college relations, stated in a letter to the editor of *Skidmore News* (2),

> There are at present three Skidmore undergraduates who were referred to the College by NSSFNS (National Scholarship Service and Fund for Negro Students).

Unfortunately, because of a combination of reasons, particularly economic and cultural deprivation, lack of motivation and segregated and de facto segregated schools, the total number of Negro candidates is understandably small, and when spread among the numbers of schools like Skidmore, which are anxious to accept them, the number on any one campus is indeed small.

NURSING STUDENTS

Over the five-year period of the project, 243 students were admitted to the department of nursing. Fifty-seven per cent, or 138 students, completed the program and graduated between 1958–1962. Five students who had been admitted during the period of the project completed their work and graduated the year following the project. Forty-one per cent, or 100 students, dropped out of the nursing program. Twelve students transferred to another department in the college, thirty-eight were disqualified, and fifty withdrew voluntarily. Thirty-two students were known to have applied to other schools of nursing, and four students returned to the Skidmore department of nursing and graduated. Of the thirty-eight students who were disqualified, at least five were known to have entered other collegiate programs in nursing, and six entered three-year diploma programs.

Of the 138 nursing students graduated during 1958–1962, 101, or 73 per cent, were Protestant; 25, or 18 per cent, were Roman Catholic; and 12, or 9 per cent, were Jewish. During the five-year period of the integration project, one Negro student was enrolled in the department of nursing; she withdrew at the end of the first semester of the sophomore year.

The Faculty

The faculty of the department of nursing was composed of the chairman of the department and all of the full-time instructional personnel. At any given time during the years 1957–1962, this faculty was composed of ten professional nurses and one nutritionist, not counting the psychiatric nurse project director. Over the five-year period, however, there were three replacements in the professional nurse group and two replacements of the nutritionist. The data on the faculty, therefore, will refer to a total of sixteen faculty members.

BIOGRAPHICAL DATA

To learn something about the general background, preparation, and experience of the faculty members, the psychiatric nurse interviewed each member in the fifth year of the project (see Appendix B).

The distribution of the faculty according to place of origin was similar to that of the total Skidmore student body. Eleven members came from the

Eastern seaboard, two from the Midwest, one from the South, and two from the West.

During the period of the project, with the exception of two members who lived within commuting distance, all members of the faculty lived in the borough of Manhattan. Seven of them lived alone, three lived with parents or siblings, four shared apartments with friends, and two were married. Of the two who were married, one was in the situation for one year and the other for a quarter and a summer session.

The age span was a wide one, ranging from the late twenties to the middle sixties. The majority of the faculty members were in their forties or fifties.

As for their religious beliefs, eight were Protestant, five were Roman Catholic, and three were Jewish. During the 1957–1962 period, there were no full-time Negroes on the faculty. However, a Negro served as a full-time lecturer during one summer session.

EDUCATION

Seven of the thirteen nurse faculty members had been graduated from a three-year diploma program; one of them had completed four years of college before entering nursing. Of the six who had been graduated from basic collegiate programs in nursing, one was in the situation for only the first year of the project, another for only the fourth year, and another for the last year of the project. Of the other three who obtained their basic nursing education in a collegiate program, two had been graduated from Skidmore College.

Nine of the nurse faculty members had master's degrees at the time of their appointment; three members completed a graduate program during the period of the project; and one member did not have a master's degree for the duration of her appointment to the faculty. Of the twelve nurse faculty members who had master's degrees, nine had completed their graduate programs within the five-year period 1953–1958. The other three had earned their degrees between 1933 and 1948. One of the members of this latter group completed a second master's degree program during the project. The three nutritionists had master's degrees. None of the members had a doctoral degree, although one faculty member had pursued full-time study and four members had pursued part-time study at the post-master's level.

Ten nurse faculty members had had from two to twelve weeks of clinical psychiatric nursing experience in their undergraduate program; the other three had had no clinical experience in this specialty. No faculty member had completed an advanced program in psychiatric nursing.

Six members had had public health nursing in their undergraduate programs—four in basic collegiate programs and two in baccalaureate degree programs for graduate nurses. Two members had had public health experience on the master's degree level: one of them had completed an advanced program in public health nursing as well as a graduate program in public health. Five members had had no educational preparation in public health nursing.

Past Professional Experience

As might be expected from the variations in age, there was a wide range in the amount and breadth of the faculty members' nursing and teaching experience. The chairman had served in this capacity since the department was established. Three other members had been in the department for ten years or more, three for between five and ten years, and nine for less than five years. Prior to joining the Skidmore department of nursing, three members had had ten or more years of professional experience which included the practice and teaching of nursing, two had had five or more years, and ten had had less than five years. Six members had taught in another school of nursing—in two instances, a collegiate program. Of the thirteen nurse faculty members, five had had experience either as a teacher or as a student in a basic collegiate program other than Skidmore.

In regard to clinical experiences in psychiatric nursing, one of the thirteen nurse faculty members had been a psychiatric aide prior to her entrance in a basic nursing program. Another member who had had no educational preparation in this field had had some experience in it as a practitioner. Four faculty members, all of whom had had educational preparation in public health nursing, had had some experience in psychiatric situations.

Rank and Tenure

Of the thirteen nurse faculty members and the three nutritionists, eight had professorial rank—three were full professors, two were associate professors, and three were assistant professors. Eight nurse faculty members had the rank of instructor, and two were promoted to assistant professor during the last year of the project.

Five of the nurse faculty members had tenure, and these members composed the executive committee, which was responsible for the administrative decisions of the department of nursing. During the last year of the project, another member received tenure, but she was not appointed to the executive committee.

The Psychiatric Team

The psychiatric nurse's experience included practice and teaching in medical-surgical nursing, public health nursing, and psychiatric nursing. Her preparation in public health nursing helped her to view psychiatry from the standpoint of the community as well as from the hospital setting. Many times this experience was a basis for communicating with some faculty members when other avenues seemed temporarily closed.

Her graduate education in psychiatric nursing had been oriented toward perceiving mental illness within an interpersonal and social framework. The primary emphasis had been on the acquisition of a large body of knowledge about psychiatric nursing and the development of skills in the practice of this specialty rather than on teaching, supervision, or consultation methods.

She had also completed a course in interpersonal psychiatry for teachers at a local psychoanalytic training institute. This course had broadened and deepened her knowledge of psychodynamics and the various schools of psychiatric thought. Her experience in long-term psychoanalysis was a vital part of her personal and professional equipment. It made it possible for her to deal more effectively with the anxiety aroused in her by the many complex problems inherent in the psychiatric integration process.

Prior to her work in the integration project, she had been on the faculty of another collegiate program for four years where she taught the course in psychiatric nursing, and in addition was responsible for integrating psychiatric concepts. Throughout this period and during her experience as director of the Skidmore integration project, she spent one day a week in the clinical practice of psychiatric nursing with individual patients and groups of patients.

The psychiatrist had a broad background of psychoanalytic practice and experience in teaching and research. He had been associated with a psychoanalytic training program for seven years and for the same period had been on the faculty of a local medical school.

Prior to joining the integration project, he had not been exposed to an undergraduate nursing curriculum, nor did he have any previous experience in teaching students in this particular age group. This lack of experience with nursing proved to be useful in the psychiatric integration project. The psychiatrist may have had fewer preconceived and stereotyped notions about nursing than would have otherwise been the case had he been more involved with nurses; he therefore was able to approach the situation with a degree of objectivity that was crucial to such an endeavor. His inquiries stimulated the psychiatric nurse and the other faculty members to explore, clarify, and formulate their ideas about nursing and nursing education. And finally, the newness of the experience fostered maximum motivation and interest on the part of the psychiatrist.

The Curriculum and Facilities

During the period of the integration project, the curriculum was undergoing extensive revision. The curriculum as described here is the one that was in force during the period 1957–1962.

The fact that the instructional facilities in nursing education and those in general education were not within commuting distance of each other to some extent influenced the pattern of the curriculum. The curriculum was so arranged that the instruction in liberal arts was given at Saratoga Springs during the freshman and senior years at which time the nursing students were housed in the same residences as the other students. The clinical nursing courses were given in the sophomore and junior years, which the students spent in New York City.

FRESHMAN YEAR

During the freshman year the curriculum consisted of courses in anatomy and physiology, microbiology, general chemistry, nutrition, English composition, introduction to general psychology, sociology, and a noncredit course in physical education—all of which the nursing students shared with other Skidmore students on the Saratoga Springs campus. In 1960, a forty-five-hour course entitled "Introduction to Patient Care" was included in the spring semester of the freshman year. Because of the problems posed by the distance between Saratoga Springs and New York City, however, this course was dropped.

SOPHOMORE AND JUNIOR YEARS

In the sophomore and junior years, as has been stated, the entire focus of the curriculum was on the study of nursing. The importance that was attached to this aspect of the educational program is illustrated by the fact that in clinical teaching and supervision the faculty-student ratio was generally about one to four. Although this small ratio created a budgetary problem, it permitted extensive use of small group and seminar experiences and enabled the faculty members to pay a good deal of attention to the personal fulfillment of the individual student and her development into a mature person. The small faculty-student ratio, the fact that when the nursing faculty and students were associated with each other the exclusive focus of the curriculum was on nursing, and the limited physical space of the department of nursing made for closely knit faculty-student and intrafaculty relationships.

The major facility utilized for clinical instruction was the New York University Hospital. This hospital also provided the classroom and office facilities for the educational program in nursing. Other clinical facilities used were those of the Cornell University–New York Hospital Medical Center, the New York State Psychiatric Institute, the Manhattan Veterans Administration Hospital, the Bureau of Public Health Nursing of the New York City Department of Health, the Visiting Nurse Association of Brooklyn, and the Visiting Nurse Service of New York.

Through arrangement with New York University the students were housed on two floors of the residence for medical and dental students. During the twenty-four-week period in which they were having their experiences in obstetric nursing and psychiatric nursing, however, they were provided full maintenance by the affiliating agency.

The nursing courses covered the full spectrum of professional nursing practice—the promotion of health, the prevention of disease, treatment, and rehabilitation. The first nursing course, taught during the first quarter of the sophomore year was a twelve-credit course entitled "Introduction to Patient Care." It constituted the students' introduction to the theory and clinical application of the medical and nursing sciences, pharmacology, and nutrition and included a twelve-hour unit in interpersonal relations in nursing taught by the psychiatric nurse project director. These units continued over the entire sophomore year, with the exception of the unit in pharmacology.

Beginning in the second quarter of the sophomore year, the students were divided into three groups and rotated through three courses (a total of 26 credits) of eight weeks each in medical, surgical, and pediatric nursing. In each course, a total of twenty hours a week were spent in clinical learning experiences, of which sixteen hours were in the inpatient services and four hours in cardiac, diabetic, vascular, and outpatient clinics. Although much of the theoretical content in medical nursing and surgical nursing was integrated, the clinical learning experiences, which included the care of both men and women, were separate. Four weeks of the surgical nursing experience were divided among the general surgical and gynecologic services, the operating room, the recovery room, and the thoracic surgery units.

The experience in pediatric nursing focused on the care of infants, toddlers, and older children and the health supervision of well children in a child health station. A three-credit course in normal growth and development was also offered in the second quarter and continued for the rest of the year.

A fifteen-hour unit in first aid and emergency care as a part of the disaster nursing project was also given at this time, as was an eighteen-hour unit in interpersonal relations in nursing as part of the psychiatric integration project.

In each of these experiences the teaching and supervision of the clinical learning experiences were the responsibility of Skidmore faculty members. About four hours a week were devoted to small group conferences. Two hours of these conferences were primarily content-oriented and two hours were spent in discussing specific clinical problems and case material. Beginning principles in public health and public health nursing, such as referral and immunization against communicable disease, were woven throughout the experiences.

In the junior year the students again were divided into three groups. Each group had twelve-week affiliations in obstetric nursing and psychiatric nursing, a seven-week course in team nursing, and a three-week course in communicable disease and long-term illness nursing.

The purpose of the three-credit course in communicable disease and long-term illness nursing was to give the students the opportunity to add to their theoretical knowledge of the prevention and control of communicable diseases and specific nursing care of such diseases when they occur and to develop beginning skill in giving nursing care to patients with long-term illness.

The seven-credit course in team nursing was directed toward helping the student to develop a broad concept of the team method of identifying and meeting the nursing needs of groups of patients. Principles, problems, and processes related to hospital organizational structure, communication, administration, and leadership were fundamental aspects of the course.

The responsibility for implementing the course in obstetric nursing was delegated to the Cornell University–New York Hospital School of Nursing, and the psychiatric nursing course was taught at the New York State Psychiatric Institute by personnel of that agency.* Communication between the Skidmore faculty and the instructors in these two subjects for the purpose of curriculum development took place at an annual meeting of the Council of Associated Institutions and Agencies, and special arrangements for small conferences were made as needed. However, real contact with students was not maintained while they were on affiliation and thus the Skidmore faculty lost the opportunity to exert its educational influence on the students during the major portion of the junior year.

The clinical curriculum was terminated with a twelve-week summer session in public health nursing, in which the total student group participated. The first four weeks included the presentation and discussion of public health and public health nursing content by the Skidmore instructor who was in charge of the course, other selected faculty members, and lecturers from other disciplines. The eight-week clinical learning experience was supervised by the personnel of the two voluntary public health nursing agencies. Students, agency personnel, and the Skidmore instructor met together two and one-half hours per week to evaluate the progress of the students and to discuss patients and their families.†

Senior Year

In the senior year, according to the *Skidmore College Bulletin,* the program included twenty-seven credits in "Electives in Liberal Arts (at least 6

* In 1962, the Skidmore faculty assumed entire responsibility for implementing the course in obstetric nursing and, in 1963, for implementing the course in psychiatric nursing.
† In 1963, the Skidmore faculty assumed responsibility for this total experience.

credits in courses chosen from the liberal arts departments, including English 6, Sociology 3, and electives in Music and Art" (2).

One nonclinical nursing course was also included in this year—a three-credit seminar which built on the liberal arts courses and in which the issues, problems, and trends within the nursing profession were identified and analyzed. The students carried out a project in which they studied one problem or issue. One of the major strengths of the seminar was that it was taught by the chairman of the department of nursing and thereby provided the students with the enriching opportunity to experience their chairman as a teacher.

REFERENCES

1. Robinson, Julius K. "Admissions Policy," Letters to the Editor, *Skidmore News,* May 5, 1960, p. 4.

2. *Skidmore College Bulletin,* 1959–60.

3. Voss, Phyllis Hermann. "Skidmore's Policy," Letters to the Editor, *Skidmore News,* May 5, 1960, p. 6.

PART II

THE EXPERIMENT

Chapter Five

SETTING THE STAGE

Men grind and grind in the mill of a truism, and nothing comes out but what was put in. But the moment they desert the tradition for a spontaneous thought, then poetry, wit, hope, virtue, learning, anecdote, all flock to their aid.

RALPH WALDO EMERSON, *Literary Ethics*

The Goals of the Project

The broad goals of psychiatric integration were identified by the faculty at the time the department of nursing applied for a grant for an integration project. During the period in which the psychiatric nurse was being interviewed by each member regarding her appointment to the faculty as project director, she and the faculty, together, clarified these broad goals. This timing was in accord with the psychiatric nurse's belief that the goals would influence the methods of integration.

The goals were as follows.

1. To foster the students' willingness and to develop their freedom to become personally involved in and committed to their professional role and, through experiencing the full awareness and impact of their own feelings, to emancipate and develop their creativeness in all aspects of nursing practice.

2. To develop the students' ability to help persons with emotional and social problems by increasing the students' awareness and understanding of the emotional, cultural, and social factors influencing illness and personality growth and development.

3. To develop the students' ability to recognize, examine, formulate, and intervene with guidance in the interpersonal and social problems of patients and personnel that they may meet in their work as staff nurses.

The psychiatric nurse recognized that these primary goals would need further refinement and that contributory goals would have to be identified after the students' specific needs with respect to psychiatric integration had been analyzed in greater detail and the resources that could be utilized for meeting these needs had been more precisely evaluated.

Opportunities for Evaluating Needs and Resources

The plans made by the faculty prior to the initiation of the integration project called for the psychiatric nurse, during the first year of the project, to be a regular faculty member with functions and responsibilities similar to those of other faculty members. During the first year, then, except for group discussions with students, none of the psychiatric nurse's activities had a direct bearing on an integration program.

Her work with students consisted of two activities. One of these activities was the clinical teaching and supervision of sophomore students. For the first quarter of the first year of the project, the psychiatric nurse participated in teaching the course in introduction to patient care to sophomore students, in which she gave demonstrations of simple nursing procedures in the classroom and supervised the students' clinical experiences. During the next quarter, she was responsible for the supervision of sophomore students on a male medical unit and in a pediatric outpatient clinic. She also taught medical nursing classes; frequently, another instructor in medical nursing and she collaborated in joint teaching. In this teaching she integrated psychiatric concepts, and through these experiences she eventually had contact in the clinical setting with all the sophomore students.

The psychiatric nurse also led a series of weekly unstructured discussions with small groups of sophomore students. These discussions were intended to provide an opportunity for the students to discuss tensions arising in their relations with patients, faculty members, nursing service personnel, and other students; to help them to become aware of how their own feelings, attitudes, and behavior influenced others; and to assist them in the problem-solving process. Another purpose was to create a relatively safe situation in which the students could begin to work out some of their unresolved attitudes toward authority figures.

A second aspect of the psychiatric nurse's activities pertained to her participation with the faculty. Her contacts with the other faculty members generally were within the context of meetings of the total faculty as a group, curriculum committee meetings, and joint teaching and planning sessions with the other instructor in medical nursing.

During this period the psychiatrist served as a consultant to the faculty when special problems arose in connection with the progress or the evaluation of the students. All his other activities were connected directly with the integration program. His principal function was to work with junior students, who were having their learning experiences in communicable disease and long-term illness nursing and team nursing, by participating in nursing care conferences devoted to problems arising from the students' relationships with patients and other clinical personnel. The goal was to help the students to become aware of their own reactions, clarify the nature of these reactions, and work out appropriate ways of handling their feelings, as well as to help them to identify and clarify the emotional aspects of patient care. The psychiatrist also gave a series of lectures for the sophomore students, which were attended by some faculty members as well. In these he presented and explored topics of special importance, such as the relationship of emotional stress to illness, the handling of pain, the nursing care of dying patients, and psychosexual development.

In her day-to-day contacts with the faculty members, the students, and the nursing service personnel, the psychiatric nurse gained significant insight into the intricate operations of the total situation—an insight which the psychiatrist did not have and could not have acquired because of the limited time that he spent in the setting and because of his different role and relationship with the faculty and students. Within the context of all her experiences, the psychiatric nurse identified the specific needs of the students that came within the scope of the integration project and appraised the department's resources for psychiatric integration.

The Students' Needs

In her previous work with other nursing students the psychiatric nurse had identified certain needs that are common to all collegiate nursing students regardless of the particular nursing program in which they are enrolled. During her experiences with the Skidmore students in the first year of the integration project, she evaluated their specific needs with respect to the goals of psychiatric integration. In this evaluation she considered the students' perception of the role of women as this impinged on their orientation toward a career in nursing, their authority-dependency conflicts in respect to their relationships with patients, faculty members, clinical personnel, and the psychiatric nurse, and their knowledge and clinical application of psychiatric content.

Perception of the Role of Women. Marriage in the United States currently occurs earlier than in any period prior to World War II. Inevitably, this trend affects the college society. According to the available records (which are not complete), at least 70 per cent of the Skidmore nursing students in the class of 1958 were married by 1960; 68 per cent of the class of 1959 were married by 1961; 40 per cent of the class of 1960 were married by 1961; and 36 per cent of the class of 1961 were married by the fall immediately following their graduation. Married students are not required to withdraw from the program. However, of the ninety students who either were disqualified or withdrew from the department of nursing during the five-year period of the project, a minimum of nineteen were known to have left because of marriage.

There is nothing to be said for or against dropping out of college to marry or, upon graduation, devoting full time to raising a family. The central issue is the extent to which the student's goal toward marriage is inner-directed. As long as the student's marriage, or any change for that matter, is accompanied by clarity about her own feelings and herself as a person, there is no basis for concern. If, on the other hand, the student's drive toward marrying is outer-directed—that is, conforming to society's pressures with respect to emphasis on marriage and a home—she is struggling to cope with her weak self-identity by belonging to someone. Instead of resolving her conflict about her dependency, she merely shifts the focus of her dependency from her parents to a husband. According to Erik H. Erikson, who stated the dilemma succinctly, "You can't get your identity straightened out by getting married and by achieving intimacy ahead of identity" (2).

The nursing student's sense of self-identify also relates directly to her motivation for nursing, her sense of commitment, her ability to exert initiative, and her desire and acceptance of responsibility to make a meaningful contribution to society. Accordingly, the psychiatric nurse, during her individual and group conferences with the Skidmore students, took pains to note any comments that reflected their attitudes toward marriage and work. Later, during the fifth year of the project, she validated her findings in individual conferences with sophomore, junior, and senior students and members of the most recent graduating class (see Appendix B).

These investigations indicated that the Skidmore student tends to view marriage as a kind of sanctuary and repository for fulfillment, some greater or lesser grail. Moreover, she is inclined to regard marriage and a career as incompatible.

This viewpoint, in the case of the Skidmore students, might be in part attributed to the fact that except for two faculty members who were in the situation for only a brief period, all of the faculty members were single. Among the students' comments about the marital status of the faculty were the following.

> I was terribly disappointed that there were no married women teaching us. I wanted to feel that a nursing career and marriage are compatible. I wondered how the instructors could ever understand our boy problems and our desire for marriage.

> All the faculty members are nurses and are single. I can't help but wonder if this means that nurses don't get married. Not only are the faculty members

nurses, but they also are teachers. And then I thought of "old maid school teachers." Maybe the instructors are single because they are so dedicated to nursing. Nurses are used to giving orders, so maybe the faculty would find it difficult to go fifty-fifty in any relationship.

The students certainly did not get caught up in the artificial split concerning marriage and career merely because the majority of the faculty members were single. Such an inference would oversimplify and distort a problem that is far more complicated. It is true, however, that the fact that the faculty members were unmarried did not help to alter or to modify the students' stereotyped views about the role of women and creative work. These views relegated the practice of nursing to the status of a short-term goal, as the following comments indicate.

From my experience of going home with some of my classmates, most of them are not oriented to the concept of working. After the first excitement of clinical experiences is over, they begin to look to and concentrate on marriage.

Many of us see a career as a necessity rather than a free choice.

There is a great deal of parental pressure for marriage. I am beginning to feel that the more education one gets the fewer opportunities there are for marriage.

The students' attitudes about marriage and their lack of orientation to creative work have a powerful impact on the teacher-student relationship. Faculty members tend to think and speak of the future in terms of a nursing career. From their own experience they have accumulated a body of content, methods, and skills that in turn they teach to students. It takes time and experience, however, to integrate and put these into practice. But generally, the student simply cannot conceive of herself as practicing nursing five or ten years hence. Consequently, she wants to achieve the same degree of expertness as her teacher, but without the time essential to do so. From this point of view, the student does identify with her teacher as a nurse and wants to be like her. The existing conflict around long-term goals, however, often leads to further conflict concerning the student's and teacher's expectations of each other; this is bound to create some frustration for both.

Implicit in the student's reactions toward marriage and a career is her search for basic values. In emancipating herself from the controls of parents, school, and church, the student is engaged in the struggle to learn how to handle her sexuality and to understand its meaning in interpersonal relationships. In this struggle the Skidmore nursing student is confronted with problems over and beyond those faced by many other collegiate nursing students.

Because the Skidmore nursing student has selected a college for women, while she is on campus her sexuality is institutionalized. However, the college campus is located within commuting distance of several ivy-league colleges for men, so that in the freshman year there is ample opportunity for the nursing student to meet and go out with men.

For many of the students the move from Saratoga Springs to New York City signifies their first experience of living in a large metropolitan area. With this move it becomes easier than on campus for the student to follow the direction of her sexuality. As her sexuality intrudes on her educational experiences and as she attempts to resolve the enormous complexities involved in realizing a sense of self-identity, the student is exposed to the danger of making artificial choices in regard to a marriage partner.

In the sophomore year, the student's first year in New York City, she is required to absorb a vast amount of theoretical material and to develop intellectual and manual skills, with the result that marriage tends to remain in the periphery of her thinking and planning. By the junior year she has acquired a clearer understanding of what professional nursing is all about, and it is then that she begins to give serious thought to marriage. Concomitantly she is apt to experience uneasiness, restlessness, and impatience about finding a steady male interest before graduation. As one student said, "The subject of marriage doesn't come up much in the sophomore year, but by the junior and especially the senior year anyone who is not engaged becomes panicky."

In returning to the college campus in the senior year, the student temporarily leaves the practice of nursing behind her. With the exception of one nonclinical nursing course with the chairman of the department, she has no other nursing experiences or nurse teachers with whom to identify. Moreover, she is exposed to and may feel bombarded by the emphasis on marriage from students in other departments and is confronted by the reality that many of her nursing classmates have moved in the direction of marriage. Students have stated that unless seniors already have boyfriends, there is little opportunity for dating because the male college students are already involved in relationships with students who have been on campus for four years. All the students agreed that the question of marriage frequently takes on a quality of urgency, if not emergency during the senior year. They felt that if a student had not yet found a male interest, she would be left behind in what by then had catapulted the group into a race for marriage.

The following student comments illustrate the mounting anxiety during the senior year on campus.

I dread coming back to school after the Christmas vacation with all of the diamond rocks that will be flashing about. I think I had better go and hide.

The college boys are interested in dating the younger students. Because of our experiences in nursing, we have matured more rapidly than other girls of the same age. Hence, by now we are more interested in older men who are out of college. We aren't interested in doing the same things we did as freshmen. As a result, if you don't already have a man, you just sit during your senior year. All of this adds up to the mounting and depressing feeling that you are forever destined to be an old maid.

The problems engendered by the interruption of the student's social life had to be taken into account in the development of a psychiatric integration program.

Authority-Dependency Conflict. As a late adolescent, the nursing student is in the full throes of resolving her ambivalence about her parental dependency. At the same time, she is trying to fulfill her needs for dependency and to clear up her uncertainty and confusion about her self-identity. She is faced with the agonizing conflict of clinging to the safety and comfort of a relatively dependent status quo or becoming engaged in the turbulent but challenging struggle of change. Her burden increases as she finds herself placed in what appears to her the precarious position of having to assume authority previously invested in parental figures; she must take care of adults, whereas up to now adults have taken care of her. There are few situations in nursing that demonstrate so dramatically the concept of role-reversal.

One way in which the Skidmore students communicated their ambivalent attitudes toward authority figures and their own dependency needs was that during the sophomore year they were primarily task-, instructor-, or doctor-oriented rather than patient-oriented. They were inclined to be more concerned with achieving a good grade or presenting a positive picture of themselves than with the welfare of their patients.

The authority-dependency conflict also was reflected in the students' discomfort with clinical supervision and their reluctance to accept help and guidance, let alone seek it on their own. The students usually were unable to discuss with the instructor those problems that arose in the teacher-student relationship. Their uneasiness with persons in authority positions was further evidenced by their rigid and irrational expectations of them. They were hard put to appraise realistically and to accept the various strengths and limitations of the faculty and clinical personnel. The majority of the students, for example, were prone to blame the instructor, the head nurse, or the physician for a situation that was not to their liking. Conversely, some other students, in the effort to create an authority image of all-sweetness-and-light, glossed over the significant authorities' limitations.

Another facet of the students' trouble in evaluating the faculty was their difficulty in identifying their own strengths. They envisaged academic and clinical evaluation as a one-way process in which the instructor focused exclusively on the student's limitations, failures, and errors and in which the student sat in passive acceptance.

Closely related to the students' lack of freedom with authority figures was their difficulty in perceiving themselves as a rational authority, specifically as this pertained to their role as a nurse. One student colorfully described her feelings about having to assume an authority role, "Just because I walk around in a nurse's uniform, the patients and the doctors assume I know what to do. But I really don't. I feel like a fraud who is posing as a nurse."

Understandably, from the late adolescent's point of view authority is based on age. One outcome of this arbitrary investiture of authority was dramatically illustrated by the repeated comment of students during their experiences in pediatric nursing in the hospital and child health station: "Who are we to make any suggestions to parents about how to handle their children, especially since they are so much older than we are? After all, they know their own kids and how to take care of them much better than we do."

As would be expected, the majority of students during the sophomore year were unable to exert initiative and leadership. There also were episodes of reality-testing and negative acting out against persons in authority positions; these occasions indicated the need for the instructor to set limits for the students.

It remained the task of the instructors to help the students to begin to perceive rational authority in terms of specialized knowledge and skills instead of viewing it as a power which is arbitrarily achieved because of age, position, and role. Such a change in viewpoint required that the students begin to identify and evaluate their own strengths and limitations within the context of their dual role of student and professional nurse. However, for the students to feel comfortable and secure enough to engage in a growth process that involves a good deal of self-exposure, it was crucial that they experience a personalized professional relationship with their instructors.

Knowledge and Application of Psychiatric Content. Although the students had intellectual knowledge of the theory of personality growth and development, their application of the concepts and principles was limited to their work with children; they were unable to utilize developmental theory in their work with adults. For example, they were likely to create a false dichotomy between meeting some of the patient's dependency needs and fostering independence. Often their own discomfort about having patients, especially adults, dependent on them was rationalized in terms of what supposedly was good for the patient, and independence was generally perceived as being good and dependency as being bad. Most of the students tended to base their judgment of how much physical care they should give to a patient on only one criterion—the patient's ability to care for himself. They did not consider that the nurse might bathe a patient who denies his illness and cannot allow himself to be dependent, in order to provide a way of helping him to accept the patient role, or that she might feed a patient to provide him with a new experience in being able to count on the willingness of the nurse to help him.

Again, the students had trouble in tolerating the anxiety that accompanies a problem-solving approach, as was manifested in their continued search for a pat answer to the resolution of problems in the nurse-patient situation. In their discussions of a patient they attached such labels to his behavior as "attention-getting," "depressed," "uncooperative," and "complaining," instead of describing his verbal and nonverbal behavior. Frequently, these abstractions represented stereotyped attitudes and responses which took the form of such value judgments as good or bad, right or wrong, superior or inferior. The development of their awareness that answers to the questions of how to handle a patient's problems evolve out of the nurse-patient interaction remained a task for the future.

One area in nursing practice that aroused much recurrent tension was the care of a dying patient. The students clung tenaciously to the hope that somehow they would be able to miraculously cure the dying patient through their nursing ministrations. Because they were not yet free enough to express their emotional responses to the situation, they camouflaged their feelings of sadness and loss by resorting to withdrawal or by blaming themselves or someone else for having failed to perform the miracle.

Then students also tended to fragment physical and emotional nursing care. There were occasions when they became so engrossed in psychologizing about some of the patient's emotional problems that the physical condition which had brought the patient to the hospital faded into the background. Perhaps the particular stage of personality development the students were going through and the kinds of unresolved problems they were having to face and handle in themselves fostered their preoccupation with the emotional aspects of nursing care; they may have hoped that knowledge of these aspects would provide the key to "What makes Sammy run?"

Moreover, within the hospital setting, the physical nursing care that was given to patients by nursing and ancillary personnel was not always of a quality that would be inspiring to students. Because of the acute nursing shortage, often much of what is labeled "routine nursing care" was delegated to nonprofessional workers. It was quite natural, therefore, for the students to think of routine nursing care as nonprofessional nursing care. For a collegiate student who is learning professional nursing, this is the unpardonable sin. To keep the students sincerely interested in what on the surface might appear to be a simple housemaid's task as contrasted with the seemingly more esoteric and therefore more challenging approaches of emotional nursing care, it is imperative for the instructor to be clear about the professional nurse's role and to have synthesized the principles of physical and emotional nursing care.

The students' emphasis on emotional care to the exclusion of physical care was not always synonymous with skill in developing a meaningful nurse-patient relationship. When a student created a physical-emotional split, she frequently was not involved with the patient on any level but, on the contrary, was temporarily leading a blinking kind of existence in which she was playing nurse instead of being one. Often her overemphasis on talking about the emotional area became a technique for avoiding the anxiety experienced in interpersonal intimacy with patients.

Caring for patients of different races, colors, and economic statuses quite naturally creates problems for nursing students. In the case of the typical Skidmore student these problems are enhanced by the fact that she comes from a tightly knit cultural, social, and religious class which places high value on economic status and defines clear cultural boundaries in regard to racial differences, mode of dress, and the role of women in creative work. Relationships with people outside her own cultural and social milieu are apt to be few and transitory. It therefore is likely to take longer and be more difficult for her to climb over these barriers than for nursing students who are from a different social and economic class. On the other hand, the psychiatric nurse observed that when the Skidmore student was successful in overcoming the biases characteristic of her social class, she appeared at times almost to transcend students from other socioeconomic groups in her ability to relate meaningfully to patients with different backgrounds. The psychiatric nurse therefore deduced that the Skidmore nursing program was achieving success in its efforts to educate students in the awareness and acceptance of cultural and social differences.

Appraisal of Resources

While refining the broad goals of psychiatric integration by identifying the students' specific needs, the psychiatric nurse was formulating the type of integration program that would help to meet these needs. The next step was to appraise the resources that were available for such a program, with particular emphasis on identification of specific factors that seemed likely to advance or obstruct progress toward the goals. The chief resources that were investigated in this way were the student services, the curriculum, the faculty, and the psychiatric team.

STUDENT SERVICES

Until the psychiatric integration program got underway, the only formal student personnel service available in the New York headquarters of the Skidmore nursing program was the student health service. Guidance with respect to emotional and professional problems was provided by the faculty members, but no organized plan of referral for counseling and guidance, psychiatric consultation, diagnosis, or treatment was in operation in the department of nursing or on the Skidmore campus.

THE CURRICULUM

If a psychiatric integration program was to evolve into anything more than a superstructure on an already existing curriculum, which in time would topple off, it was essential for the psychiatric team to participate actively in curriculum development. The available resources and the curriculum pattern affected the integration project and what the psychiatric team members would be able to accomplish. Two characteristics in particular had a bearing on the project: the geographic separation of the department of nursing from the college and the fact that not all the nursing courses were being taught by Skidmore faculty members.

Because the department of nursing was so far from the campus, it was impossible for the project personnel to collaborate with members of the other departments of the college. In particular, there were no social scientists with whom they could consult about the project. Nor could the psychiatric team utilize the liberal arts courses for the project or effect any basic changes in these courses. In short, the project was confined to the nursing courses in the curriculum.

Even within these boundaries the project was limited by the fact that obstetric nursing and psychiatric nursing and the clinical learning experience in public health nursing—three areas that are particularly fertile fields for the integration of psychiatric concepts—were not taught by Skidmore faculty members, so that it was difficult to establish a reasonable degree of continuity of psychiatric integration in the nursing curriculum. The separation of the course in psychiatric nursing from the rest of the curriculum had a special impact on the integration project. Such a separation made it difficult to establish the connection between normal behavior and responses to illness and other crises in living on the one hand and psychopathology on the other. Moreover, because of this separation, the Skidmore faculty members had had little opportunity to collaborate with specialists in the psychiatric field.

THE FACULTY

The psychiatric nurse believed that the faculty members of the department of nursing constituted the most important resource in the psychiatric integration efforts—that the goals of psychiatric integration would be achieved only to the degree that every nursing instructor was able to identify emotional and social problems that arise in nursing situations and to apply psychiatric concepts, principles, and processes in exploring these problems with students while teaching them the physical aspects of nursing care. Accordingly, the psychiatric nurse took particular pains in appraising this resource and identifying the areas that might be further developed. In this appraisal, she gave consideration to the faculty members' knowledge of psychiatric concepts and ability to apply them to teacher-student, intra-faculty, and faculty-psychiatric team relationships.

Knowledge and Application of Psychiatric Content. The theories and problems of psychiatry and psychiatric nursing are generally seen as being the common property of all specialties in nursing. However, the impression that all nurse teachers share with the psychiatrist and the psychiatric nurse an acquaintance with basic principles of gestalt psychology, psychoanalysis, learning theory, social structure, and processes of group interaction proved illusory in the case of the Skidmore faculty. The faculty members were inclined to create an artificial split between "mental health" and "psychiatry." Generally, they viewed mental health as dealing with so-called normal behavior and the prevention of emotional breakdown, whereas they perceived psychiatry as being concerned exclusively with psychopathology and the treatment of patients with serious emotional disorders.

Although all but one faculty member had a masters degree, with the exception of three instructors the faculty members' theoretical knowledge of psychodynamics, communication theory, theory of the unconscious, and principles of interactional process seemed minimal. The concepts regarding the development of man which are basic to understanding his behavior were frequently not applied in the teaching-learning process. Some faculty members were able to verbalize about the impact of cultural, social, familial, and psychological forces on the individual, but they often seemed to have little genuine understanding of the significance of these forces and their implications for the students' and the patients' adaptive and maladaptive modes of behavior.

What the faculty members did know of psychiatric content was more likely to be used to describe a patient and a student than to gain insight into the dynamics of their behavior. When helping students to care for a dying patient, for example, the instructor found it difficult to identify that the student's withdrawal from the situation, instead of being an expression of her not caring about the patient, more frequently represented a nonverbal expression of her feelings of hopelessness about the patient and her sense of helplessness because of her inability to alter the dying process. Although the majority of the instructors gave a good deal of emotional support to patients and students, it appeared that they were guided largely by their intuition and experience rather than by a conscious identification of the psychodynamics of the situation. Most of them appeared to have difficulty in conceptualizing what they had done to help a patient or a student.

There was a wide range of psychiatric knowledge and skill among the faculty members. The instructors in pediatric nursing and public health nursing were at the upper level of theoretical knowledge, and the instructors in public health nursing had the greatest skill in transferring their knowledge to nurse-patient relationships.* Although the instructors in pediatric nursing were highly skilled in verbalizing the principles of normal growth and development, all but one of them appeared to have difficulty in using these principles in the exploration of nurse-patient relationships in action. Some of the faculty who were members of the Executive Committee and the instructors in medical-surgical nursing seemed to have the least psychiatric knowledge and skill in its application.

Certainly, the Skidmore faculty was much too small a sample on which to make any broad generalizations about the significance of this distribution; nevertheless, one can pose some questions about it and speculate about some possible explanations. Why did the specialists in public health nursing have a broad knowledge and awareness of psychiatric concepts accompanied by skills in applying them? One reason may be that because public health nurses work not only with patients but also with their families, and not only with sick patients but also with well persons within the community setting, they are likely to be more versed in dealing with the principles of human motivation, verbal and nonverbal communication, group dynamics, and cultural and social differences.

The fact that the instructors who taught in the medical and surgical units seemingly had minimal psychiatric knowledge and skill might be accounted for in part by the complexity of medical-surgical conditions, treatment, and nursing care. Because medical-surgical conditions require the use of elaborate diagnostic tests, a wide variety of medications, special diets, and complicated procedures, treatments, and techniques, the specialist in medical-surgical nursing not only must learn a vast amount of content relating to the disease process and its treatment, but also must develop considerable manual dexterity. The burden of learning hangs even more heavily when one considers that medical-surgical nursing is the foundation on which the nurse learns to handle all of the physical problems she encounters in every area of nursing practice.

At least one distinguishing aspect of surgical nursing may contribute to the surgical nurse's paucity of psychiatric knowledge and skill. Once the climax of excising a diseased organ is reached, it seems almost as though the patient should no longer have other major concerns. Such a conclusion involves the risk that a much more complex problem has been oversimplified. In surgical nursing there is the serious issue of the nurse's learning how to recognize and handle the patient's feelings of assault to his body image and the affect-laden processes of convalescence and rehabilitation.

---

* The instructor who was appointed to the faculty to teach the course in obstetric nursing in the sixth year of the project (which is beyond the purview of this book) came with a broad knowledge of psychiatric concepts and with highly developed skill in applying them.

Several reasons might account for what appeared to be the meager psychiatric knowledge and skill of some of the faculty members of the Executive Committee. They had limited contact with patients and in some instances had minimal teaching responsibilities and so may have lost touch with the kinds of problems that patients, students, and nurse teachers face and must handle. Again, some of them had no preparation in psychiatric nursing in their undergraduate programs and no exposure to it as nurses. It is questionable, however, that the kind of course in psychiatric nursing that was being taught at the time they were studying nursing would have facilitated the integration process. This point was demonstrated by the fact that the instructors who had had an undergraduate course in psychiatric nursing apparently had just as much difficulty in applying psychiatric concepts as did the faculty members who had had no course. A fascinating but also disturbing aspect of this question of the relationship between the psychiatric knowledge of faculty members and the recency of their education was that there seemed to be little difference in the degree of psychiatric knowledge and skill possessed by the six nurse faculty members who had completed their graduate programs between 1953 and 1958, the one member who did not have a masters degree, and the three who had earned their masters degrees between 1933 and 1948.

Faculty-Student Relationships. During the psychiatric nurse's attendance at curriculum and various other committee meetings in which the students were discussed and evaluated and in the course of her work with students in individual and group situations, she had ample opportunity to identify the factors in faculty-student relationships which facilitated progress toward the goals of integration and those which seemed to impede such progress.

There were numerous assets in the faculty-student relationships. The faculty's philosophy of nursing education was completely educationally oriented; there never was any problem of the student being used for service in the courses taught by the Skidmore faculty. The faculty was very much concerned with the fullest growth and development of the student as was illustrated by the faculty-student ratio of one to four.

The motivation to help students was one of the key forces among the faculty group. For the majority, no effort to assist students was too great and no proposal for their personal welfare was rejected. When, for example, the psychiatric nurse, prior to her appointment to the faculty, suggested that time be allotted in the curriculum for her to have group conferences with students, this proposal was immediately and enthusiastically approved.

One of the most positive characteristics of the faculty members was their unabashed enjoyment in being nurses and their pleasure in being able to practice clinical nursing themselves. There can be no question that this devotion and commitment to nursing were communicated to the students.

From the time of the establishment of the department of nursing, a great deal of emphasis had always been placed on the emotional and social aspects of nursing care. Undoubtedly, the faculty's unusual appreciation of the importance of applying psychiatric concepts to all aspects of nursing care was a result of sustained leadership during the pioneer work of preparing students for public health nursing. The department of nursing provided a truly educational situation.

One of the limitations in the area of faculty-student relationships that was uncovered during the first year of the project pertained to the instructors' tendency to emphasize the negative aspects of the students' performance and to show insufficient recognition of their strengths. The instructors were especially critical during their day-to-day supervision of the students' clinical experiences. This behavior was in direct contrast to their approach in the structured evaluation conferences, in which they took cognizance of both the students' strengths and their deficiencies.

Closely tied to the instructors' tendency to emphasize the students' mistakes in clinical performance were their unrealistic and unclarified expectations of the students. Sometimes the faculty members seemed to expect the students to be now what they should eventually become. For example, they often expected the students' clinical performance during the sophomore year to be at a level that might more realistically have been expected during the junior year. Because of these expectations, a great deal of pressure was put on the students to reach a certain degree of maturity within the first clinical year. Some students could achieve the goal; others could not.

Unrealistic expectations reflect some lack of clarity about the learning process as well as preoccupation with what goes on between the student and a patient. When a nurse teacher overemphasizes the interaction between a student and a patient, she frequently does not teach the student what to do, but still expects her to do it. Such an expectation leaves the student feeling as if "I am being watched all the time."

Unrealistic expectations of students results in both the instructor and the students feeling aggressive, hostile, envious, and demoralized. The nurse teacher may be inclined to rationalize these feelings on the grounds that all she is trying to do is to upgrade nursing education and practice. This rationalization, however, does not compensate for her feeling of failure as a teacher when the students do not meet her expectations. It is a miserable experience for the nurse teacher to put herself through, and by making herself miserable she manages to make the students and the other faculty members miserable also.

The most reasonable explanation for these unrealistic expectations pertains to the nature of the curriculum design. Because the students had their affiliation experiences during the junior year, and received instruction from the Skidmore faculty only in communicable disease and long-term illness nursing, team nursing, and the theory in public health and public health nursing, the faculty members' responsibility and influence were largely limited to the sophomore year. Consistently, all the faculty members verbalized their feelings of frustration because of these built-in limitations of the curriculum. One cannot help but ponder the influence of this frustration on the instructors' expectations of themselves, each other, and the students during the sophomore year. One faculty member summed up the issue succinctly when she said, "When we are responsible for all the experiences in the two clinical years, many of our problems will be lessened."

Undoubtedly, also, many of the instructors' expectations of students evolved from their experiences as students and their exposure to unrealistic expectations in a program which emphasized giving service and which utilized the apprenticeship method of teaching. It is difficult for an instructor to give to students what she herself has not experienced. The faculty members' unrealistic expectations of each other may also have had a bearing on their attitude toward students. Achieving the goals of nursing education is contingent not only on the nature of faculty-student relationships but also on the extent to which the faculty members experience a positive professional relationship with each other.

Insufficient clarification of all expectations to the students usually went hand in hand with having unrealistic expectations. The students habitually felt that they were not coming up to standard, and they were constantly afraid of failing. Was it possible that the problems in communicating expectations to students arose partly from the teacher's awareness that some of her expectations did not make much sense and that if she were to be explicit about what she expected she would risk running head on into student and faculty disapproval, student rebellion and utilization of various modes of escape, and the loss of her role as a helper of students?

A third area of limitation in faculty-student relationships concerned the teacher's vacillation between overprotecting students and giving them insufficient guidance when they needed it. Overprotection of students sometimes served as a way for the teacher to maintain her position as a powerful authority figure by keeping the students dependent on her. When, for example, an instructor's need to feel needed by students was intense, the more mature students who required only minimal help and guidance from her ran into interpersonal difficulty with her. Insufficient guidance was inextricably bound up with unrealistic expectations, as was illustrated when an instructor, instead of seeking out a student to help her and to clarify how she was performing, waited until the student initiated the contact.

Inconsistency between overprotection and giving insufficient guidance may have stemmed in part from an instructor's conflict between having students dependent on her and assuming her rightful role as an authority.

Perhaps both behaviors may have arisen from the instructor's discomfort with the students' dependency needs as well as her own. The faculty members' conflict in regard to unresolved attitudes toward authority and dependency penetrated every aspect of their professional functioning and therefore had to be given serious consideration in the development of an integration program.

Communication, Power, and Intrafaculty Relations. During the various meetings in which the psychiatric nurse participated as a regular member of the faculty (not as project director), she observed the quality of intrafaculty relationships and the impact of the interaction on herself. It was within the framework of these meetings that she was able to identify some of the assets of the faculty members (those factors which fostered group cohesiveness and thereby advanced the integration process) and the problems among the faculty members (those factors which led to group divisiveness and obstructed the integration process).

The faculty members' deep and sustained motivation to help students, coupled with their skill in working with them, was one of the predominant forces that led to group cohesiveness. Their recognition of this shared motivation resulted in mutual trust in decisions pertaining to students. For example, although the total faculty made the formal decision as to whether a student passed or failed, the group always accepted the recommendation of the course instructor. There was little attempt on the part of the other instructors to influence her judgment or to change her decision, and her evaluation was upheld by those faculty members who had authority for administrative decisions. Though administrative support of a faculty member's decisions is basic to successful evaluation, such support is not automatically forthcoming in all educational settings.

Another asset was the faculty's genuine desire and effort to create a democratic environment. Cooperation had a high value within the group, as was manifested in the assumption that each member would participate in all aspects of curriculum development, decision making on educational policies, student evaluation, and psychiatric integration. All the faculty members, for instance, had a voice in the appointment of new personnel, as when the psychiatric nurse was interviewed individually by each instructor and the final decision concerning her appointment was made by the group. Total participation in matters like this was possible most of the time because the faculty was small enough for all the members to work together as one group.

As for the factors that led to divisiveness in the faculty group, a brief description of how the faculty members interacted during many of their meetings will help to clarify the major trends that were operating at the time and that later played an essential part in determining one of the focuses of the integration program and the methods utilized in it. Because no specific experiences had been organized for faculty participation in the project during the first year, the data for all the descriptions of the intra-faculty and faculty-psychiatric team interactions that follow are limited to the psychiatric nurse's and the psychiatrist's observations and written recordings of what occurred. In their weekly conferences together the team members explored some of the psychodynamics that seemed to be operating within the faculty group, and the descriptions are based on the data from these conferences. Beginning with the discussion of the second year of the project, concrete examples of interaction will be given. It is hoped that these vignettes will serve as validation of the current description.

Early in the first year, it became apparent to the psychiatric nurse and to the psychiatrist (at those times when he was asked to attend a meeting) that the faculty members had divided themselves into two factions which they categorized as the "younger group" and the "older group." This division was not based on age; it referred to the individual faculty member's real or perceived place within the educational hierarchy, which was determined by the length and breadth of her experience in the Skidmore program, the degree of her authority, her academic rank, and her immediate and long-term goals.

Included in the older group were those five faculty members who, because of their greater experience, length of time in the situation, higher academic rank, and tenure, had more status and authority than did the others. These members composed the executive committee, which was the decision-making body of the department of nursing with respect to administrative matters, such as those pertaining to the budget, the evaluation of faculty members, the granting or withholding of certain rights and privileges, and the establishment and implementation of arrangements with cooperating agencies. In varying degrees the older members had been responsible for the development of the department into what it was. They were deeply committed to the program and to the department and were likely to raise questions about administrative matters in the executive committee meetings rather than in meetings of the total faculty.

The term *younger group* was applied to the nutritionist and the five nurse faculty members who had less experience than the others and were without tenure. These members frequently were dissatisfied with several aspects of the current situation and their position in the hierarchy. They behaved as if they were powerless to take any constructive action. The primary roots of the younger members' cohesiveness were implanted in their status needs, their conflict about authority and dependency, as illustrated by their ambivalent attitudes toward authority figures, their tendency to blame the older members for all the existing problems, and their feelings of impotence in dealing effectively with authority relationships on either an individual or a group level. The following incidents illustrate the characteristic pattern of interaction between the younger and the older faculty members and demonstrate some of the behavioral responses to the introduction of change.

In a curriculum meeting the psychiatric nurse raised several questions regarding the faculty's goals for the educational program and the relationship of these goals to the instructors' expectations of the students' academic and clinical performance and to the criteria and methods of student evaluation. The younger members remained silent, and the topic was bypassed; however, some of the older members returned to it later in the meeting. This incident represented a beginning of acceptance on the part of some faculty members that the psychiatric nurse's contribution was of value.

The curriculum meetings gradually provided the opportunity for the psychiatric nurse and the other faculty members to share ideas about curriculum development which were less threatening than suggestions for implementing psychiatric integration. On several occasions the psychiatric nurse introduced the question of the advisability and possibility of exploring ways to improve the affiliation experiences in psychiatric nursing. The ways in which the two faculty groups handled the ideas that pertained to psychiatric matters or that held some implications for change were essentially different. All the younger members tended to remain silent, not seeking information, raising questions, or expressing agreement or disagreement. On the other hand, some members of the older group, who rejected the possibility that anything could be done currently about the psychiatric nursing experience, would prematurely close off further investigation of the subject by focusing almost exclusively on such concrete matters as time, teaching loads, schedules, curriculum design, and intra-agency policies and underscoring these matters as the predominant obstacles to change. These pressures frequently did not pertain to the main issues, but seemed to be used as rationalizations. The younger members, who probably felt excluded from the discussion of these matters, withdrew further.

On occasions when a question suggestive of some dissatisfaction was raised by the younger members, the older members frequently responded as if the question were intended as a personal criticism—which sometimes it was—and became defensive, withdrew, or became entangled in concrete details. In such instances it may have appeared to the younger members that the older group seemed impervious to what mattered most to them. The younger members· then proceeded underground by passively resisting change through silence and withholding any question or comment during the meetings.

The members of the younger group attempted to regain some of the power they had relinquished through their withdrawal by increasing their membership. When a new instructor joined the faculty, they would attempt to add to their forces by indoctrinating her to their side. Although, by definition, the new instructor automatically was a younger member, the chief requirement for admission to the younger group consisted of being "against" the older members. It also excluded being for change or taking any constructive action directed toward change.

Thus, the younger members helped to perpetuate what by now had become an obvious faculty schism by withdrawing from any effort directed toward change. They were just as opposed to innovations as were the older members, with whom they were struggling for approval and recognition. The two groups, each in its own fashion, were equally resistant to change, and each group also managed to sustain the fantasy that change was impossible.

In the course of her participation with the faculty members in group and individual situations, the psychiatric nurse identified four major behavioral patterns that were disruptive to intrafaculty relationships. These were (1) conformity and difficulties in decision making; (2) difficulties in direct confrontation and intervention; (3) unclarified and unrealistic expectations; and (4) the pattern of scapegoating.

Despite the faculty members' desire for freedom and their ability to frequently establish a democratic give-and-take with each other, there tended to be an implicit expectation that all faculty members should resemble each other with respect to role and function. The role and activities assigned to the psychiatric nurse during the first year of the project constituted a case in point. This expectation of sameness was by no means limited to the psychiatric nurse, however.

A great deal of stress was put on the value of faculty collaboration in all areas of endeavor. This asset also embodied the belief on the part of some faculty members that any instructor should be able to function equally well in more than one clinical area, regardless of the scope of her specialized preparation. The practical application of this philosophy created a paradoxical situation. On the one hand, a faculty member might find herself in the peculiar position of having to teach in an area for which she was not adequately prepared and in which she was not primarily interested. Often she was treated as if she had become an expert in this field by virtue of her assignment to it. On the other hand, she might be given little recognition as an expert in the field in which she had specialized preparation. For example, it was because of the psychiatric nurse's position as an instructor in medical nursing rather than because she was an expert in psychiatric nursing that the faculty members accepted suggestions from her.

The communication of the faculty's stereotyped notion that equality of faculty members is synonymous with uniformity was a predominant theme throughout the integration project. It underscored certain unresolved attitudes toward authority-dependency which created problems related to the democratic process and decision making. To the degree that any individual

instructor felt helplessly caught in the field of whatever forces were operating at the time, her sense of professional autonomy was blocked. The
faculty member who felt like a nonentity as a person scrabbled incessantly
to try to raise her status. The result was competition, reluctance to give
individual recognition, difficulty in taking responsibility for decision making,
and a breakdown of the communication process.

The competitiveness of the faculty members was demonstrated in the
issue about whether student confidences should be held or shared. When
the psychiatric nurse withheld from other faculty members the content of
her unstructured group conferences with students, she became a target for
suspicion, even though from the outset she had stressed to both the faculty
and the students that confidentialness was a prerequisite to the development
of free communication. The psychiatric nurse's individual interviews with
students were also surrounded with mistrust on the part of some faculty
members because she had not kept them informed about the problems that
were affecting the students' academic and clinical performance. The key
issue in the integration project was that the psychiatric nurse was unable
to develop a positive relationship with the other faculty members as long
as she maintained a highly private and confidential relationship with students and individual faculty members.

Although a high value was placed on collaboration in making a decision,
intrafaculty relationships were frequently disrupted in the process of
decision making. Generally, the faculty had difficulty in utilizing a problem-
solving approach in reaching decisions. Upon analysis of the group interaction, the following pattern was identified.

When the group was faced with the task of reaching a decision, there was
first a strong tendency to avoid having to make the decision by talking all
around the issues involved. The next step was the reaching of what appeared
on the surface to be a consensus on common problems. Recurrently, however, this consensus seemed to be a matter of some of the members yielding
an opinion in the sincere effort to create a polite, pleasant, and democratic
atmosphere. Such premature consensus frequently led to rash decisions
which later misfired. When a decision miscarried, some faculty members
denied their responsibility for their part in making it and were inclined to
blame others for the miscarriage. In these circumstances the faculty was
likely to change the decision—without, however, employing a problem-
solving approach. By blaming each other and shifting the task of decision
making to some higher authority, such as the older members or the college
administration, some faculty members relinquished their responsibility and
power to make decisions.

Generally, premature consensus and decision making are defense maneuvers for avoiding the anxiety of dealing with the various interpersonal
conflicts which, upon deeper exploration, might come into the open. This

anxiety was further expressed in the faculty members' avoidance of direct confrontation, intervention, and limit setting with each other.

Among the faculty members there was a generalized fear of, and a tendency to avoid, confronting an instructor with whom one had interpersonal difficulties or who was not effectively fulfilling her professional responsibilities to the rest of the faculty, the students, or the clinical personnel. There were instances when every faculty member but the one who was most directly involved seemed to be aware of an interpersonal problem. For example, on the occasions when some younger members acted out inappropriately, the older members found it difficult to intervene in their behavior and to define realistic limits. The younger members, on the other hand, found it difficult to stand up to the older members when something they believed in and cherished appeared to run counter to the older members' interests and values. The faculty members channeled much of their unsteady passion into the narrow field of student contact and gave vent to their feelings by pouring them out in secret conclaves with members of their own subgroup.

The faculty members' avoidance of direct confrontation may have been a way of trying to "maintain the peace"; at the same time, however, the peace was being undermined as negative feelings about individual faculty members were stirred up but remained underground and were therefore left unresolved. The central problem was not that the faculty members sometimes reacted negatively to each other or to a situation, but rather that they did not discuss their reactions with the person involved. The result was that instead of becoming circumscribed, current problems became diffuse. Under these conditions, the lines of authority became blurred and communication was short-circuited.

Interwoven with this absence of directness among the faculty members was their reluctance to state their expectations of each other clearly and explicitly and to follow through on these expectations. Directly and indirectly, many faculty members, both younger and older, in informal groups and singly, expressed to the psychiatric nurse the feeling that they were repeatedly placed in the untenable position of having to try to divine what was expected of them. All the faculty members expressed some uncertainty about where they stood in relation to members of both their own subgroup and the other one. This uncertainty was also demonstrated in their behavior. In group meetings some participants were prone to emphasize their successes and hide what might appear to others to be their failures. Much of this need for approval and oversensitivity to criticism and rivalry with each other for a place in the sun seemed to be founded on their feelings that somehow they were not measuring up—but to what they were not sure.

The faculty's difficulties in the evaluation of students were symptomatic of the unrealistic and unclarified expectations and breakdowns in communication. Several stumbling blocks in the evaluation process became evident during the first year of the project.

There was a tendency on the part of some instructors to assign a higher grade than seemed warranted by either their oral or their written evaluation of a student. This practice created a troublesome situation both for the student and for her instructor in her next nursing course. During one clinical experience, for instance, a student received a higher grade than either the written evaluation or her performance called for. In her next experience she was given a lower grade, which was more consistent with her performance and the instructor's evaluation. This discrepancy in the evaluation of the same student by different instructors happened with enough frequency to warrant concern. The instructor who gave lower grades worried about her reputation among students as one who had unrealistically high expectations and "was out to fail students." (There may have been some justification for this fear, because one instructor, whose course followed that of a "high-marker," failed a fairly sizable proportion of students.) The instructors who found themselves in this position were displeased with certain other instructors who they felt had evaded their responsibility by passing on to someone else the task of failing a student.

Another problem in the area of student evaluation was the discrepancy that often occurred between the instructor's oral and written evaluations of a student. Many times the written evaluation did not communicate clearly enough the degree of the student's limitations. This practice created serious problems for the faculty members high in the administrative hierarchy when they tried to give the parents evidence that would justify the decision to fail the student.

The most serious problem related to the instructor's role in regard to students who were failing in their clinical learning experiences. Before a student had completed a particular clinical experience the instructor might neglect to communicate the possibility of the student's failure either to the faculty member who had the administrative responsibility for communicating with the student and her parents or to the student herself. In these instances, the outcome of the final evaluation sometimes came as a shock to the student, the rest of the faculty members, and the student's parents. The faculty members with administrative responsibilities were then placed in the embarrassing position of having to face parents with a failure that appeared to be unforeseen by everyone in the situation, with the possible exception of the instructor in the course. It was extremely difficult to justify the failure, especially when it appeared that the student's position had not been sufficiently precarious to have required some kind of warning.

On such occasions intrafaculty relationships were seriously disrupted. Rather than examine the roots of the existing problem so that it might be

managed more effectively in the future, the faculty members adhered to
a pattern of attaching blame to someone. Those in administration, who felt
that they had been put in an untenable position with both the student and
her parents, tended to blame the instructor for not keeping them informed.
In response, the instructor blamed the administration for what she felt to
be the unrealistic expectation that she should always be able to predict a
failure. In some instances the student was blamed for being unable to
identify when she had performed poorly. Frequently the instructor, instead
of examining the possibility that she had relinquished her leadership responsibility for taking a stand regarding the student's failure, reacted to
the understandable but not always realistic fear that the faculty would
reject her, and consequently she blamed herself for being a failure as a
teacher and a colleague.

Placing blame is, of course, a defense operation that is used to circumvent
the anxiety of having to face one's personal feelings of helplessness in certain
situations and of having to deal with the very human but irrational aspects
of one's fear of losing face with significant persons. The process through
which placing blame is generated follows a definite pattern—there are
personal reactions (frequently negative) to a person or a situation; fear of
directly communicating these reactions at the time and in the context of
their occurrence; frustration and feelings of hopelessness about being able
to alter the situation; feelings of helplessness; and abdication of personal
responsibility for asserting leadership, accompanied by guilt feelings and
the relinquishing of one's own realistic expectations, needs, and aspirations
through ingratiation or withdrawal. Finally comes the displacement of all
these unidentified feelings onto other persons and situations through the
seemingly magical operation of creating a scapegoat. And so the process,
if uninterrupted, continues.

During the first year of the project this pattern of placing the blame on
some person or group or even thing—one's self, those with administrative
authority, professional colleagues, the psychiatric nurse, nursing service
personnel, the physicians, the curriculum design, or available resources as
these pertained to heavy schedules, insufficient time, and inadequate physical facilities—became evident among the faculty members, particularly in
group situations in which they interacted with each other.

Faculty and Pyschiatric-Team Relationships. During the entire first year
of the integration project the relationships between the faculty and the
psychiatric nurse were colored by circumstances surrounding the employment of the team members and the activities which the faculty had planned
for them. In the early stage of the project the faculty, upon the advice of
selected physicians and psychiatric nurses, had decided that the project
should be conducted by an interdisciplinary team consisting of a psychiatric
nurse as project director and a psychiatrist. Finding it difficult to secure

a psychiatric nurse who was qualified for the position, the faculty had gone ahead and employed the psychiatrist on a part-time basis before employing the project director.

The psychiatric nurse was extremely ambivalent about participating in the project on a regular basis with any psychiatrist, and if the choice had been left to her, it is possible that she would not have had one as a participant in the project. Many of her past professional relationships with physicians had been more or less superficial. In the large mental hospitals in which she had worked, doctor-nurse collaboration had been difficult because of the scarcity of available psychiatrists. In smaller hospital settings and in the community, her relationship with physicians had consisted of short-term contacts while she was giving nursing care to a patient. Working closely with a psychiatrist was a relatively new experience for her.

Her feelings about the project also entered into the situation. For a long period before she joined the faculty as project director, she had been interested in the integration of psychiatric concepts in generic baccalaureate programs in nursing. Many of her experiences had been consciously geared toward preparing for this pioneer endeavor. When she learned that a psychiatrist would participate as a team member, she feared that he would take over the project.

She also was apprehensive about his psychiatric philosophy and theoretical orientation. Would he be descriptively or dynamically oriented? Would he be concerned with categorical diagnoses and attaching labels instead of dealing with the steps in problem solving? Would he be threatened by the expanding role of the nurse and attempt to relegate the psychiatric nurse to a state of subservience to him? Or would he concur with the broad concept of professional nursing that recognizes the psychotherapeutic relevance of the psychiatric nurse's role?

The psychiatric nurse also felt resentful about her immediate role. With the exception of her group conferences with students (which she had suggested to the faculty and which it readily agreed to), all the activities in which she was to participate had been planned by the faculty before her arrival. In these plans, as has been stated, the predominant focus of the team members' activities was the students. No experience had been planned for working with the faculty in relation to the integration project. The psychiatric nurse, on the other hand, had expected that during the first year she would be sufficiently free of teaching responsibilities to have an opportunity to study all aspects of the situation as a basis for developing an integration program.

Despite her expectations, when she was being interviewed for the position the psychiatric nurse acted as if she had accepted the role predetermined for her by the faculty. She equated her lack of directness, leadership, and guidance with avoidance of telling the faculty members what to do; at the same time she expected them to use her as a specialist without clarifying this fact for them.

The psychiatric nurse's reluctance to take issue with the faculty's concept of the role of project director was perhaps related to at least three dynamics. First, she had the unrealistic expectation of herself that she should have been able to identify in advance her role and functions as project director and the methods of integration to be used instead of allowing them to evolve from a study of the situation and from work with the students and the faculty. The second dynamic pertained to her response to the faculty's anxiety about differences in role and status. Because her previous experiences had taught her how the whole area of psychiatry and the psychiatric nurse can threaten other members of a nursing faculty, the psychiatric nurse compromised her own uniqueness by putting herself in the vulnerable position of permitting the faculty members to cast her into whatever role they saw fit. Third, her intense and long-standing desire to participate in a psychiatric integration program was attended by the fear that if she allowed her conflict with faculty members to come into the open, she might not be employed.

As for the faculty's attitude about having a psychiatric nurse on the faculty for the first time, not unlike business management, it acted as if it felt compelled to put a new person through the various ranks, irrespective of any special knowledge and skill that she might have to offer. The combination of the faculty's attempt to carve the psychiatric nurse's role within the context of the existing status quo and the psychiatric nurse's failure to communicate her reaction to this attempt resulted in resistance to change on the part of the faculty members and a reduction of the possibility for change to occur.

The background in experience and education which the psychiatric nurse and the psychiatrist brought to the project and their role in psychiatric integration were different from the background and roles of the other faculty members, which were fairly similar with respect to the integration project. Therefore, the members of the psychiatric team were frequently perceived as outsiders who had interloped in the affairs of the faculty. Having had no previous experience with a psychiatrist and a psychiatric nurse on the faculty, the rest of the faculty members responded to them in terms of the roles they did know, such as authority figures—be they tender hearts or martinets, chums, or peers (4). The fear that the psychiatrist and the psychiatric nurse would somehow manage to "fool around" with their unconsciouses reflected a stereotyped perception of psychiatry, the psychiatric nurse, and the psychiatrist.

In their relationships with the psychiatric nurse, the faculty members were likely to handle her differences in knowledge, skill, and experience by denying their existence through casting her into the role of a peer. In contrast to their perception of the psychiatric nurse, the faculty members tended to feel that greater knowledge could be achieved from a higher authority, preferably the physician. They therefore ascribed ascendancy in status to the psychiatrist. This concept of status differences was reflected in the faculty's charismatic view of the psychiatrist. Such a view of the doctor-nurse relationship prevented them from making a realistic appraisal of the psychiatric nurse's unique value as well as their own.

Because in the early period of the project the psychiatrist seldom met with the faculty as a group, the faculty and psychiatric-team relationships consisted primarily of interaction between the psychiatric nurse and the rest of the faculty. In certain situations the psychiatric nurse resembled the rest of the faculty members in her role and functions, and it was within this context that she was accepted by them. When, however, she shifted to her other role and assumed leadership for developing an integration program, as has been pointed out, her suggestions were rejected with such responses as silence, preoccupation with a myriad of details, and refusal to talk to the group at large.

Because she had the vague foreboding that she was a potential scapegoat among the faculty members, she was reluctant to intervene in the blaming process that was going on within the group. As a way of coping with her frustration and her anger toward the faculty members, she removed herself from the anxiety-laden situation by employing the transitory measures of withholding and withdrawing from them. For example, she kept the faculty in the dark about what was happening in her group conferences with students. Aside from her belief that whatever students divulged should be kept in confidence, she harbored the notion that because this was her only activity which was geared specifically to the goals of psychiatric integration and the only one which she had had any part in creating and developing, she was not "about to give it away."

Instead of striving to work through the problem with the faculty, she side-stepped it by focusing all her attention on the students and by spending more time in her office, using the excuse that she was writing up "all these pertinent data." In order to avoid disappointment and achieve an island of security, it seemed safer, at the time, for her to exclude the rest of the faculty members from her activities. As much as possible she avoided contacts with them. Through her withdrawal she relinquished her strategic position for handling the faculty members' autistic perceptions of and reactions to her.

As for the psychiatric nurse's behavior with respect to the faculty schism, instead of taking a bifurcated stance, she temporarily joined sides with the younger members against the older members, whom she viewed as obstructing her leadership role. In her desire and search for support from some direction, she often confused a younger faculty member's explicit statements of dissatisfaction with an implicit acceptance of herself. She had yet to learn that to take sides with an instructor is in no way tantamount to receiving the instructor's genuine support in efforts directed toward introducing change.

In the face of the faculty's generalized antipathy toward the psychiatric nurse whenever in the curriculum committee meetings she moved from her role of peer to that of leader, her most urgent problem was to avoid feeling helpless and hopeless and thereby to become immobilized because her unrealistic expectations of introducing change without struggle remained unrealized.

Many of the communication problems among the faculty members, and between them, the students, and the psychiatric nurse, arose from unexpressed attitudes or silent areas in interpersonal relations, which were covertly communicated in a multitude of ways that periodically disrupted relationships and were deleterious to the educational program. The pressure caused by the beginning of the integration project, plus the addition of two psychiatric experts to the faculty, understandably served as a catalyst in uncovering the unresolved interpersonal problems among the faculty group. In response to the anxiety that was aroused by the threat of change, the faculty members' characteristic responses, especially as these were triggered off by defense operations, were brought into full play. During this period of exploration, therefore, the forces that led to group divisiveness overshadowed, at least temporarily, those forces that might have led to group cohesiveness.

THE PSYCHIATRIC TEAM

The presence of the psychiatric nurse and the psychiatrist on the faculty compensated for certain deficiencies in the educational program. The faculty members were provided with the opportunity to work with experts in psychiatry and psychiatric nursing and thereby to become oriented to psychiatric matters as well as to begin to alter their stereotyped image of psychiatry and the people working in the field. The team also functioned as a bridge between the affiliation in psychiatric nursing and the rest of the nursing curriculum.

Another asset was that professional persons who had been prepared to work within a broad range of behavior problems were available for the counseling and psychiatric referral of students. In line with these guidance activities a major strength was that, unlike the psychiatric nurse, the psychiatrist had no responsibility for evaluating student performance or assigning grades. Consequently, the students' fear of being penalized for exposing themselves, especially in regard to the revelation of some negative attitudes toward their educational experiences, was reduced considerably in their contacts with the psychiatrist.

One of the obstacles to achieving the goals of the integration project pertained to faculty, psychiatric-team relationships, especially with respect to the assigned activities of the team. Although the first-year activities of the psychiatric nurse, as planned by the faculty, gave her an opportunity to assess the particular needs of the Skidmore students and to appraise the resources of the Skidmore program, the psychiatric nurse's and the psychiatrist's activities had some serious deficiencies both as an orientation experience for the team members and as an opportunity to plan and organize an integration program.

The psychiatric nurse, who had had considerable experience in teaching in collegiate schools of nursing and who was therefore familiar with their practices, did not need so much orientation. The psychiatrist, who had never had any experience with nursing instructors or nursing students and who had never been associated with an undergraduate program of any kind (except as a student), was only minimally exposed to a few aspects of the nursing program. As a consequence, his real orientation, under the guidance of the psychiatric nurse, had to be extended well beyond the first year, and it was some time before he could contribute to any great extent to the problem-identification function of the psychiatric team.

As far as the planning and organization of the psychiatric integration project were concerned, some major disadvantages accrued from the psychiatric nurse's service as a regular faculty member. Because of her full-time responsibilities for clinical teaching and supervision, it was difficult, and often impossible, for the psychiatric nurse and the psychiatrist to work together in developing an integration program. During the time the psychiatrist was having clinical discussions with a group of students, the psychiatric nurse, much to her frustration and disappointment, was involved either in supervising students in the clinical area or in demonstrating and supervising nursing procedures in the classroom.

Another disadvantage was that although the students were exposed to a concentrated dose of psychiatric concepts in their medical nursing experiences with the psychiatric nurse, no provision had been made for faculty exploration of the methods that might be used to develop the students' ability to utilize their knowledge of psychiatric concepts in their experiences in other areas of clinical nursing that were under the direct guidance of the Skidmore faculty.

One of the most serious disadvantages of the psychiatric nurse's role during this first year pertained to her responsibility for evaluating the students' clinical performance and assigning grades. This function reduced the students' sense of freedom in discussing with her their subjective responses to the problems that arose in their relationships with her, with the psychiatrist, with clinical personnel, and with other faculty members.

Another initial limitation of the team as a resource was the relationship between the psychiatric nurse and the psychiatrist. As has been stated, the psychiatric nurse was not the least bit happy to find a psychiatrist already in the situation. This problem, coupled with the fact that the psychiatric nurse and the psychiatrist had not chosen each other, made it extremely difficult for them to begin their work with much in the way of a teamlike feeling. The process by which the psychiatric nurse and the psychiatrist worked through their relationship and became synthesized into an inter-disciplinary team is analyzed in step-by-step fashion in Chapter 13.

During the first year the psychiatric nurse and the psychiatrist did have a one-hour weekly conference during which they identified some of the psychodynamics and sociological principles that may have been operating in the meetings attended by the psychiatric nurse. Much of the time, how-ever, was consumed by the psychiatric nurse's expression of her feelings of frustration concerning the role in which she had allowed herself to be cast by the faculty, with the result that the team members did not fully utilize the one experience that afforded them the opportunity for collaboration.

On one occasion, after the psychiatric nurse had told the psychiatrist about how the other faculty members had responded negatively to one of her suggestions, he asked, "Why do you present suggestions for an integra-tion program to the faculty on your own? By now, we both have some ideas about how they probably will be received. Why don't you use me? That's what I'm here for—for us to work together as a team."

This incident became a turning point in the team members' relationship. Together, the psychiatric nurse and the psychiatrist formed a plan for an integration program.

Methods of Psychiatric Integration

In the team members' efforts to formulate an integration program, the psychiatric nurse assumed the leadership role. The psychiatrist gave full recognition to her special knowledge of the total setting, which evolved from her professional identification with the other faculty members, from her previous experience in teaching in a generic baccalaureate degree pro-gram in nursing, and particularly from her role as a full-time faculty member.

The methods and activities which the psychiatric team formulated for the first year of the project were chosen with a view to making full use of the assets and overcoming the limitations of the existing resources. The methods also reflected the psychiatric nurse's and the psychiatrist's belief that their function was to help the faculty members and the students to recognize the roots of interpersonal difficulties within the framework of their profes-sional relationships and to perceive the complexity of the issues underlying group behavior. This meant that the faculty members and the students had to give up the strongly held conviction that problems in a given situation are directly related to a single cause—usually the inept behavior of some contending person or group (1). In other words, the psychiatric nurse and the psychiatrist perceived psychiatric integration as an ongoing educational and re-educational process, and they viewed their role in the project as that of change agent.

This perception of the project also led the psychiatric nurse and the psychiatrist to decide that the integration program should have a double focus —the students and the faculty in individual and group settings. They also concurred that they would jointly participate in as many experiences as possible.

Focus on the Students

From the beginning of the integration project the psychiatric nurse recognized that a vital part of the team's role would be to work with the students. She also knew that in order to meet the goals of integration, some new learning experiences would have to be set up to meet the students' needs, and certain of the existing learning experiences would have to be modified or expanded.

Because there were no guidance facilities for the students, the team members realized that the responsibility for individual student guidance, counseling, and psychiatric referral should constitute an important part of the integration program. They agreed that the psychiatric nurse's weekly unstructured conferences of one hour each for the four groups of sophomore students should continue.

Because there were no social scientists available in the department of nursing, it was planned that the psychiatrist would teach a twenty-hour course in social science concepts, "The Self in Society," to sophomore students. Because of the necessity for the students to acquire a knowledge of psychiatric content, the team members agreed that the psychiatric nurse should teach a forty-four-hour course in psychodynamics, also to the sophomore students.

The psychiatrist and the psychiatric nurse decided that because the psychiatrist would be moving into other areas, the psychiatric nurse probably should assume responsibility for the clinical conferences with the junior students who were having experiences in team nursing under the guidance of the Skidmore instructors. The number of hours could not be determined until after discussion with the faculty.

Focus on the Faculty

In the psychiatrist's opinion, and to a certain extent in the opinion of the faculty, the students were to be the major focus of the project. However, the psychiatric nurse pointed out that for any pervasive and continuing change to take place help must be provided for the faculty who were responsible for developing the educational policies and the curriculum and for teaching students. As a way of furthering faculty growth, the psychiatric team planned two experiences for the faculty members—work with the individual instructors in clinical conferences and work with the faculty as a group in one-hour discussions every week.

In their work with the individual instructors, the team members planned to work with one instructor at a time for a series of the three regular weekly clinical conferences which each instructor held with her students. The purpose of this experience was to help the instructor to increase her knowledge of and ability to apply psychiatric content and to develop her skills in teaching this knowledge and its application to small groups of students.

The plan for the work with the faculty as a group was developed as a result of the psychiatric nurse's recognition that the most important contributory goal of the integration project was to help the faculty members to grow in their ability to communicate, their ability to conceptualize, and their willingness to change their professional behavior. The team believed that the first effort they should make toward facilitating this change and growth was to work toward a higher order of explicit communication among the faculty members. In selecting a method for bringing about such change, they recognized the principle enunciated by Floyd C. Mann, namely, that in trying to reduce conflict and create a different system of communication, it is seldom if ever possible to bring about the desired change by dealing with one person or with members of a group individually (3). Because many of the intrafaculty conflicts seemed more related to both the formal and informal organizational structure of the department of nursing than to the personal characteristics of the individual faculty members, the psychiatric team believed it was necessary to deal with the whole complex of relationships within the department as simultaneously as possible. Accordingly, the team decided to utilize a technique directed toward facilitating and obtaining sanction for the expression of private attitudes and feelings through the gradual exposure and exploration of problematic behavior insofar as it intruded on the faculty member's role as a nurse, a teacher of nurses, and a professional colleague, *at the time of its occurrence* within the group setting, rather than through a didactic and more traditional approach.

The technique the team planned to use involved the concept of interactional process. It provided for the faculty members to live through various professional experiences together under the joint guidance of the psychiatric nurse and the psychiatrist. The subject matter in this method of teaching included the faculty members' professional conflicts and harmonies, their identifications with each other, and the interaction of ideas.

The formulation of a plan for these meetings marked a change in the psychiatric nurse's and the psychiatrist's original conception of the integration project as a curriculum study which would include some teaching of the faculty but would focus almost entirely on the students. The project as they now envisioned it had broadened to a participant-observational study of faculty interaction.

The psychiatric nurse and the psychiatrist also realized that the methods of integration that they formulated at this time were based on a preliminary assay of the situation. In a project as dynamic as this one, all the methods that were to be used could not be predetermined, especially because more assets and obstacles would be uncovered in the ongoing process of problem solving. Table 1 shows all of the team's various activities during the first five years of the project.

PRESENTATION OF THE PLAN TO THE FACULTY

An inherent and vital component of the plan was that the psychiatric nurse would cease to function as an instructor in medical nursing. The psychiatric nurse and the psychiatrist were faced with a crisis in the current life of the project. Its survival depended solely on whether or not the faculty would accept at least the basic structure of the plan for implementation. This acceptance required some change. Even though the first spell cast on her by the appearance of faculty group solidarity had faded away, the psychiatric nurse's restless hopefulness remained undefeated.

At the request of the psychiatric team members, they met with the faculty as a group for the purpose of presenting their plan for an integration program to begin in the second year. Behind a palisade of pens and pencils and note taking the other faculty members listened as the psychiatric nurse gave the report. The atmosphere was oppressive. Members of the older group were the first to respond by asking questions which focused on the availability of time, schedules, the proper or improper use of language and terminology, the goals of teaching psychodynamics, and the meaning and validity of certain psychiatric assumptions. The younger members' participation consisted almost exclusively of intramural communication in which one member muttered enigmatically to another.

The psychiatrist participated actively by refocusing the discussion and by clarifying what was said. He reduced some of the mounting tension by injecting bits of humor at appropriate times. The faculty members repeatedly acted out their view that the physician is superior to the nurse by dismissing any idea or suggestion the psychiatric nurse offered, only to accept, at least on the surface, the same idea when it was repeated by the psychiatrist. The psychiatric nurse also became enmeshed in the false superior physician, inferior nurse concept of status and for the time being relinquished her leadership role to the psychiatrist. This abdication was to have a marked effect on the progress of the project, particularly insofar as the faculty group meetings were concerned.

After two stormy sessions, during which negative attitudes toward psychiatry and the psychiatric nurse, and opposition to change were revealed,

Table 1. Activities of the Psychiatric Team During the First

	FIRST YEAR 1957–58 PsyNs-Psych-Team
PROJECT ACTIVITIES	
Work with Students	
Teaching Psychiatric Content	
Series of lectures on psychodynamics	+
Course in psychodynamics	
Course in social science concepts	
Cliincal conferences in psychiatric nursing	
Leading Unstructured Group Discussions (Sophomore Students)	×
Serving as a Resource in Nursing Courses	
Normal growth and development	
Communicable disease and long-term illness nursing (clinical conferences)	+
Team nursing (clinical conferences)	+
Pediatric nursing (child health station)	
Public health nursing (family care conferences)	
Disaster nursing (seminars)	
Medical-surgical nursing (consultation in clinical area)	
Conferring with Individual Students	×
Making Psychiatric Evaluations and Referrals	+
Work with Faculty	
In Clinical Conferences with Students	
In Faculty Group Discussions	
In Individual Conferences	
Collection of Data for Book	
OTHER ACTIVITIES	
Orientation	
Teaching	
Fundamentals of nursing (theory and clinical supervision) ..	×
Medical nursing (clinical teaching and supervision)	×
Pediatric nursing (supervision in outpatient department)	×
Team nursing (clinical supervision)	×
Participation in Regular Faculty Activities	
Participating in Faculty Meetings	×
Serving on Faculty Committees	
Psychiatric and mental health nursing (chairman)	
Curriculum	
Disaster	
Serving as Consultant	
To faculty, in evaluation of students' presenting behavior problems	× +
To Executive Committee of the faculty	
To Faculty-Student Council	
To student health nurse	
Supervision of Graduate Student in Psychiatric Integration Field Experience	

Five Years of the Skidmore Psychiatric Integration Project

Second Year 1958–59			Third Year 1959–60			Fourth Year 1960–61			Fifth Year 1961–62		
PsyNs	Psych	Team	PsyNs	Psych	Team	PsyNs	Psych	Team	PsyNs	Psych	Team
X			X			X					
	+										
			X		✻	X		✻			
X			X			X					
	+				+						
X			X								
X			X								
X											
			X			X					
						X					
X			X			X			X		
X			X			X					
	+			+			+			+	
		✻			✻			✻			✻
		✻			✻			✻			
X	+		X	+		X	+		X	+	
									X		
X			X			X					
X						X					
X			X			X					
X			X			X					
X	+		X	+							
			X								
			X			X					
			X			X					

implementation of the plan with only one minor change was agreed to. This change required that the psychiatric nurse's course in psychodynamics for sophomore students be reduced from forty-four to thirty-six hours. It was also decided that the psychiatric nurse would have eight hours of group discussion with each group of junior students who were having their seven-week experience in team nursing. This passive agreement to the plan for the integration program was, of course, not tantamount to acceptance of it. Nonetheless, it provided a starting point for the next year—the year of impact.

Summary

The first year of the project was a time during which the psychiatric nurse and the psychiatrist identified the goals of integration and some of the assets and obstacles to the achievement of these goals. It was a period which was punctuated by the faculty's resistance to change and which gave portent of a split between the younger and older faculty members, and between the faculty and the psychiatric team.

For the psychiatric nurse and the psychiatrist the first year was a time characterized by a struggle to identify and formulate their respective roles in relation to the faculty and the students and to coordinate themselves as a team. Interdisciplinary collaboration was a terrain not to be traversed for some time to come.

Toward the end of the year the psychiatric team formulated a plan of activities involving work with both students and faculty. This plan expanded the original scope of the project to include a participant-observational study of faculty interaction. The plan received the formal approval of the faculty.

The stage was set. The prologue had been completed. The play was about to begin.

REFERENCES

1. Elliott, Jacques. "Interpretive Group Discussion as a Method of Facilitating Social Change," *Human Relations*, **1**, 533–549 (1948).

2. Erikson, Erik H. "Youth: Fidelity and Diversity," *Daedalus—Journal of the American Academy of Arts and Sciences*, **5–27** (Winter, 1962).

3. Mann, Floyd C. "Changing Superior-Subordinate Relationships," *Journal of Social Issues*, **7**, 56–58 (1951).

4. Zaphiropoulos, Miltiades L. "Tender Hearts and Martinets: Some Varieties of Countertransference," unpublished paper, read at the William Alanson White Psychoanalytic Society, New York, March 16, 1961.

Chapter Six

THE WORK WITH STUDENTS

Youth is life as yet untouched by tragedy. . . . When youth
has once grasped where Beauty dwells—with a real knowledge
and not as a mere matter of literary phraseology—its self-surren-
der is absolute.

ALFRED NORTH WHITEHEAD, *Adventures of Ideas*

In line with the original conception of psychiatric integration as a curriculum study that would focus primarily on the preparation of
those who in the future will provide nursing care to patients, from the beginning of the Skidmore project a major emphasis was put on the students.
Even after the concept of the project was expanded to include work with the
faculty members, the focus on students continued throughout the five years
of the first grant (See Table 1, pages 110–111).

Because the psychiatrist was a part-time participant in the project, the
limitations in time made it necessary for priorities to be established in utilizing his knowledge and skill. Therefore, in contrast to the work with the
faculty, which was largely a team endeavor, the work with students became
primarily the responsibility of the psychiatric nurse.

As has been pointed out, during the first year of the project, the psychiatric
nurse identified three broad areas of student problems. Immediately evident
was the students' difficulty in applying their knowledge of psychiatric concepts to nurse-patient situations—a difficulty that was related to their reluctance to acknowledge and express their subjective reactions to their
educational experiences and to employ the steps in the problem-solving
process. Another problem area involved the students' numerous misgivings
about embarking on a nursing career, which they perceived as being incompatible with marriage. Other problems emerged from the students' unresolved
attitudes toward authority and dependency, particularly as these attitudes

were associated with the students' relationships with patients, the faculty, the clinical personnel, and the psychiatric team.

For dealing with the needs of the students, the psychiatric team designed a two-pronged approach. First, activities were planned to help students to learn and apply psychiatric concepts in their care of patients. A second series of activities was organized to assist the students to effectively handle the problems arising in connection with their own change and growth. Except for the questions proposed by the psychiatric team for the general examinations, no course of assignments or grades were given in any of these experiences, a fact which, as has been emphasized, helped to eliminate some of the students' fear of punishment or failure, to reduce their need for seeking approval and reward, and to develop a sense of freedom in participating spontaneously.

As the plans for these activities with the students were developed, they were presented, discussed, agreed to or rejected, and evaluated in the faculty group conferences.

Teaching Psychiatric Concepts

In instructing the students in psychiatric concepts, the members of the psychiatric team assumed several roles. First, they planned and taught two courses in which psychiatric content was presented to the students. Second, they participated in the teaching of the psychiatric nursing course by holding group conferences with the students in connection with their clinical experiences in this course. Third, in the other nursing courses they served as resource persons with respect to the psychosocial aspects of the subject matter being taught.

COURSES IN PSYCHIATRIC CONTENT

The two courses for which the psychiatric team members assumed responsibility were a course in social science concepts, taught by the psychiatrist, and a course in psychodynamics, taught by the psychiatric nurse. These courses were for sophomore students. The primary emphasis of both of the courses was on helping the students to acquire a body of theoretical knowledge which would assist them in identifying, understanding, and effectively handling the range of emotionally disturbed behavior commonly experienced in any clinical situation. Lectures plus experiential teaching were utilized in both courses. The students were encouraged to raise questions, express opinions, and react to the material presented.

Content and Method. The twenty-hour course entitled "The Self in Society," taught by the psychiatrist, was introduced in the second year of the project. The classes met once a month for ten two-hour sessions. The psychiatric nurse and the majority of the faculty members attended the classes.

For the purpose of creating a background of knowledge from which to approach problems associated with emotionally disturbed behavior, students were oriented to the sources of personality within the framework of the cultural, social, and idiosyncratic life experiences of an individual. The development of personality was perceived as an evolving process. Reactions to illness were viewed against the screen of sociocultural influences and within the range of individual modes of adaptation to emotional stress.

For the most part the students did not appear to be inhibited by the presence of the faculty members, who, because they were auditing the course, did not contribute or respond to the discussions. The psychiatric nurse participated with the psychiatrist by calling attention to the nursing implications of the students' comments and questions and by further clarifying the meaning of the subject matter under discussion through giving concrete illustrations.

Some of the broad areas of content that were discussed were the following.

1. The role of institutions in molding human needs and the ways in which they aid or abet the meeting of these needs.

2. Cultural factors which tend to play down, maximize, or exploit illness.

3. How society induces anxiety by establishing certain taboos, how it relieves anxiety, and how these anxiety-inducing and anxiety-relieving measures influence health, illness, and treatment.

4. The hospital as a social institution and the ways in which cultural attitudes conflict with hospital practices.

5. The origin of language with particular emphasis on the two modes of organizing language: the referential mode, in which the meaning of words is rooted in objective reality, and the experiential mode, in which personal meaning transcends the objective meaning.

To enable the psychiatrist to participate in other activities that were initiated in the third year of the project, this course was discontinued after one year.

The course in psychodynamics taught by the psychiatric nurse was entitled "Interpersonal Relations in Nursing" and was referred to by the other faculty members as the "mental health classes." Originally this was a thirty-six-hour course; after one year, to permit the inclusion of other experiences in the curriculum, the classes met every other week for fifteen two-hour sessions. So that the other faculty members might be oriented to what the students were being taught, all the instructors were invited to attend the classes. Two instructors, one older and one younger, attended regularly, and two instructors, one from each group, attended sporadically.

A central theme of the course was the nursing student's role as a participant-observer in nurse-patient relationships. Therefore, besides the orientation of the student to understanding the meaning of patient behavior, a great deal of emphasis was put on the student understanding her own behavior and learning how to use it in resolving a felt difficulty and in modifying her professional relationships with others. The meaning of behavior and its implications for the communication process were analyzed against the backdrop of the impact of culture, subculture, and social system on attitudes, feelings, thoughts, ideas, values, and modes of communication.

In the classes the students worked on tasks especially designed to develop their ability to conceptualize (a skill which requires moving back and forth from the abstract to the concrete and differentiating referential from experiential language), their ability to formulate theoretical ideas, and their ability to utilize a problem-solving approach. Such tasks included exploring the perceptions of illness in the United States through the analysis of get-well greeting cards (2); desymbolizing familiar adages; and exploring an author's meaning of such concepts as love, democracy, and dependency through the identification and analysis of the central themes in extracts taken from poetry and popular songs. To facilitate maximum participation and group interaction, the students were divided into small groups of five or six.

The students' experiences with patients and personnel were used to illustrate the various concepts and principles under discussion. A bibliography was provided, and the students were encouraged to read selected material, although such readings were not required.

In the third year of the project many of the concepts and principles that had been included in "The Self in Society" course were incorporated into the course taught by the psychiatric nurse. Some of the broad areas of content that were discussed were the following.

1. The hospital as a social system and its bureaucratic structure.

2. Illness as a process and as socially deviant behavior; body image, integrity, and assault, and their relation to self-identity.

3. Dying as an interpersonal process; psychological alienation, and the concept of "cure" versus "caring for."

4. Unconscious motivation.

5. The concept of anxiety and such security operations as selective inattention, dissociation, denial, malevolent transformation, and somnolent detachment.

6. Frustration-aggression: aggression as a way of relating with others as opposed to a feeling.

7. Conflict: the concept of choice, and principles of decision making.

8. Communication theory especially in terms of verbal and nonverbal communication; referential and experiential language; body language, such as symptoms of illness, and physical nursing care and the critical use of

touching as an instrument in developing a nurse-patient relationship; and the principles of interviewing.

9. Steps in the problem-solving process, including the identification and formulation of theoretical concepts and the recurring ideas that are basic to every interpersonal relationship.

Although no separate course credit or grade was given, at the end of each semester the psychiatric nurse and the psychiatrist were charged with the responsibility of preparing an examination question to be incorporated in a general examination which covered some areas of medical-surgical, pediatric, and emergency nursing, and the content of the courses taught by the psychiatric nurse and the psychiatrist (see Appendix E for examination questions used during project). The psychiatric team constructed the questions, and the psychiatric nurse graded the responses; the grade on the question constituted about 10 per cent of the overall grade of the general examination.

Problems and Issues. This course posed several problems for the students, the faculty members, and the psychiatric nurse. Insofar as the students were concerned, the problems generated by the course were related to the unique nature of psychiatric content and to the experiential method of teaching. Many of their questions and responses indicated that much of the anxiety that was aroused in connection with the content stemmed from their concern with the implications of the content for their own behavior, especially in terms of "good" and "bad." The emphasis on the students' revelation of their feelings and attitudes, rather than the use of a more didactic approach to the study of psychiatric concepts, constituted an additional threat.

Another problem was that in spite of the numerous clinical illustrations that were used in teaching the course, the students found it extremely difficult to relate the theory to their clinical practice. As with most nurses, in the early period of the course the students were almost exclusively action-oriented, and unless they could immediately grasp the significance of the content either for their own behavior or for the solution of a clinical problem (which they conceived of in terms of a pat answer), they were likely to become uninterested in it. Consequently, some students absented themselves from classes, but within the limits of the number of total absences permitted by the department of nursing.

As has been pointed out, as the course progressed into the second semester, there was a marked tendency on the part of most of the students to become preoccupied with the emotional aspects of illness and nursing care, to the exclusion of the physical aspects. As with the case of too much of anything, such preoccupations were symptomatic of some underlying anxiety and conflict. In this situation the anxiety seemed, on the one hand, to be tied to the students' reluctance to become involved with patients, and on the other hand, to be related to their perception of physical nursing care as demeaning.

The first faculty problem engendered by the course involved an examination question that had been prepared by the psychiatric team. During the first year of the course, this examination question became the justification for an internecine struggle between the psychiatric team and the rest of the faculty (see Chapter 8, May 19 and June 30, 1959). The faculty's reactions revolved around such issues as the appropriateness of the clinical situation presented in the question, the criteria for grading it, and the effect that the grade on the question might have on the student's score on the total examination. Also the instructors had intense and negative reactions about not knowing which patients were being discussed in the course—reactions that were fortified by the view of some instructors that the material which students were presenting in class was a distortion of what actually had occurred in the clinical situation. Some instructors assumed that the psychiatric nurse's analysis of the situation, including the identification of possible ways of handling it more effectively, was based exclusively on a distorted picture, and presumed that therefore whatever insights and guides to action evolved from the analysis were all for naught (see Chapter 9, July 2, 1960).

Another problem was connected with the strong feelings on the part of some instructors that students automatically should be able to apply their newly acquired knowledge of psychiatric concepts to their work with patients. The psychiatric nurse believed that the individual instructor had the responsibility to help students transfer their knowledge to the clinical setting. However, there was the problem of insufficient knowledge of psychiatric concepts and skill in applying them on the part of most of the instructors. Although this problem might have been modified if the instructors had attended the classes, because the majority of them did not avail themselves of the psychiatric nurse's invitation to do so, they were not in a position to know what the students were being taught and were expected to apply.

The psychiatric nurse had not given sufficient consideration to the critical point that for an instructor to be able to use the course as an experience in learning psychiatric concepts she had to become a learner—a situation which involved a role reversal for her and one that understandably aroused much anxiety about loss of esteem (see Chapter 7). She also had overlooked the advantages of utilizing some of the instructors as resource persons in the course.

As a result of the faculty members airing their dissatisfaction with the course, some modifications were made in it in the fourth year of the project. One change that was introduced was that the instructor was requested to attend the class at which her students were to discuss their patients. Having been in direct contact with the students, the patients, the visitors, and the personnel, this instructor was in a unique position to help the students to identify those experiences for which the theory under discussion had particular relevance. An instructor in medical nursing, one in surgical nursing, and one in public health nursing also participated in selected classes by functioning as resource persons.

This course continued to be taught beyond the duration of the first grant.

CONDUCTING CLINICAL CONFERENCES IN PSYCHIATRIC NURSING

Beginning in the third year of the project, the psychiatric team conducted weekly two-hour clinical conferences for the junior students during their twelve-week psychiatric nursing course. These conferences were held at the affiliating agency at which the psychiatric nursing course was given. All the sessions were tape recorded.

The essential purpose of the conferences was to create a bridge between the course in psychiatric nursing and the rest of the curriculum by providing an opportunity for the students to discern more clearly the continuity between normal behavior and psychopathology. Another purpose was to add greater depth to the psychiatric nursing experience.

The content of the conferences consisted of the dynamics underlying the behavior of patients and their families, the students' feelings in response to the patients' behavior, their relationship with authority figures in the psychiatric facility, and their modes of adaptation to the total experience. This content was derived from a student's case presentation of a patient.

Participating Personnel. The psychiatric nurse project director met with each of the three groups of students at all meetings—a total of thirty-six meetings per year; the psychiatrist met with the group once a month. In addition, beginning in the second year of the conferences, upon the request of the project director, the head nurse from the unit where the student presenter was having her experience and an instructor at the agency attended every conference. The participation of the agency personnel helped to round out the patient's history and to clarify his problems; it also facilitated the transfer of suggestions for dealing with the presenting difficulties to the clinical settings.

As a means of closing the hiatus between the psychiatric nursing course and the rest of the curriculum, the psychiatric team, in the second year of the conferences, recommended that the other Skidmore nurse faculty members participate in the conferences on a rotation basis. This recommendation was not accepted by the faculty on the grounds that the majority of the instructors felt that they did not have the time for such participation. However, one of the older faculty members volunteered to participate and attended all the conferences throughout two of the twelve-week affiliations, and another older member attended three conferences.

These two instructors contributed significantly to the bridge-building function of the conferences in several ways. They assisted the group to give more attention to the personality growth and development aspects as these pertained to the age group of the patient who was being discussed. This emphasis helped to clarify further the relationship between normal behavior and psychopathology. Much more consideration was also given to the physical status and needs of the patient and to the significance of these considerations in the total nursing care of the patient. Lastly, but perhaps of most importance, was the fact that the participating instructors shared their reactions to this experience with the rest of the Skidmore faculty members.

Methods. For the purpose of creating a laboratory in participant-observation and problem solving, a double focus was utilized in the teaching method. First, in each session a student who either had volunteered or was selected by the group gave a case presentation of a patient with whom she had worked. Besides including the patient's medical and social histories, the student was helped to put emphasis on her feelings and thoughts about the behavior and the verbal communications of the patient, the clinical personnel with whom she worked, the instructor at the affiliating agency, and her compeers. Thus, by airing these feelings she could identify her modes of adaptation to the experience. The accent on the self was based on the psychiatric nurse's belief that students could develop their understanding of the meaning of patient behavior to the degree that they gained insight into their own behavior. Although the self was not the exclusive focus of the conferences, it provided some of the necessary groundwork for the students to take a long look at the behavior of psychiatric patients and to identify how they related with them. All this material was used as the basis for the identification and discussion of specific and general issues in psychiatric nursing.

On several occasions in those conferences in which the psychiatrist participated, the patient who was to be discussed was brought into the classroom and was interviewed by the psychiatrist, the psychiatric nurse, or the student who had been nursing him. The interview was a way of helping the students to experience the patient more completely as a person and, through the discussion of their observations and reactions to him, to derive a clearer picture of his problems, to experience the impact of his behavior on themselves, and thereby to achieve greater awareness of his impact, on the other personnel.

As a way of further building on, deepening, and expanding the students' earlier experiences with the psychiatric nurse during the sophomore year, the second point of emphasis was on the quality of the student leadership in the conferences and, specifically, on the observation and discussion of the interaction among the group members. The students rotated as leaders of the discussion and as observers of the group process, the report of which included the student observer's own subjective responses to the group interaction and to the case presentation. Under the guidance of the psychiatric nurse, the students were helped to identify, analyze, and summarize such points as shifts in group participation, role taking, feeling tones and nuances, and steps in the problem-solving process. For fifteen minutes before the end of each conference, this material was presented by the student observer, discussed by the group, and used to demonstrate the principles underlying individual and group dynamics as well as to relate these whenever possible to the interaction within the psychiatric setting.

Feelings of Hopelessness and Helplessness. The initial impact of the psychiatric nursing experience on the students resulted primarily in their feeling hopeless about the prognosis of the psychiatric patient and helpless about being able to help him. The following discussion, which took place early in the experience of one group of students, illustrates feelings which in varying degrees were pervasive throughout the experiences of all groups of students.

October 16, 1959
This is the first group of students to have this experience with the psychiatric nurse, and this conference is the first in the series; therefore a student leader and process observer are not assigned. The students have been involved in psychiatric nursing for ten days.

PSYCHIATRIC NURSE. It is good to see all of you again. It's been so long.
[*Members of the group smile, doodle, and appear uneasy.*]
PSYCHIATRIC NURSE. I am eager to hear all about your experiences and your reactions to psychiatric nursing. It has been a long time getting to this place.
[*There is a tense silence. The students look at the psychiatric nurse almost as if she were a stranger.*]
PSYCHIATRIC NURSE. I admit that psychiatric nursing is my real love, but that doesn't mean you have to fall in love with it too. I am much more concerned with what is going on with all of you.
[*Silence.*]
PSYCHIATRIC NURSE. A sadder, more down-mouthed group I have never seen.
[*A burst of nervous laughter.*]
[*Christine DuBois looks up at the psychiatric nurse as if to say something.*]
PSYCHIATRIC NURSE. What is it, Christine?
CHRISTINE DUBOIS. The patients. They keep returning to the hospital. Regardless of what we do they always get sick again. You can be sure they will always come back.
[*Several heads raise and some students exchange furtive glances.*]
PSYCHIATRIC NURSE. Hmm. How do the rest of you see the situation?
VALERIE BENHAM. How can mental patients ever get married and have children?
PSYCHIATRIC NURSE. What about you, Janet?
JANET SMOLER. Mental illness is much more frightening than physical illness, I guess because it is closer to us. There is such a fine line between normal behavior

and going off your rocker. Are we really normal? At least when a patient has a physical disease—even cancer—as a nurse, I know what to do about it.

PSYCHIATRIC NURSE. You seem to be saying two things: that, "There but for the grace of God go I," and that you feel you don't know how to help the patient.

EDITH HULL. The onset is so insidious. Will this ever happen to me?

LOUISE ATKINS. I feel like a disciplinarian with the kids. I'm nothing but a policeman, and I feel anybody can do what I'm doing.

[Several students nod in agreement.]

CONNIE VAHN. I spend most of my time trying to look busy. In desperation I talk to patients because I am sick of talking just to my classmates on the unit. But most of the time a classmate and I end up playing ping-pong together.

[All the students are alert. Most of the side comments have ceased.]

MARCIA MANNING. Women are much more out in left field than men.

PSYCHIATRIC NURSE. Yes?

MARCIA MANNING. So where does this leave us?

PSYCHIATRIC NURSE. Like Janet and Edith, you are wondering if this will happen to you?

[Marcia Manning looks up at the psychiatric nurse as her eyes fill with tears. Janet Smoler squeezes her hand.]

PSYCHIATRIC NURSE. It's not easy but I think it is important to get all of your feelings aired. And you are doing a good job. Let's continue for a bit.

NANCY SPIEGEL. What's the point of this whole experience anyway? Patients don't want to talk to us. They just say, "Hello" and "Goodby." They don't want to get involved with us, and why should they? Most of them are sick in the first place because they were rejected over and over by their parents. They will only be hurt all over again when we leave the service. I can see why they won't have anything to do with us.

PSYCHIATRIC NURSE. You feel if you become important to the patient he will get sicker?

EDITH HULL. I don't know. I don't know what the answer is. Whenever I try to get close to my patient he tells me not to bother because he is never going to get better.

PSYCHIATRIC NURSE. One of the issues that all of you have been raising is that hopelessness is greater in psychiatric disturbances. With respect to the patient's feelings about his hopelessness, it is important to recognize that his feelings do not exist in a vacuum. People exist only in relation to other people; for example, if a person is totally isolated for a protracted period of time, he will start hallucinating. Therefore, the only way to cut through the patient's feelings of hopelessness is to establish contact with him. You have made some faltering attempts to do this, but the patient cuts you off. Whenever a person interferes with our contact with him, anxiety is always aroused within ourselves. Trying to relate to psychiatric patients stirs up anxiety not only in the nurses, but in anyone. This is how psychiatric illness is qualitatively different from physical illness. The physical components of illness are more "in" the patient, so that if these could be isolated from the whole complex of the patient's problems (which they cannot be), the relationships on the clinical unit would matter very little.

In the case of the patient with a functional psychosis, however, the illness does not exist in the patient, but in his interaction with the people around him. This does not make emotionally disturbed behavior less tangible. It is more difficult to deal with, but there are also more possibilities for dealing with it. Since psychopathology grows out of interaction there is more opportunity to change.

As I see the problem, there are at least two main issues involved. One issue is that as a late adolescent you haven't yet dealt with your own fear of being rejected and therefore you are so easily rejected. The psychiatric patient is sensitive to your rejectability, and he is frightened by it and so he drives you away. Psychiatric patients make the late adolescent face her own incompetence in interpersonal relationships. What happens in these circumstances is that then you want the patient to make you feel good about relating to him. And when he doesn't do this, you perceive the patient as being hopeless. In this kind of a situation the student's ability to relate to the patient is at fault, not the patient's ability.

The other issue is that you have been unable to draw a line between the patient's estimate of the situation and what the situation really is. In evaluating illness, as a nurse you need to ascertain the source of that illness. There are many illnesses in which the symptoms are not a reliable indicator of the severity of the illness, as for example, a skin rash. In mental illness the patient also has symptoms, and hopelessness about his condition is one of his symptoms.

When a patient complains of palpitations, for example, the physician considers and examines all aspects. But the patient's feelings of hopelessness provide only an amateur estimate of the degree of his pathology. He may be hopeless and he may not be. To realistically estimate the severity of the patient's illness and the degree of hope for his recovery, you have to arrive at an objective picture of the patient. What kind of a person was he before his illness erupted? What are his resources? How well did he function before he became ill? This is where the physician comes in. You cannot come to a reliable estimate of the patient's condition without his help.

NANCY SPIEGEL. But some of the sickest patients functioned well.

PSYCHIATRIC NURSE. You are leading into the question: What are the conditions under which a person becomes ill? Any person can take stress only up to a certain point. The central issue in estimating the severity of mental illness is whether there is a balance between the pathologic symptoms and the healthy aspects. The issue is not whether the pathologic symptoms are ruling the roost for the time being, but rather, what positive resources can be brought to bear. The concept of cure is not the elimination of the illness but getting on top of it. A well-adjusted person is not one who is without problems but one who can get on top of them.

LOUISE ATKINS. No one seems to care about the patients, so why should we care either. There's no consistency. One minute we are told to get involved, and the next minute we are told not to get involved.

CONNIE VAHN. The head nurse who sees the patient as hopeless relays this message on rounds when she says, "He is not making any progress."

PSYCHIATRIC NURSE. In order for the patient to be hopeless he has to convince

the outside world that he is. There is the element of struggle in seeing the
hope in a total picture. Why make mental illness a scapegoat for tragedy? There
are physically handicapped persons who are in institutions for life also. You
have even taken care of some of these patients. The vagueness about mental
illness is not in the illness itself; it lies in the nurse's vagueness about it and
how to help the patient.

It is true that there are some mentally ill patients whose condition is irreversible. In organic illness, as for example the child with cerebral palsy, we don't
give up when the child isn't normal. We need to get at his potential. This can
be done only in terms of where the patient is, not in terms of where I myself
want him to be.

As a consequence of their unresolved fear of and vulnerability to rejection
from people in general, the students made the irrational demand of psychiatric patients to make them feel comfortable and competent. In essence,
they expected the patients to take care of them, and when a patient did not
meet this expectation he was viewed as hopeless by the student.

The students' intense feeling of hopelessness concerning the ultimate prognosis of psychiatric patients also was entrenched in failure to appraise the
total picture of a patient's life situation. Their concept of cure excluded a
realistic estimate of a patient's assets; instead it was based exclusively on his
pathology in terms of his presenting symptoms, especially his own feeling
of hopelesness about himself. This unidimensional picture of psychiatric
patients as drawn by the students was not a product of attitudes that existed
in a vacuum but was a mirror of the stereotyped view held by society as a
whole.

The inevitable sequel to the student's sense of hopelessness was their
feeling of helplessness about being able to contribute in any way to a reversal of the patient's illness. Withdrawal from further contact with patients
became their most characteristic mode of adaptation to the problems. However, their withdrawal not only reinforced but increased their sense of
hopelessness and helplessness by creating guilt feelings for not having fulfilled their professional responsibility to the patient.

The central problem with which the project director had to deal was not
the fact that the students felt hopeless and helpless about caring for the
psychiatric patient, but that they had to be helped to uncover their feelings
and identify their distortions and thereby to pave the way toward a more
realistic picture of the patient.

One overall problem emerged in conjunction with the clinical conferences
in psychiatric nursing. The students expressed the feeling that frequently,
from their point of view, the psychiatric nurse's and the psychiatrist's perception of a patient in terms of the degree of hopefulness or hopelessness
about his course of illness seemed to be diametrically opposed to the agency
personnel's appraisal of the situation. The students' comments and their

reactions to their experiences revealed that on numerous occasions they felt torn between what they interpreted as conflicting conceptions of the patient's situation and the role of the nurse.

The issue involved was not whether such a disparity existed, but rather it was a problem in which the students' perception of the situation pointed up their need for much more continuous supervision and help as well as far greater depth in the psychiatric nursing experience.*

Generalized Fear of a Patient Explosion. Another problem that frequently arose during the affiliation in psychiatric nursing was the students' fear that a patient would "blow up" and hurt himself or them. Coincidental to this fear was the students' expectation that they had the responsibility to do something about the explosion if it occurred. During the following conference this problem was explored.

October 29, 1960

This conference takes place in the second year of this activity. It is the psychiatric nurse's sixth meeting with this group of students. A student presents the case of a patient with whom she has worked. Another student functions as leader of the discussion, and a third student observes the group process.

PSYCHIATRIC NURSE. I think we should get started, Evelyn.

EVELYN SAUNDERS [*leader*]. Okay. Selma, would you please start to present your case?

SELMA KRUTHERS [*presenter of case*]. My case is about a seventeen-year-old girl named Lois. Her case history consists of the following:

Lois is a white, Jewish, single female, she lives with her mother, who was born in Poland, and her father, who was born in Germany. She completed the eleventh grade in high school and went to Jewish camps during the summer. She has had a good deal of physical illness. At the age of twelve, after she returned from camp, her parents discovered her masturbating, and they talked it over with her. Ever since then she has been obsessed by guilt. She is very depressed, although she denies suicidal thoughts or wishes. She is on 50 mgm. of thorazine. [*Pause.*] Oh, before I forget it, she is completely dependent on her mother, who is domineering and punitive.

EVELYN SAUNDERS. Selma, tell us something about your reactions to the patient.

SELMA KRUTHERS [*talks rapidly and her face is flushed*]. I was struck by her seeming sweetness; she isn't boisterous. She appears young and untouched. On one occasion I was sitting with her alone and we both were silent. Then all of a sudden, like a bolt out of the blue, she said, "I won't get better until I stop thinking about me." I should have given her reassurance and told her that she

---

* In 1963–1964 the Skidmore faculty assumed full responsibility for teaching the course in psychiatric nursing, and a psychiatric nurse was appointed to the full-time faculty to teach the course.

didn't have to get better all on her own. At the time I should have said something to help her.

[*Long silence.*]

[*Evelyn Saunders looks pleadingly at the psychiatric nurse.*]

PSYCHIATRIC NURSE. It sounds, Selma, as if you feel you aren't moving as fast with the patient as you think you should.

SELMA KRUTHERS. It is so difficult to get to know the patient—to get her to talk. I tend to push her and I'm trying my darndest to hold back. [*Her voice is high-pitched and then cracks.*]

[*All eyes are on Selma Kruthers. Some students look to Evelyn Saunders for direction and then look to the psychiatric nurse.*]

PSYCHIATRIC NURSE. Tell us some more about what has been happening.

SELMA KRUTHERS. It was my turn to observe all the patients who are on suicidal observation, including Lois. She kept pacing up and down and said, "I'm running away from myself." She also told me that she is afraid the hospital won't keep her and will send her away. She said, "Everyone is so kind. I don't deserve your special attention."

I told the patient that suicidal observation was to protect her, and I pointed out that I do this also with other patients. The patient answered, "I want so much to have someone to trust. I don't want to bother you." She's so paranoid and is afraid people are listening to our conversation. Sometimes she ignores me.

PSYCHIATRIC NURSE [*looks at Evelyn Saunders, who has withdrawn from leading the group*]. Maybe if we could find out how Selma feels about the patient. . . .

EVELYN SAUNDERS. What are your feelings about the patient's behavior, Selma?

SELMA KRUTHERS. I want so terribly to help her. She is intelligent, and she seems to have a certain warmth, even though it is buried.

PSYCHIATRIC NURSE. How do the rest of you view the patient?

EVELYN SAUNDERS. At times I think she is very hostile but she can't express it.

SELMA KRUTHERS. I'm afraid if she lets go I won't know what to do about it. And as a result, I'm afraid I'm closing her off.

VIOLA BECK. She didn't want to take her medication. She vacillates between wanting help and not doing what she should. She's off the thorazine now.

PSYCHIATRIC NURSE. What do you see happening if Lois "let's go"?

SELMA KRUTHERS. I think she is ready to go on a tirade. When she does, everything is going to pop. I'm scared she may want to commit suicide. [*Pause.*] I guess what I'm really scared of is that she will attack me.

ELSIE BLAKE. I'm frightened of her. She is so controlled that I have the feeling if she ever loses control there will be trouble.

PSYCHIATRIC NURSE. What kind of trouble?

ELSIE BLAKE. That there will be an explosion. That she will kill herself or us or both.

PSYCHIATRIC NURSE. Hmm. [*Pause.*] How do you regard the patient? Do you see her as sick? Or do you see her as nervous, unhappy, but not necessarily sick?

GAIL FURST. I think Lois is sick, although she has many attributes. There is a discrepancy between reality and how she interprets it. She is ambivalent and hostile.

SHIRLEY COOPER. It seems as if everyone on the staff is against Lois. I don't think her feelings are so unique. All of us feel conflicted and hostile at times.

SELMA KRUTHERS. I think she feels unworthy.

PSYCHIATRIC NURSE. What do you feel Lois is frightened of?

VIOLA BECK. I don't feel the patient will lose control.

HEAD NURSE. We have had other patients who have let go and nothing so terrible happened.

GAIL FURST. Wouldn't the nurses feel better if Lois did let go? At least all of us would know what we are dealing with.

PSYCHIATRIC NURSE. Why is Lois' desire for suicide abnormal? Why do we interpret suicide as being sick within this situation? Suicide is a solution that won't solve anything because it doesn't include a reliable estimate of other possibilities.

You need to be more specific. I think it is important to clarify the specific areas where you feel the patient may "let go" and may cause trouble instead of getting caught up in the generalized fear of an explosion. As long as the nurse treats Lois as a fragile doll that will break, she plays into her illness which is, in essence, the result of distance between herself and people.

In the nurse's relationship with the patient, it is crucial for her to bring understanding of the patient's problems and of the danger areas. The patient is different from a piece of fragile machinery. She does have touchy areas, but she also has untouchy ones. She has made it very clear to Selma [*Kruthers*] that she wants a relationship and wants to communicate. It is true that she is ambivalent, but this too is healthy. We need to focus on the patient's acceptance.

In a professional nursing relationship, the nurse must evaluate what needs to be known about the patient. You are responding to Lois as though the problem were a one-way street—as if the problem is exclusively a case of the dam bursting. But the nurse participates with the patient and the way she does this will influence what comes from the patient.

And what if there is an "explosion"? The issue here is that the patient has to know your capacity to understand her and her problems and your capacity to handle your own anxiety. And incidentally, from some of our past experiences together, I think you are inclined to underestimate your own capacities. [*The group is thoughtful and attentive. Some students smile; some nod in ageement.*]

PSYCHIATRIC NURSE. The patient must be able to experience you and know how you handle your anxiety. Will you, for example, withdraw from her? This does not necessarily mean that you get into personal facts about yourself or the patient. It does mean that whatever you bring to the relationship with the patient, you bring in terms of its effect on her.

GAIL FURST. I think she is guilty about masturbating. Then I think another raw area is her parents.

ELSIE BLAKE. I think she is afraid of hurting people.

PSYCHIATRIC NURSE. You see what I mean about how you underestimate your capacities? You have put your finger on the problem. [*Nervous laughter; several students doodle; some shift their positions.*]

PSYCHIATRIC NURSE. Lois' conflict is related to problems centered around masturbation, her mother's attitudes about her masturbating, and her feelings that what she does is hurtful to other people. What are some of the less sensitive and safer areas?

SELMA KRUTHERS. She does participate in many of the activities.

HEAD NURSE. She isn't allowed to leave the building, but all the activities are open to her.

SHIRLEY COOPER. She was a counselor at camp.

SELMA KRUTHERS. She tries to knit, but she feels she can't do it well enough. If she just could see some progress. Lois says she has poor manual dexterity.

HEAD NURSE. Does she?

ELSIE BLAKE. At first she was very tense while dancing, but then she loosened up. Now she relaxes. She did some interpretive dancing alone and she has a good sense of rhythm.

PSYCHIATRIC NURSE. All of this information is important, and it can be extremely useful in relating to the patient. However, in putting your major emphasis on what activities the patient might engage in, you have gotten away from your interpersonal relationship with her. You have an awareness of the patient's hunger for closeness and you sense her dependence on becoming engaged with you, and then somewhere along the way you become frightened of getting engaged with her. What would you do if you were with a stranger on a desert island?

SELMA KRUTHERS. I don't know how much to give of myself.

PSYCHIATRIC NURSE. Two strangers on a desert island would have to find out about each other. A relationship can only get started as people get to know each other. In the case of the patient, what is it that is appropriate to know? It is appropriate to know one's feelings about the situation. Knowledge of the patient and the nurse comes about in several ways—directly, by giving and telling and by reacting to what is happening in the relationship. Lois told the nurse (*Selma Kruthers*) how important it was to have someone to talk to. She probably was also saying something like, "I have no one I can tell what kind of person I really am. I am afraid to let myself be known."

People in general tend to overlook the fact that they had no decision about who their parents are, about what century and what culture they were born into. In other words, they overlook that they had no say in determining the central factors that influence their whole lives. Instead, the dominating feeling is "I hate myself because I am bad—because I have these feelings."

[*Several students lean forward in their chairs. Everyone appears more relaxed.*]

HEAD NURSE. The patient has to be pushed. She gets guilty from all the extra attention.

SELMA KRUTHERS. But it seems to me that the point of all our discussions is that as nurses we have to understand her guilt from her point of view. And I guess that means I have to become comfortable enough with it so that she will feel like telling me about it. [*Sighs deeply.*] Oh, dear.

PSYCHIATRIC NURSE. How come, "Oh, dear"?

SELMA KRUTHERS. I don't know if I will ever be able to get to that place.

PSYCHIATRIC NURSE. You already have taken the first step by recognizing the nature of the problem.

The patient most likely had put the students in touch with their own potential for hostility as well as their repressed hostilities. Aside from the contagion of anxiety, the students' potential for destructiveness might well have been the real source of their anxiety in this situation. This patient, in turn, had fantastic ability to suck the student into her problem and to make her feel guilty.

Many of the students' difficulties in working with this patient also stemmed from their problem in understanding the patient and her world as she saw it. It was especially difficult for them to understand that it may be more important for a patient to resist all their approaches than to relate with them. The psychiatric nurse's goal in this conference was to bring the students to the awareness that understanding this fact and some of the reasons for the resistance is the only tool the nurse has for dealing with her own frustration.

SERVING AS RESOURCE PERSONNEL IN OTHER NURSING COURSES

The psychiatric nurse and the psychiatrist functioned as resource persons in various aspects of courses taught by the rest of the faculty. Unlike their work with individual instructors in clinical conferences where the focus was on the learning of the instructor, in these activities the students were the central point of concern. In all of the situations, the team member participated upon the invitation of the instructor who was responsible for the course.

Because the psychiatric nurse was a full-time member of the faculty, she was more available to the instructors than was the psychiatrist. One of her leading roles as the project developed was as a resource person to the faculty. Her resource activities were of several kinds. She participated in the classroom presentations, in seminars, and in learning experiences in the clinical units. In some instances her participation was arranged in advance; in others, she was called on as specific problems arose. By the end of the fourth year of the project, she was participating in all the nursing courses except for the twelve-week course in obstetric nursing taught at an affiliating agency—an exception that occurred because the faculty and the psychiatric nurse recognized that the psychiatric nurse could spread herself only so far without jeopardizing the goals of the project and agreed that in allotting her time participation with the Skidmore instructors should be given priority.

In the second year of the project, which was the first in implementing the integration program, the psychiatric nurse participated with the instructor who was responsible for the learning experiences in the child health station and with the instructors who taught the courses in long-term illness, team, and public health nursing, all of whom were members of the older faculty group. Consequently, during the second year of the project, the older instructors and the psychiatric nurse had the opportunity to experience each other and to learn the special areas of knowledge and skill each had to offer. On the other hand, except for the bits and pieces of second-hand information that filtered through from students and the older instructors, the younger instructors were pretty much in the dark about the psychiatric nurse's activities during this period. This situation had powerful repercussions on the integration project (see Chapter 8).

The activities with students in which a member of the psychiatric team participated as a resource person were as follows.

1. Course in normal growth and development.
2. Learning experiences in the child health station.
3. Clinical conferences in communicable disease and long-term illness nursing.
4. Clinical conferences in team nursing.
5. Family-care conferences in public health nursing.
6. Seminars in disaster nursing.
7. Psychiatric nursing consultation with adult patients on medical surgical units.

The structure of the clinical conferences in which the team participated was similar to those in psychiatric nursing. In each session one student presented a case in connection with her work either with a patient and his family or with clinical personnel. Students rotated as leaders of the discussions and as observers of the group process. Many of the conferences were tape-recorded.

Course in Normal Growth and Development. In the second year of the project, the psychiatrist collaborated with the instructor of the normal growth and development course for sophomore students in several sessions on psychosexual development. Some of the areas that were explored were: (1) the meaning of the word *sex*, its human aspects, and how it is differentiated from sexual experiences on other levels of life; (2) romantic love; (3) sexual deviations and maldevelopment such as sexual pleasure through pain, control and submission, exhibitionism, homosexuality, autoeroticism (masturbation), substitution of sexual organs (as displacement of sexual activities to the skin because of guilt and taboos), and complete alienation of all sexual activity; (4) common problems in the acculturation of sex; (5) biological factors and cultural pressures that impinge on the adolescent and such methods of handling these as increased fantasies and dreams, increased curiosity, experimentation through necking and petting (frequently accompanied by guilt), masturbation and nocturnal emission, virginity, premarital intercourse and the social implications of pregnancy outside of wedlock;

(6) sexual problems such as premature ejaculation and frigidity; and (7) the role of parents, teachers, and nurses in sex education.

All the sessions were marked by lively exchanges among the students, the psychiatrist, and the instructor of the course. There was great freedom and spontaneity in expressing opinions and raising questions. Some superstitions and incidents of incorrect information were uncovered and clarified. In the third year of the project another faculty member was responsible for the course, and the psychiatrist no longer participated.

Learning Experiences in the Child Health Station. In the second year of the project the psychiatric nurse collaborated with the instructor who was responsible for the sophomore students' learning experiences in the child health station, which were part of the course in pediatric nursing. The emphasis of these experiences was on helping students to begin to develop skills in interviewing, in health teaching and supervising, in applying the principles of normal growth and development in their work with children and parents, in collaborating with other members of the health team, in making referrals, and in recording significant observations and recommendations for the future.

For the most part the children and parents who came to the child health station were of different cultural backgrounds and lower socioeconomic status than the students. Many of the problems and issues stemmed from the students' attitudes, values, and biases. For example, their attitudes toward the unwed mother and contraception, toward persons with a language barrier, and toward health care and treatment on a clinic basis rather than with a private physician had to be uncovered and worked with. In the students' work with parents the problem of their unresolved authority-dependency conflict stood out in bold relief. Then also, the emphasis on health teaching and prevention of illness required the students to reorient their thinking in terms of the expanding role of the nurse outside of the hospital setting.

Clinical Conferences in Communicable Disease and Long-Term-Illness Nursing. In the first year of the project, before a psychiatric integration program had been designed, the psychiatrist participated with the instructor of the three-week course in communicable disease and long-term-illness nursing for junior students. All the patients with whom the students worked were veterans of World War I or World War II. Many of them were homeless men who had pulmonary tuberculosis, a condition which was further complicated by a high incidence of chronic alcoholism.

When working with these patients the students were also confronted with the problem of sexual acting out which, although not uncommon among adult male patients on any clinical service, is often regarded as a psychiatric or psychiatric-nursing problem and therefore selectively inattended in the clinical instruction in other nursing courses. The resource services of the members of the psychiatric team were of particular value in helping the students to deal with this problem. To illustrate with an example,

> During one of the conferences attended by the psychiatrist, the problem of a twenty-eight-year-old, single, white, male patient overtly masturbating in front of the student who had taken care of him was analyzed. The student's reaction to this episode consisted of feelings of embarrassment, fright, surprise, disgust and repulsion, anger, resentment, and pity. The student who had had the unpleasant experience had evaded and denied it by turning away from the patient and energetically remaking a corner of an empty bed.

For the purpose of helping the students to cope with their own responses, their characteristic modes of adapting to anxiety-laden situations were uncovered by eliciting their suggestions for handling the situations. The students' suggestions were as follows.

1. Evasion and denial by turning away from something unpleasant and using energy in carrying out an unthreatening function which is unrelated to the problem, as in the case of the student remaking the corner of the bed.

2. Escape from the situation as quickly as possible by fleeing from the room and allowing the behavior to continue.

3. Diversion by talking about something else with the patient, such as the weather.

4. Some recognition of the need to abort the behavior, but through attacking the patient by expressing a value judgment and dislike, for example, "Tell the patient not to do this as long as I am around."

After having elicited the students' modes of adaptation to the problem, the psychiatrist stressed the necessity for the understanding of the meaning of the patient's behavior. He stated,

> What might the patient's behavior mean? There is an exhibitionistic flavor about it, for since he was off standing in a corner there is little basis for concern about physical danger. Showing his sexual organs or using them in a public way can be a serious malignant end-point of self-interest. The way in which he handles his sexual needs is unique because it is a way for him to handle his anxiety and tensions. His acting out is not primarily a response to a provocative situation. What he is doing is seeking relief from anxiety. His behavior also is his way of establishing a moment of masculine dominance— the female, the nurse, flees and is helpless. There also is a hostile element of taking advantage of another person. It also is an unconscious way of flaunting authority and social conventions.
>
> In a roundabout way, the patient is asking for help. The method of handling the situation must consider the nurse's feelings, the patient's feelings, and the values of the culture. The goal in dealing with the problem is to help the patient to feel less horrible so that he will be in a better position to handle the problem. Some of the principles to keep in mind are: Avoid depreciating the

patient, for his behavior is based on guilt and self-depreciation. Get across to him that there are other things in him that you like. Come back to the patient. As for the principles in methods of handling, the action should be aborted because you do not want to reinforce the patient's neurotic drives. You have to understand the various meanings of the patient's behavior such as his chalking up another victory. It should be recognized that the hospital and the nurse herself help to trigger off the patient's anxiety.

This is seriously disturbed behavior that may warrant further medical treatment. The nurse's use of denial or aggression can bring about a psychiatric emergency. Arresting the behavior in a manner that lets the patient know you understand him and care about him most likely will result in the patient's relief and cooperation. You have to let the patient know that his behavior interferes with your taking care of him and other patients. The work you are doing is for him. Just as the patient who pushes away his tray of food or pulls out his Levine tube puts an obstacle in the way of the nurse taking care of him, in this situation the obstacle is the patient's sexual behavior.

Because of the students' overwhelming positive responses to this discussion, the psychiatric team thought it would be of value if they could provide a similar learning experience for other students earlier in their educational program. With this goal in mind, in the following year, the psychiatric team utilized this episode as the basis for the examination question which was challenged by the rest of the faculty (see Chapter 8, May 19 and June 3, 1959).

In the second and third years of the project the psychiatric nurse participated as a resource person in the course in communicable disease and long-term-illness nursing. She gave a two-hour lecture discussion on some of the psychodynamics that operate in alcoholism and their relationship to some of the psychogenic factors in tuberculosis. For the purpose of orienting the students to patients' problems of adjusting to long-term hospitalization and to the way these problems are reflected in the social structure of the clinical unit, the psychiatric nurse discussed Skid Row, from which many of the patients came, as a particular kind of social system.

In addition, she participated in three weekly two-hour clinical conferences in which problems arising in the care of chronically ill patients were explored. In addition to the problems of sexual acting out, other problems that were discussed were fear of contracting tuberculosis; the mask as a barrier in establishing interpersonal contact; conflict about establishing a professional or a personal relationship and the differences between them; a patient's attitude of resignation toward his illness and his cooperation with fate to be put out of his misery by not following the plan for his treatment and care.

In the fourth year of the project the instructor responsible for the course in communicable disease and long-term-illness nursing, on her own initiative, assumed the responsibility for integrating the psychiatric concepts in her clinical conferences and for presenting the material on the sociological analysis of "Skid Row." One of the contributory goals of the integration project thereby had been realized with one instructor. Although the psychiatric nurse no longer attended the conferences, the instructor used her as a consultant from time to time, conferring with her about handling problems that arose.

Clinical Conferences in Team Nursing. In the first year of the project, the psychiatrist met with the junior students who were having the seven-week course in team nursing. In the second, third, and fourth years, the psychiatric nurse assumed the responsibility as a resource person and met with junior students and their instructor in the course for four two-hour clinical conferences.

The content of the discussions evolved from the exploration of the tensions and obstacles concerning the student's functioning as a team leader. Many of the student's difficulties were related to the nature of the organizational structure of the hospital and of the clinical unit where she was assigned, and to the effect of this structure on communication and decision making. Of even greater significance, however, was the student's conflict about taking a rational authority role, especially with those staff members who had directed some of her activities during the sophomore year. This was most pronounced when, as a team leader, she was called upon to intervene in patient and personnel situations that required change.

The following comments made by students during the group discussions illustrate some of the problems they encountered in their relationships with the nursing personnel.

> The sophomore students are the only ones who really use us as team leaders. We communicate with the head nurse and assistant head nurse, but they don't always tell us what is happening, such as informing us about new orders that have been written for a patient.

> I think there is a status problem. Some of the staff seem to feel threatened by us because we are in a collegiate nursing program, whereas the head nurse, assistant head nurse, and many of the rest of the staff have no degree.

> It is depressing to find out that the head nurse and the supervisor make mistakes and that they are human beings with problems.

Family-Care Conferences in Public Health Nursing. In the second, third, and fourth years of the project, the psychiatric nurse participated in the weekly two-hour family-care conferences with junior students during the eight-week period of the clinical learning experiences in public health nursing. The purpose of the conferences (led by the Skidmore instructor but held at the public health nursing agency) was to provide an opportunity for the students as a group to identify the total health needs of a particular family, to formulate a plan for future action, and to identify means for implementing it. Each week a student presented a family situation for discussion. The supervisor of the office where the student was having her experience also attended the conference. Her participation helped to expose some of the distortions that arose in the students' perception of a situation, to identify the short- and long-term goals for the family, and to facilitate the incorporation of the group's suggestions into the agency's future plans for care.

As has been pointed out, during the first year, the psychiatric nurse had identified that the sophomore students' evaluation of whether they should give routine nursing care to a patient or whether they should encourage the patient to do so for himself generally was based exclusively on a patient's physical ability to do so. The student's rationale for this position was that it was a nurse's role to foster a patient's independence and to discourage dependence. From the viewpoint of the psychiatric nurse, the students' tendency to create an artificial split between physical and emotional nursing care came into sharpest focus during the public health nursing experience. It was during the conferences in public health nursing, therefore, that the psychiatric nurse and the instructor had the best opportunity to work on the problem with students and agency personnel. The following description of a family-care conference illustrates a situation in which a student fragmented nursing care and in which the psychiatric nurse's handling of the problem miscarried.

August 8, 1961

The students are discussing the problem of a fifty-five-year-old arthritic woman who, although she manages to get out of bed and to care for herself in between the nurse's visits, refuses to do so when the student calls. Expressing great impatience and open annoyance at the patient, the student who is presenting the case says, "Even though she is perfectly capable of getting out of bed with some help, she refuses to do so. She is able to wash herself, but I have to hand her the wash cloth and the soap and stand there while she does it."

Repeatedly, the psychiatric nurse and the instructor try to help the students to examine the meaning of the patient's behavior in terms of what she might be needing and asking for from the nurse, but to no avail. The psychiatric nurse states that she feels the patient needs an experience in being physically cared for by the nurse and that some of her dependency needs will have to be met before she can move to independence. She further points out that the student and the patient appear to be caught in a power struggle with each other, and that, when the chips are down, the patient is the one who is in the best position to win this battle.

The psychiatric nurse then throws out a few possibilities which might enable the student to begin to establish a positive relationship through meeting some of the patient's needs for dependency, such as washing the patient's back and giving her a backrub. These are unceremoniously rejected on the grounds that, "Her family does all this for her between visits." Sticking tenaciously to her point, the psychiatric nurse asks the student presenter if she has considered combing the patient's hair, which, as later was revealed, is badly in need of attention. The student responds as if the psychiatric nurse has taken total leave of her senses; in disdainful amazement, she spurts out, "Comb—the patient's——hair?"

In guiding the students in the problem-solving process, the psychiatric nurse moved too quickly to suggestions about the activities the nurse might use as a means of becoming engaged with the patient. This information can be extremely useful when it is properly timed, but in this case it took the students away from the nurse's relationship with the patient. Had the psychiatric nurse spent more time and exerted more effort in helping the students to understand the meaning of the patient's behavior and the way the patient perceived her world, the resolution which the psychiatric nurse had prematurely tried to engineer most likely would have occurred. Instead, however, the suggestions which she had forced the students to swallow were just as forcefully ejected by them. Not unlike the student and her patient, the psychiatric nurse and the students became immured in a power struggle over the position each had taken.

In the psychiatric nurse's less-than-skillful negotiation of this conference, her negative feelings had interfered. She had become angry at the students for considering only their own feelings and leaving the patient out of the picture. She was disappointed in them for what she perceived to be their intolerance of the patient's viewpoint. Lastly, she wondered how she had failed to bring them to the point of being able to put themselves in the position of a patient by identifying unmet needs and of being able to synthesize the emotional and physical aspects of nursing care.

In spite of the fact that the psychiatric nurse might have handled the conference more skillfully, the fact still remained that, as far as some students were concerned, physical nursing care was being, or already had been, relegated to an inferior position within the total scheme of professional nursing practice. This attitude may have been enhanced by their association with practitioners of public health nursing—a field of nursing in which great emphasis is put on helping the patient to become as independent as possible and on delegating nursing care to other members of the family when it is feasible to do so. However, whether or not the agency personnel were inclined to de-emphasize physical care as an important vehicle for meeting patients' emotional needs in selected situations was not the central issue; the primary matter of concern was that the students were apt to use defensively whatever attitudes they may have picked up to support their own position regarding physical nursing care. This problem had powerful implications for the Skidmore nursing curriculum in general and specifically for the course in public health nursing and pointed out the need for more continuous guidance of students and for the psychiatric integration project.*

Seminars in Disaster Nursing. Shortly after the initiation of the psychiatric integration project, the department of nursing became involved in a project to prepare students for nursing in disasters. At the request of the disaster nursing project director, the psychiatric nurse participated with her in two two-hour seminars with small groups of junior students. The purpose of the discussions was to analyze the dynamics of collective behavior under the impact of severe stress associated with disaster and to identify the leadership role of the nurse, especially in terms of intervention in such modes of response as apathy, withdrawal, and panic.

In her final progress report of the disaster project, the project director vividly described the experiential teaching-learning process as it evolved in the first of these seminars, illustrated the role of the psychiatric nurse as a resource person, and identified some implications of this seminar for the course in disaster nursing (1).

> Over the past three years of many such discussions, it has been noted by the disaster project director that the students become anxious and often display a helpless and fatalistic attitude at some point. In May, the faculty member who directs the integration of mental health project agreed to participate in these discussion classes. The two faculty members planned a flexible structure for discussion and certain areas of content.
>
> The discussion class started with an intellectual exploration of certain behavioral responses to disaster situations. The project director [*disaster nursing project*] then told several personal experience stories, which created an atmosphere of suspense and some anxiety. The students were then presented with a disaster problem in a familiar setting and asked to set up a plan of action to meet the situation. There were a few questions and a few generalized nonoperational suggestions, but the prevailing attitude among the students was one of apathy.
>
> At this point, one student expressed the opinion that the situation was hopeless, that actually nothing effective could be done. The student group became restless; there was a great deal of shuffling and changing of positions. The apathy changed to active anxiety, with almost everyone in the group contributing opinions, judgments, and rationalizations to the effect that the situation was hopeless and, in reality, nothing could be done. Then a general silence prevailed; a few leading questions evoked no constructive response.
>
> Then one faculty member [*the psychiatric nurse*] described a similar disaster problem in another setting and gave a rather dramatic account of how she would behave if confronted with it. This account of specific action seemed to mobilize the students. They responded with specific problems and took issue with the faculty member's choice of action as a leader in a disaster situation.

* In 1963–1964, the responsibility for teaching the course in public health nursing was taken over by the Skidmore faculty.

From then on, the two faculty members took leadership in bringing the students to the point of utilizing their knowledge of the disaster scene, going back to the facts in order to define the original problem, and using knowledge, judgment, and constructive action in a problem-solving framework.

The final plans and alternatives worked through by the students, as well as the philosophical approach, were realistic, practical, and in operational terms. Later, the faculty members reviewed the experience in the class and were excited by the progress in interaction and in the behavior patterns exhibited by the group. We were of the opinion that we had created a stress anxiety reaction that had immobilized the students and that we had been able to lead them back to a state of considered action. This experience had opened up a whole field of possibilities in the area of teaching methods, applicable to small groups in a classroom setting, that could result in actual experiential learning. Arrangements were made for the mental health project director to have another class with the same group of students in order to review with them the interaction processes and assist them to recognize and analyze the group experience.

Psychiatric Nursing Consultation with Patients on Medical and Surgical Units. Beginning in the fourth year of the project, the psychiatric nurse worked with selected patients who had medical or surgical conditions and whose behavior was creating nursing care problems for the sophomore students, their instructor, and the clinical personnel. One purpose of this activity was to provide an opportunity for the psychiatric nurse to have more direct exposure to students' problems as they emerged in the clinical setting and to observe the impact of a patient's behavior on the student. Another purpose was to elicit the student's feelings about a patient and to help her to identify the problem and alternative ways of handling it.

The following structure was developed for this activity. A patient was referred to the psychiatric nurse by the instructor, often at the request of a student or a head nurse. The psychiatric nurse went to the clinical area and had a joint conference with the instructor, the head nurse, and the student who was responsible for the nursing care of the patient and helped the student to uncover her feelings about the patient and to identify and formulate the problems the patient presented to her and the nursing staff, her expectations of the psychiatric nurse, and her own goals for the patient.

Then, for the purpose of identifying some of the patient's needs and problems and the ways in which these problems were influencing the nurse-patient relationship in action, in many situations the psychiatric nurse gave the prescribed nursing care to the selected patient. She then was in a strategic position to experience the patient firsthand and the impact of his behavior on herself and thereby to better understand the effect of his behavior on the student and the nursing staff, including their perception of the problem and how it emerged. In identifying herself to the patient, the psychiatric nurse would tell him that she was a Skidmore instructor, that she was getting to know some of the patients whom students were taking care of, and that on this occasion she would be taking care of him. So that the psychiatric nurse might get a clearer picture of the patient's impact on the student and would not usurp the student's role with the patient, whenever possible the student participated with the psychiatric nurse in giving various aspects of nursing care.

Next, the psychiatric nurse had a joint conference with the instructor and student in which she shared her impressions about the patient, identified some of the possible meanings of the patient's behavior, and made suggestions for intervention. The student, her instructor, and the psychiatric nurse then had a conference with the head nurse and members of the nursing team who were responsible for the care of the patient. In this conference, the psychiatric nurse helped the student to function as team leader. To avoid contaminating the nursing personnel's automatic responses to the patient under study, the psychiatric nurse shared her impressions and findings only after this student had attempted to elicit the staff's feelings about the patient, had formulated the problem, and had sought suggestions for handling the situation. The psychiatric nurse and the instructor functioned as resource persons. Under the guidance of the head nurse and the instructor, the student implemented the various recommendations, as for example, referral to the social service department or to a public health agency.

The following are examples of patient problems that were referred to the psychiatric nurse.

A fifty-two-year-old insurance salesman who had a severe myocardial infarction and was left with extensive residual damage but who refused to remain on bed-rest. In spite of numerous warnings by clinical personnel, whenever the nurses seemed to be out of clear view he continued to do everything for himself.

A nineteen-year-old woman who was in the terminal stage of a rare and irreversible disease and who experienced severe pain when she was touched or moved. The nurses were uncomfortable about taking care of her.

A nineteen-year-old man with diabetes mellitus who appeared to have more theoretical knowledge about his disease than many of the nurses who took care of him, but who nevertheless continued to spill 3 to 4 plus sugar in his urine during his hospitalization. None of the students wanted to take care of him because, owing to his greater knowledge, he supposedly was in a better position to care for himself than were the nurses.

A thirty-six-year-old mother of three children with a severe case of subacute bacterial endocarditis who became clinically depressed.

A thirty-eight-year-old man who, prior to his hospitalization, had made a suicide attempt while intoxicated by drinking lye and who, as a result, had a stricture of the esophagus. He was recovering from surgery. He expressed a great deal of anxiety about his alcoholism and whether or not he would be able to "stay off the bottle." He also complained that no one really wanted to take care of him.

In all her consultation work with patients, the psychiatric nurse's principal goal was to identify a specific need of the patient which had been left unmet and to demonstrate how a nurse might meet it. To illustrate the way in which she established a relationship with a patient and how she identified an unmet need and went about meeting it, three vignettes which illustrate these aspects of her work with patients are presented. These incidents, it will be noted, were not specific to psychiatric nursing. Whatever the psychiatric nurse did with patients was not a matter of her descending from rarefied psychiatric atmosphere to shed her light on the students, the instructor, and the nursing staff, with the implication that they had been remiss. What the psychiatric nurse did, the Skidmore instructors frequently did with patients on an intuitive level. It is important, however, for a nurse teacher to be able to communicate to students her perception of a patient's needs and how to deal with them. The chief value of the following vignettes and the purpose in presenting them, therefore, is that they provide material from which to tease out the principles that apply to a professional nurse's work by conceptualizing a patient's problems and complaints into teaching concepts.

In the first clinical situation, Mr. Gianesi, a forty-six-year-old patient who had had a spinal fusion and who, because he was required to lie flat in bed, was not permitted to do anything for himself that entailed extensive movement, was referred to the psychiatric nurse at a student's request to her instructor. The presenting difficulty was that throughout the ten days following his surgery the patient had consistently refused to allow a nurse to give him a bath. The reason he gave for his refusal was that his wife bathed him when she visited him.

Upon preliminary investigation of the problem, the psychiatric nurse learned that no one on the staff had ever seen Mr. Gianesi's wife give him a bath. She also learned that in their approach to the patient, the student and the nurses would walk into the patient's room each morning and as they stood by the doorway would ask, "Do you want a bath, Mr. Gianesi?" His response, of course, was always, "No."

Efforts to collect more information about the patient and how the nurses felt about him yielded a fuzzy picture. No one seemed to know much about him except that he continued to have some pain, that he was pleasant enough, and that he was easy to take care of because he made so few demands. Through arrangements with the instructor and the head nurse, the psychiatric nurse took care of the patient for one morning.

June 21, 1961

The psychiatric nurse walks into Mr. Gianesi's room and finds a tall, powerfully built, and attractive-looking man lying, uncovered and without a pillow, partly on his side and partly on his back, in a bed that barely is long enough to permit him to lie fully extended. He is reading an Italian classic. The psychiatric nurse calls him by name, bids him good morning, refers to the unbearably hot weather, and introduces herself. He looks up at her and comments on her Italian pronunciation of his name. As they talk about various Italian cities, including his place of birth, and some of the Italian classics that are on his bedside table, the psychiatric nurse notes that he is perspiring profusely and that his pajamas and sheets are damp.

Ten or fifteen minutes later the psychiatric nurse says, "I want to hear all about your surgery, how it came about, and your hospitalization, but first I want to go and get the bath water and fresh linen so I can freshen you up; you don't look very comfortable." As she holds her breath and waits for his reply, he answers "Okay. Fine. I'll be waiting."

While the psychiatric nurse bathes the patient, occasional comments about the just-right temperature of the bath-water and about how good it feels to have his back washed and rubbed break the silence. As the psychiatric nurse starts to make his bed, the patient assures her that it will be all right if he gets out of bed just while she makes it. She responds, "I don't think that would be such a good idea. I know you must get terribly fed up with having to lie flat and to be waited on hand and foot, but it is important for your recovery. Thanks anyway." As she leaves the room to discard her equipment, Mr. Gianesi says, "When you come back, I have something I want to talk to you about."

Upon the psychiatric nurse's return, the patient tells her that he is a mason and that because of his bad back he is concerned about whether he ever will be able to work at his trade again. He pours out his worry about not being well soon enough to visit his aged and seriously ill mother in Italy as planned. Lastly, with much anguish, he tells her about his oldest daughter who has epilepsy and who is having frequent seizures again, even though she is on medication. He reveals that he is especially concerned that she has become a serious behavior problem and that he despairs of being able to handle her.

The patient's refusal of nursing care was his way of denying his current state of helplessness and dependency on others. He needed to refuse to be dependent so as to deny his reality problems—the possibility that he might not be able to return to his former job as a bricklayer—and also to deny his fear of the inability to function sexually. In having left choices about his care up to him and in having accepted his refusal on face value, the nurses had placed him in the untenable position of making decisions which were the responsibility of the nursing personnel. As a consequence, not only had the patient not received the nursing care he required, but meaningful contact had been cut off and he had been left alone to ruminate on his numerous personal problems. When the psychiatric nurse took the responsibility for the decision of giving the patient a bath, she made it clear to him that she wanted to take care of him. Her directness relieved him from having to make a decision at this time; nor was he required to test her to find out if she would accept him in his dependent state and if it was safe to expose himself to her.

The crucial factor in the nursing care was that such concrete reality problems as the patient's loss of his job and the care of his daughter had been identified. If these problems had not been elicited no steps could have been taken for handling them, such as referral of the patient to a social worker for the purpose of clarifying problems of retraining for a new job. Bodily care provided a direct route to dealing with those reality problems which the patient had denied.

In another situation a fifty-five-year-old patient, Mr. Rogers, had not been referred to the psychiatric nurse, but he came to her and a student's attention while the two of them were talking to another patient who shared his room and who had been referred to the psychiatric nurse. As a result, neither the psychiatric nurse nor the student knew anything about Mr. Rogers at the time the following episode occurred. Subsequently, however, they learned that he had carcinoma of the prostate and had had a prostatectomy which had been carried out in two stages.

October 5, 1960

Mr. Rogers is sitting up in bed with his luncheon tray before him on the overbed table. The psychiatric nurse feels his gaze and looks over at him. He has not touched his food. He looks frightened and as if he wants to ask a question. The psychiatric nurse suggests to the student that she go to him and find out if he needs help. The student comes back to the psychiatric nurse and tells her, "He wanted to know if it is all right for him to eat now, and I told him to go ahead."

Sensing some intense anxiety on the patient's part, the psychiatric nurse and the student go over to Mr. Rogers' bedside.

PSYCHIATRIC NURSE. Mr. Rogers, Miss Elgin tells me that you are wondering if it is all right for you to start eating your lunch now.
[*Patient nods as he searches the psychiatric nurse's face.*]
PSYCHIATRIC NURSE. You seem hesitant about eating.
PATIENT. My stomach feels funny.
PSYCHIATRIC NURSE. You feel nauseated?
[*Patient nods "yes."*]
PSYCHIATRIC NURSE. Well, let's take it easy then. How about your trying some of the soup? It might help to settle your stomach.
[*No response. Patient continues to stare.*]
PSYCHIATRIC NURSE. Some of the milk and ice cream would be good for you too.

[*No response. Patient has a tense and worried expression on his face. He makes no move to eat.*]

[*Psychiatric nurse picks up a spoon and begins to feed the patient, who physically is quite able to feed himself.*]

[*Student stands on the opposite side of the bed and intently watches what is going on.*]

PATIENT. [*accepts being fed, all the time studying the psychiatric nurse's face; he seems to enjoy it. Halfway through his meal, he takes the spoon out of the psychiatric nurse's hand and finishes his lunch by feeding himself*]. Thank you, nurse. Thank you. Thank you so much.

[*Psychiatric nurse says nothing but nods and stays.*]

PATIENT [*a whole stream of words pours out*]. I don't know what is going to happen to me. This is my sixth time in the hospital. And all the pain. But I don't want to tell the nurses because I am afraid of bothering them.

The patient was immobilized by some conflict which was unidentified. His fear of acting for himself, derived perhaps from a fear of doing some harm to himself, was symbolized by his desire to be fed by someone else. When the psychiatric nurse was willing to meet this infantile need, the patient was able to move to the next developmental era and to use language to communicate some of his problems more directly and appropriately.

The last vignette concerns a fifty-eight-year-old woman, Mrs. Weinberg, who was in the terminal stage of carcinoma of the uterus with metastasis to the spinal cord. She had had numerous hospitalizations and extensive surgery. She had a good deal of pain and required a moderate amount of narcotics. Although she still could do a few things for herself and could get out of bed with help, she was becoming progressively weaker.

The principal nursing problem was that Mrs. Weinberg was very demanding, particularly about being given her pain medication promptly when she asked for it. She also was extremely critical of the nursing personnel, whom she felt really did not want to take care of her, a reaction which only increased her complaints.

Some of the nurses responded to Mrs. Weinberg's requests, complaints, and demands by completely withdrawing from her. Because of the impasse that had been reached in the nursing personnel's relationships with the patient, the case was referred to the psychiatric nurse, who recognized the need to intervene in the situation on two levels simultaneously. First, she had to experience the patient and to explore the meaning of her behavior. Second, she had to work directly with the staff nurse assigned to the patient not by alienating her but by helping her to face her needs and recognize how these inhibited her productivity and satisfaction.

On one occasion when the psychiatric nurse was on the unit she witnessed an explosive interchange between the patient and the nurse. Mrs. Weinberg criticized the nurse for supposedly having made her wait a long time for her medication and because her bath water was cold; the nurse responded by being rude and sarcastic and by severely reprimanding Mrs. Weinberg in front of the other patients and personnel in the open unit. Shortly afterwards, the psychiatric nurse walked over to the nurse, who was busily making the patient's empty bed. The following conversation took place.

PSYCHIATRIC NURSE. Here, let me give you a hand with Mrs. Weinberg's bed.

STAFF NURSE. [*with flushed face, looks up with an expression of surprise*]. Oh, you don't have to bother.

PSYCHIATRIC NURSE. But I want to. [*Pause.*] As you probably know, I couldn't help but overhear your trouble with Mrs. Weinberg. What was it all about? She seems to present quite a problem to everyone.

STAFF NURSE. [*at first she is quite tentative, but then she speaks quite openly*]. I have had it right up to here [*puts her extended hand under her chin*] with her. Nothing we do is ever right as far as she is concerned. I swear she watches the clock when it comes to getting her Demerol, and when we try to postpone it for her own good so she won't become addicted, she says the nurses are just being cruel. That's the thanks you get.

PSYCHIATRIC NURSE. There is no question that this kind of patient can be terribly trying to the staff, to the other patients, and most of all to herself. [*Pause.*] I don't know if you know why I am up here.

STAFF NURSE. Something about helping the students to take care of patients who are mental.

PSYCHIATRIC NURSE. Something like that. I am up here to help the students work with patients like Mrs. Weinberg whose behavior interferes with the students' taking care of them. What do you think about you and me working together with Mrs. Weinberg? I don't understand yet all of what is going on with her either. And I don't know if I will come up with anything that will be very useful. But maybe between the two of us we can get some ideas about how to get her off the nurses' backs.

STAFF NURSE. There's nothing to lose. What do you want me to do?

PSYCHIATRIC NURSE. You already have been helpful by giving me some idea of how you see the situation. But I haven't had to go through any of these experiences with Mrs. Weinberg as you have, and for that reason I think it would give me a better feel of her if I took care of her just once.

STAFF NURSE. [*breaking into a broad grin*]. Be my guest. She's all yours.

PSYCHIATRIC NURSE. Of course, I'll be needing to talk with you from time to time so we can compare notes with each other about what is happening with both of us.

STAFF NURSE. [*turns away as she starts to leave the unit, and then turns back*]. Thank you for helping me make the bed.

The psychiatric nurse had paved the way for her own work with the patient and at the same time had forestalled the staff nurse's withdrawal from Mrs. Weinberg by engaging her in a collaborative endeavor. This approach was a face-saving one for the staff nurse inasmuch as it helped to reduce some of her guilt about her encounter with the patient. (From that point on and whenever the psychiatric nurse came to the service to work with other patients, this staff nurse sought her out.) Many of the staff nurse's negative feelings about Mrs. Weinberg were neutralized.

The following day, as planned, the psychiatric nurse took care of Mrs. Weinberg. The physical care consisted of giving her an enema, bathing her, applying medication to areas of her skin that were irritated from x-ray therapy, massaging her back where she experienced most of her pain, giving her her medications, combing her snarled hair, and encouraging her and helping her to get out of bed.

> As the psychiatric nurse washes and massages the patient's back, Mrs. Weinberg talks with much bitterness about her altercation with the staff nurse and her feeling about the other nurses. Then she says, "This is the first decent bath I have had since I have been in the hospital. I can feel your hands. I know you are really here. And I feel clean for a change. The way these nurses slop the washcloth around, it's nothing more than a bird bath." The psychiatric nurse does not answer.
>
> After all the care is completed, Mrs. Weinberg takes the psychiatric nurse's hand and kisses it. Her eyes fill with tears.

PSYCHIATRIC NURSE. Tell me. What is it?

PATIENT. [*begins to cry*]. It is two months now since I have been in the hospital, and I don't seem to be getting any better. [*She grabs hold of the psychiatric nurse's hand. The intensity of her sobs increase.*] I wonder if I will ever get out of here. I am so discouraged and fed up. [*She wipes her eyes and nose.*] I'm sorry. I don't mean to be such a baby.

PSYCHIATRIC NURSE. You know, Mrs. Weinberg, with all you have been through—the numerous hospitalizations, all the surgery, all the pain, all the pills—I don't wonder that you become discouraged and heart-sick and wonder if you will ever get better. As a matter of fact, under these circumstances, I would be worried about you if you didn't feel like throwing in the sponge from time to time. As for you being a baby, you seem to feel that you shouldn't have these feelings or at least that you shouldn't express them. From where I stand as a nurse, your tears seem pretty normal and just plain human to me. Of course you are going to have more bad days, lots of them, as you improve. But you will have good days too, just as you have had them all along the way.

PATIENT. [*has stopped crying. Her red eyes are opened wide*]. You mean the way I feel is natural? Really? [*Pause.*] I never thought of it in this way before. Then all this is just a part of getting better, isn't it?

[*Psychiatric nurse smiles and nods in the affirmative.*]

PATIENT. I would like you to do one more thing for me. Lower the bed. I think I'll take a nap now. [*The hour at which the patient was allowed to have medication for pain had long since passed unnoticed.*]

PSYCHIATRIC NURSE. Fine. And if you are awake before I leave, I'll get you up in a chair so you can eat your lunch.

[*Patient nods sleepily. She already is dozing.*]

The patient's behavior—her demanding, her complaining, her criticizing, her crying—were all symptoms of regression in illness. Regressive behavior in adults is extremely difficult for nurses to handle because it tends to arouse irritating reactions. To deal effectively with the regressive behavior of a patient requires a highly personalized nurse-patient experience.

The change in this patient's behavior was not the result of long, drawnout psychotherapy or esoteric approaches. Rather, it was due to the deepening of a professional relationship, which means the nurse must have both the predilection and the skill to change her professional relationship from an impersonal to a personal one. Such an alteration of a professional relationship requires the nurse be able to sense a patient's bottled-up need to cry, to explode, to give vent to his feelings. Inherent in the art and science of providing a psychotherapeutic experience for Mrs. Weinberg was a nurse's ability to help her both "to take the cork out of the bottle" and to unfreeze her congealed terror about dying. Until the time of the psychiatric nurse's intervention, Mrs. Weinberg had not had with any nurse the kind of a relationship that would allow this to happen.

One of the most important aspects of the psychiatric nurse's consultative work was that in all her experiences she did not encounter any undue resistance among the nursing personnel or the medical staff to her work with patients. She was free to move from one patient to another and from one clinical unit to another, as well as to function on whatever level seemed advisable to her at the time. The majority of the head nurses were interested and cooperated to their utmost.

Several circumstances may account for the relative absence of barriers to the psychiatric nurse's work in the clinical setting. One reason pertained to the positive relationship that the instructor who was involved and the psychiatric nurse had established with each other; the instructor automatically communicated her own acceptance of the psychiatric nurse, including the value of psychiatric nursing consultation, to the head nurse. Another reason was that the positive relationship which the instructor had developed with the nursing staff paved the way for the psychiatric nurse to enter the situation. A further possible reason was the psychiatric nurse's point of emphasis. Because she was not principally concerned with studying, evaluating, and improving the quality of the care given by the nursing service personnel, she did not expect any change to occur, except perhaps as a by-product of her work with the students and the instructors. Consequently, there probably was less need for the nursing personnel to feel threatened by her.

Helping Students to Change and Grow

In line with the belief that an essential goal of baccalaureate nursing education is to assist the student to use the self in a therapeutic way with patients and families, the psychiatric team designed two experiences to help the student cope with the problems which interfered with her freedom to use the self.

In the main, the problems that arose did not pertain to lack of information or knowledge; rather, they stemmed from the student's emotional limitations and the anxiety inherent in these limitations which frequently clouded her innate capacities. Many of the presenting problems in using the self therapeutically were tied up with the student's attitudes toward authority, with her willingness and ability to take responsibility, and with her use of judgment and initiative.

To facilitate the development of freedom in use of the self, experiences were organized for dealing with student problems within the context of student group discussions and within the context of individual student conferences. As in the case of her other activities with students, in these two experiences the psychiatric nurse stripped herself of the usual pedagogical power of assigning grades. This alteration in the traditional teaching role and function was particularly essential in these endeavors because their success hinged primarily on the student's ability to learn to trust the psychiatric nurse, who was more closely identified with the other faculty members than was the psychiatrist.

EXPERIENTIAL TEACHING IN UNSTRUCTURED GROUP CONFERENCES

The unstructured group discussions with sophomore students were introduced into the curriculum in the beginning of the first year of the project, and they continued throughout the first five-year period of the project. Once a week the psychiatric nurse met for one hour with all the sophomore students in small groups of from eight to ten. The purpose of these group meetings was to provide opportunity for the students to discuss the tensions arising in their relationships with patients, other students, clinical personnel, instructors, and members of the psychiatric team and to help them become aware of their own feelings and values and the way in which they were communicating these. This activity was also designed to help them to analyze the effect of their behavior on their professional relationships and to assist them in utilizing the problem-solving process. Another purpose was to create a relatively safe situation in which the students could begin to work out some of their unresolved attitudes toward authority and dependency as these affected their educational experiences.

Methods. The first point of emphasis in the conferences was on the analysis of the emotionally disturbing experiences that had been selected for discussion. In each session the students had the responsibility of choosing the topic to be discussed. The subject chosen was discussed for one or several sessions, depending on its depth, the students' investment in it, the problems raised in connection with it, and the readiness of the students to grapple with these problems. In the discussion of a particular topic, the initial emphasis was put on the students' own emotional responses to their experiences, and they were encouraged to air their feelings about the various persons involved. This approach to problem solving is the reverse from the one in which the primary focus is on the behavior of other persons and which generally results in the failure to consider one's own behavior. This concentration on the self was only the first step in the process of helping the student to understand the behavior of other people.

As in the case of all the clinical conferences in which the psychiatric nurse participated as a teacher or a resource person, the second point of emphasis was on the observation and discussion of the interaction process among the group members in terms of the students' subjective reactions to the topic under discussion and what had occurred in the group. Whenever possible the psychiatric nurse used this content to clarify the role of the student nurse and to identify the role of the professional nurse.

It was in this experience that students first were exposed to a double focus in the teaching-learning process and first were introduced to taking the roles of leader and observer of the group interaction process. This assignment of students to leader and observer roles, however, was not an innovation in the Skidmore program, for prior to the initiation of the psychiatric integration project this experience had been provided for students in some of their courses.

Topics Discussed. Some of the topics chosen for discussion by the students were as follows.

Factions within the sophomore class.

Expectations of the faculty and the criteria for evaluation of students; fear of dismissal from the nursing program.

Fear of an instructor.

Anger at the psychiatric nurse.

The purpose of examinations and how to prepare for them.

The role, function, and effect of rumor.

Clarification of the goals of the student health service.

Adjustment to the interruption of social life on campus and to living in New York City and in the residence hall.

Inadequate opportunity to meet men and have dates.

The social versus the professional role with patients.

Discomfort in talking with patients.

The male patient who demonstrates provocative and seductive behavior.

The patient who gives gifts to the nurse.

The patient who is of a different color.

The complaining patient.

The crying patient.

The dying patient.

The head nurse who derogates students.

The relationship between Skidmore students, the nursing service, and the medical personnel.

Lack of understanding of the purposes of the conferences.

Negative attitudes about having to take the roles of leader and observer in the group conferences.

Anxiety about the use and purpose of the tape recorder in the group discussions.

As the choice of the subjects for group discussion indicates, one of the ground rules of the conferences was that the selected topics were to be limited to the context of the students' educational experience. To avoid traversing into group psychotherapy, the psychiatric nurse focused exclusively on those experiences that impinged on the student's role as a student and as a nurse.

Analysis of the experiential teaching-learning process revealed that each group of students passed through three successive stages of group development. These stages in learning were similar to the eras of personality growth and development.

The Stage of Dependency. During the first phase of the group's development, which might be described as a stage of relative helplessness or dependency, the student's task was to learn to trust her peers and the psychiatric nurse. In the case of a few students, dependency was reflected in initial curiosity, budding interest, and a desire for new experiences. In most of the students, dependency covered up anxiety that was related to their feelings of poor self-esteem, fear of exposing themselves, and fear of criticism from their peers and the psychiatric nurse.

Frequently during the first semester of the group discussions, the students acted out their dependency on the psychiatric nurse by coming to the conferences with the expectation that she would feed them pearls of wisdom, which they would uncritically swallow and regurgitate at strategic times. They communicated this expectation by addressing their comments and questions to the psychiatric nurse instead of to the student leader. Recurringly, they came to the conference without having thought about a topic for discussion and asked the psychiatric nurse to suggest some for them. Over and over they asked the psychiatric nurse what it was she wanted, what she expected from them, and what she thought they should do.

When the psychiatric nurse left the decisions up to the students, they became anxious, frustrated, and angry. They communicated these feelings in various ways. Some students dozed, some doodled, others chain-smoked. Some giggled, some daydreamed. Others formed their own little "kaffe klatch." The students' behavior during this period can best be described as testing. Certainly their behavior tested the attitudes of the psychiatric nurse—those of which she was aware as well as those which were unconscious.

By their reality testing, the students most likely were trying to ascertain whether the psychiatric nurse could be trusted. Did she really mean what she said about expressing their thoughts and feelings? Was it safe for them to feel free with her or would she punish them for exposing themselves? Did she really believe in their capacity for growth? Would she respect their views even when they differed from her own? Would she continue to love them even on those occasions when they seemed unlovable?

As long as the psychiatric nurse was not made unduly anxious by this behavior, she did not intervene actively. Understanding what the students were revealing about their feelings helped to reduce her anxiety. For achieving this understanding, however, it was necessary to allow the students' behavior to go on long enough for the psychiatric nurse to identify what was happening. The proper timing for intervention differed with each group and with the psychiatric nurse's ability to withstand her own anxiety. On occasion she moved in prematurely, thereby preventing the students from becoming aware of what they were doing. At other times she waited too long; by the time she intervened the students had become too anxious to focus on the problem at hand. Their anxiety in turn made the psychiatric nurse more anxious.

These errors in judgment were not catastrophic, for the psychiatric nurse's feelings about the students served as a safety valve; her attitudes always got across to them in one way or another. Another safety valve was the students' desire and capacity to look at and discover themselves. Besides alerting her to some of her own unresolved attitudes, the psychiatric nurse's awareness of her anxiety and her feelings of frustration and anger also functioned as a barometer of what the students were feeling.

The psychiatric nurse's interventions generally consisted of her open response—approving or disapproving—to the students' behavior. On one occasion after about four weeks of the students' negative acting out—by mumbling to each other, coming late for the conferences, and spending the entire conference time in searching for a topic for discussion—the psychiatric nurse's annoyance and impatience with them reached a peak. She told them how she felt about their behavior.

> I think it is time for us to talk about what is going on in the group. For several weeks now you have been acting like naughty children. What disturbs me most is that not only are you rude to me but you are disrespectful to each other. You cut each other off, and some of you have made snide comments about your peers when they try to pull the group together.
>
> I appreciate the fact that these meetings are a new kind of experience for you and are therefore bound to arouse anxiety. But as professional nurses you

will constantly be exposed to similar situations. Therefore, I think it is crucial that we try to understand what you are doing to each other and, even more important, what you are doing to yourselves. This is by no means an easy or painless endeavor. However, I have never promised you an easy time. Learning involves change, and change is never easy. I for one have had just about enough of this tugging and pulling at each other. So let us get back to what we are here for in the first place.

How did the students react to the psychiatric nurse's intervention? Immediately following her intervention, the psychiatric nurse elicited the students' comments, among which were the following.

We knew we were acting like spoiled brats, but we just couldn't seem to stop ourselves.

Part of us wanted to stop but the other part wanted you to stop us.

When you didn't stop us it made me feel that maybe you didn't really care enough about us after all.

The psychiatric nurse's reaction to the students' behavior was a potent force in helping them to come to grips with the realization of how their behavior affects others.

In response to the students' comments, the psychiatric nurse asked them, "If I had moved in sooner and interrupted your behavior, what do you think might have happened?" At first glance, their responses appeared startling.

In allowing us to behave the way we did for so long you forced us to look at what we were doing.

We have acted like babies, and yet we complain bitterly whenever we think we are being treated like them.

If you had jumped in sooner, we would have felt you really didn't mean that this was to be a safe place to try out our different ways of solving problems.

In calling the students' attention to the problem within the group, the psychiatric nurse evoked independence and self-expression, which is what the students were struggling to achieve in the first place.

It was from this point that the group began, dramatically, to grow. The students and the psychiatric nurse had taken a giant step in learning to trust and count on each other. After going through this crisis together, they had something of substance to share. They came out of the experience with newly awakened feelings of closeness with and tenderness for each other.

The Stage of Independence. The second stage of the group's development might be described as the period of independence. Some students manifested independence by rejection of their peers' and of the psychiatric nurse's help; by lack of interest; and by silence, and it masked their need to control and manipulate people and situations. Other students reflected a potential readiness to reveal both their strengths and their weaknesses.

The students' attempts to emancipate themselves from their dependency were communicated in numerous ways. They now chose the topics for discussion. They became annoyed with any and every suggestion made by the psychiatric nurse. The student leader cut off the psychiatric nurse whenever she raised a critical question. The rest of the students glared at her with black looks as if to say, "Whose group discussions are these anyway?" Some students actually turned their backs on the psychiatric nurse. It was as though she had been relegated to the status of a piece of furniture. She was perceived as an intruder.

Once again the psychiatric nurse tried to wait it out, remembering it was necessary to keep in mind the meaning of the students' behavior. When she began to feel unappreciated and rejected, she intervened, for as long as she kept her hostile feelings to herself she could be of no constructive use to the students.

By this period in the group's growth process, most of the students felt safe enough to talk about their feelings toward the psychiatric nurse and about what was happening. Most of the time, they were able to be quite open and free about their reactions. Their comments were somewhat as follows.

> We want you to be here, but we want these meetings to be our conferences.

> We want you to stay but go over there [pointing to a corner of the room outside of the group circle].

The psychiatric nurse explored with them again, for what seemed to her to be at least the hundredth time, the purposes of the group discussions. She and the students analyzed her role. The students' independence now expressed a beginning willingness to test out new ideas.

Some of the comments that came out of this discussion were as follows.

> It kills me to admit it, but I guess we are acting like adolescents.

> In wanting to try out our own wings, we have pushed you out. Now that I think about it, I do the same thing at home.

> We want you to be here, but at the same time we don't.

> Since we have pushed you away from helping us, we must do the same thing with our mothers and fathers. No wonder they lose patience and become angry.

> Good heavens! Do you think we have been doing the same thing with our instructors?

At this phase of the group experience, the students had made considerable progress in resolving the authority-dependency conflict.

Because the students' attitude of independence was apt to function as a barrier to seeking or accepting help from the psychiatric nurse, this attitude often was more difficult for the psychiatric nurse to work with than those attitudes associated with the students' dependency.

The Stage of Interdependence. Toward the end of the semester the students moved into the third stage of the process—the stage of interdependence, or collaboration. Many of the students were able to take a large share of the responsibility for the group discussions. At the same time they were more aware of when they needed help and guidance from the psychiatric nurse. Because they were better able to seek assistance from her, it became less necessary for her to intervene in the discussions.

The students began to raise critical questions with each other. They could disagree with each other without considering disagreement as a personal attack. One by one the students were able to listen to those whose opinions differed from their own. They could tolerate higher levels of anxiety, as manifested in their increased ability and willingness to sit out silences. They began to take a second look at those whom they had earlier rejected, as is illustrated by the following group discussion, in which the students struggled to work through some of the problems arising in student-instructor relationships. Prior to this conference a great deal of meeting time had been spent venting strong feelings against a particular instructor with whom the students had experienced numerous interpersonal problems but with whom they also had frequent contact.

April 24, 1959

Four students have arrived and are animatedly chitchatting with each other. The students already have arranged the chairs in the usual circle. About five minutes before the group conference is scheduled to begin, the psychiatric nurse walks into the seminar room, lugging the tape recorder with her. She greets the students. One student quips, "I don't think I would know you without that tape recorder," to which the psychiatric nurse responds, You know, I don't think I would know myself either." The students giggle. As the psychiatric nurse hooks up the recorder, the students continue to talk to each other. The rest of the students arrive.

The meeting is a somber one. The many silences are pregnant with thoughtful introspection. Nervous giggles and occasional side comments break through the serious tenor of the meeting. Though there is much tenseness, a tone of openness and frankness not heretofore achieved permeates the discussion.

MERCEDES CLARIDGE [*the leader, addresses the psychiatric nurse*]. We decided before we came to this meeting that we would like to talk about our clinical experience.

[*Some students groan; others mutter to each other.*]

PSYCHIATRIC NURSE. Fine, if this is what the rest of the group wants to talk about.

MERCEDES CLARIDGE. The problem is with our instructor. She is so dogmatic. Students are always in the wrong regardless of what they do.
[*Long silence; several glance across the room.*]
PSYCHIATRIC NURSE. How about the rest of you?
STEPHANIE MASTERS. She seems uninterested in us. She is so cold. She doesn't even talk to people on the clinical unit.
PEGGY REISMAN. I feel as if she isn't a human being. I can't feel close to her.
[*Long pause.*]
[*Mercedes Claridge doodles, a faraway look in her eyes.*]
PSYCHIATRIC NURSE. What about you, Judy?
JUDY WHITBY. I agree. I am afraid of her.
[*Stephanie Masters looks up and stares at Judy.*]
PSYCHIATRIC NURSE [*to group*]. What is there about the instructor that frightens you?
JUDY WHITBY. I'm not sure.
DORIS THOMPSON. I think I am afraid that I can never come up to her expectations. I always have the feeling that even when I do something right, it is never enough. [*Long pause.*] It has to be one way—her way.
[*Judy Whitby and Stephanie Masters nod in agreement. Karen Becker and Joyce Scarpitti mumble to each other and giggle.*]
PSYCHIATRIC NURSE. What's the giggling about?
KAREN BECKER. It's a funny situation.
JOYCE SCARPITTI. It's not funny. All of this makes me nervous.
PSYCHIATRIC NURSE. Probably you are not alone in your feelings. I don't think we should let them slip by unnoticed. Any ideas as to what your nervousness is about?
[*Karen Becker doodles.*]
DORIS THOMPSON. It just doesn't seem right to talk about an instructor this way.
PSYCHIATRIC NURSE. Hm, hm. [*Pause.*] What about you, Karen?
KAREN BECKER. When I said it was a funny situation, I guess I really mean—I feel funny.
PSYCHIATRIC NURSE. Would you try to elaborate?
KAREN BECKER. I don't know exactly how to say it. I know we are supposed to discuss our problems here, but I feel odd talking about the instructor.
[*Silence.*]
PSYCHIATRIC NURSE. What about you, Joyce?
JOYCE SCARPITTI. Who are we to criticize our teachers anyway? After all we are only students.
STEPHANIE MASTERS [*eying the tape recorder*]. Maybe if the tape recorder weren't taking everything down. . . .
[*The spontaneous reaction of the psychiatric nurse is to turn off the tape recorder, but instead, she waits. The group struggles to keep a straight face.*]
DOLORES NOVICK. Oh, come on, Steve. Let's not start beating that dead horse again. We all know by now that the tape recorder isn't what is our trouble.
PSYCHIATRIC NURSE [*to the group*]. What we seem to be talking about are your guilt feelings about discussing your negative reactions toward faculty members.

The purpose of bringing your feelings—positive and negative—into the open is not merely to let off steam and gripe. Rather, the purpose of exposing your feelings is to help you understand them and to put them into proper perspective so that you are able to appraise an instructor on a more rational basis. However, before you can understand your feelings and change them you first have to know what they are. Keeping your negative feelings to yourself doesn't change them or cause them to magically disappear. They continue to operate underground, outside of your awareness and therefore beyond your control. Unidentified feelings can wreak all kinds of havoc. Your concern is understandable, but it is not realistic. Nevertheless, it says a lot for your growth that you have been able to talk about your feelings instead of sitting on them.

[*The group is pensive; some students look at the psychiatric nurse and nod in agreement; deep sighs punctuate the thoughtful mood.*]

JUDY WHITBY. Does the instructor appear aloof because she always is so terribly busy?

PEGGY REISMAN. Yet when the resident calls, she runs on the double.

JULIA FERRIS. She bawled me out for my interest in the pathology of the patient.

STEPHANIE MASTERS. She always seems to pick on some students.

[*The psychiatric nurse looks at Mercedes Claridge, the student leader, who appears to be in a reverie.*]

Maybe we had better try to pull some of these ideas together. An important question we must wrestle with is: What does this instructor do to make students feel "picked on"?

From your comments, it seems as if she makes you feel inferior. You have stated that she closes you off, and you feel that clinical content appears to be more important to her than the students as people. You seem to feel, for example, that her prime concern is with the manner in which she presents the material to you and the way you give it back to her. Then there also is the point that your curiosity about anything other than her focus seems to be pushed by the wayside. All of this behavior contributes to your feeling that you can't measure up to her standards.

[*Much nodding; some doodling. One student exhales her cigarette in a large cloud of smoke.*]

PSYCHIATRIC NURSE. What does the instructor's behavior communicate to you regarding her feelings about students? How does it make you feel?

PEGGY REISMAN. I think she is distrustful of us. Since she is always emphasizing what we don't do right, I don't think she respects us for what we are able to do.

MARJORIE MOSLEY. She was astounded when she found me in another instructor's office, where I had gone to borrow a book. She wouldn't take my word that I had permisison, and so she went to the other instructor to check.

[*Several knowing glances are exchanged.*]

PSYCHIATRIC NURSE. This is an interesting point you have raised. If, as you believe, the instructor does not trust you or respect you, what do you think her distrust and disrespect might be about?

[*Long pause.*]

DOLORES NOVICK. I'm not so sure it is a matter of distrust and disrespect. I think some of the problem is that she is so shy. Maybe she is uncomfortable with people.

DORIS THOMPSON [*in an almost inaudible voice*]. Could it be that she is scared of getting close?

PSYCHIATRIC NURSE [*thinks to herself, "Out of the mouths of babes!"*]. I don't think everyone heard you, Doris, and it is important. So come on, say it again.

DORIS THOMPSON. Maybe the instructor is frightened of closeness and that's why she acts so aloof.

KAREN BECKER [*nods in agreement*]. She always shows interest and concern when students are ill. I think that she would like to get close to us but she doesn't know how to go about it.

MARJORIE MOSLEY. One day I forgot my purse and left it in the seminar room, and the instructor called me at the residence to tell me she had it so I wouldn't worry.

PSYCHIATRIC NURSE. Our time is almost up so we have to stop soon. What did you think of today's meeting?

STEPHANIE MASTERS. I wondered if we were going to wander all around the barn in this discussion as we do so often.

JUDY WHITBY. Even though we didn't come up with any answers, I think maybe I understand the instructor a little better. Maybe I won't be quite as scared of her.

PEGGY REISMAN. Just talking about it makes me feel better. The whole group has been sitting on this problem for weeks. We wanted to bring it up but felt it wasn't right.

PSYCHIATRIC NURSE. How about you, Mercedes [*Claridge*]? How do you feel about the situation now?

MERCEDES CLARIDGE. The instructor doesn't dig me, and I'll never dig her.

PSYCHIATRIC NURSE. My, but you sound awfully pessimistic about the situation.

MERCEDES CLARIDGE. It's just that we're not each other's cup of tea.

JOYCE SCARPITTI. And yet, yesterday the instructor came over and stood next to me so she could say "hello" to Mercedes.

[*All eyes are on Mercedes Claridge.*]

[*Mercedes Claridge doodles and shrugs her shoulders.*]

PSYCHIATRIC NURSE. It is true that talking over a problem once doesn't guarantee a magical solution. But we have taken the first step in the resolution of a problem by bringing it into the open. What impresses me most about today's meeting is that after airing all your negative feelings about the instructor, you spontaneously began to point out some of her positive qualities. The central principle of today's seminar is that once you were encouraged to ventilate your negative feelings without any pressure from me to humanize the instructor, you were able to begin to consider her feelings. In exploring how she might view the situation you came to a more realistic appraisal of her on your own.

This experience has important implications for your work with patients. If you can personalize your relationship with a patient by allowing him to express his negative attitudes directly, whether they are in response to the staff, to his family, or to yourself, without prematurely closing him off, the way is paved for him to come to a more realistic evaluation of the problem that confronts him.

JUDY WHITBY [*laughs; turns to Marjorie Mosley*]. We'll have to try this out on
  Mr. Valloni.
  [*Several students giggle.*]
PSYCHIATRIC NURSE. What?
JUDY WHITBY. He has the whole staff in an uproar—but mostly me—with his com-
  plaining.
PSYCHIATRIC NURSE. We might discuss this patient next week. In the meantime
  try to get beyond the static of his complaining and your reactions of irritation
  by listening to him so you can begin to hear what he is trying to tell you.

Problems and Issues. The problems that emanated from the student group
discussions were related to the nature of the structure of the conferences,
to the students' preoccupation with themselves, to student-teacher relationships, and to the faculty's responses to the experience.

The provision of a group structure that was sufficiently flexible to give
the students the freedom to discuss any and every aspect of their educational
experiences, including the persons involved, resulted in the students' temporarily becoming very self-centered as compared to being patient-centered
This phase in the students' development did not create undue hardship
for the psychiatric nurse, but it frequently was extremely disconcerting to
the instructors who were concerned with helping students not only to learn
to take care of patients but to *care about* taking care of patients.

Another area of difficulty that emerged pertained to student-teacher
relationships. As the student began to trust the psychiatric nurse, who had
no power in grading them, many students identified strongly and positively
with her. In the process of resolving their authority-dependency conflicts,
some students began to compare the psychiatric nurse with some of their
other instructors. In some situations this comparison led a student into
temporarily estranging herself from her instructor. As long as the psychiatric
nurse could allow her own positive and negative feelings about faculty
members to come into her full awareness and could recognize her unrealistic
needs for the students' admiration and approval, this troublesome phase also
passed without undue disruption and in time the students' trust in the
psychiatric nurse was extended to other faculty members.

The third, and by far the most complicated, problem with which the
psychiatric nurse had to deal evolved from the faculty members' attitudes
about and their responses to this kind of learning experience for students.
From the beginning of the experience in the first year of the project, the
psychiatric nurse had emphasized to both the faculty and the students that
for her to be able to help students to establish a higher order of explicit
communication it was crucial that she keep in confidence what was discussed
in the conferences. At that time the faculty verbally concurred with this
principle. Accordingly, during that year the psychiatric nurse withheld the
content of her unstructured group discussions.

At the end of the first year, however, the faculty members reversed their stand. The psychiatric nurse had prepared a written analysis and summary of each group's activities in addition to a compilation of the activities of all four student groups. These summaries contained a listing of the topics discussed by the students, some of the highlights of group interaction, the key problems identified by the psychiatric nurse, including her own functions, and an evaluation of the progress in all four groups. Copies of these summaries had been distributed to all the sophomore students and the faculty members. In spite of this attempt to keep the faculty informed about the broad and general aspects of the conferences, the psychiatric nurse became the butt for the faculty's distrust, suspicion, competitiveness, hostility, and overt aggression (see Chapter 8, July 14 and 21, 1959).

Changes in Structure. In an endeavor to counteract the divisive effects of the student group conferences on the faculty–psychiatric nurse relationships, at the psychiatric nurse's suggestion, in the third year of the project two instructors from each clinical area attended all the conferences of their group of students (see Chapter 8). A total of eight instructors—five younger and three older—two in medical nursing, two in pediatric nursing, and four in surgical nursing, participated in this activity. The instructors' attendance in the conferences almost immediately created serious problems which eventually reached a point of crisis. Some of the younger instructors used their attendance in the conferences as an opportunity to try to sabotage the psychiatric integration program (see Chapter 9, pp. 251–252).

As a result of several more faculty group discussion of the student conferences, during which still more problems engendered by some of the faculty members' negative attitudes were uncovered, a compromise was effected and introduced in the fourth year of the project (see Chapter 9, April 12, 19, and 26, 1960). The compromise consisted of the following changes in the structure and focus of the conferences.

1. The psychiatric nurse had the weekly unstructured conference with students for twelve weeks in the fall instead of having them throughout the sophomore year. The focus of the discussions and the teaching methods remained the same. The other faculty members no longer attended the conferences, except by special invitation of the psychiatric nurse or the students.

2. For the remainder of the sophomore year, the focus of the conferences was shifted to the students' expression of their attitudes toward any of their educational experiences to exclusive emphasis on problems associated with the clinical situation. One instructor from each clinical area met with her group of students and the psychiatric nurse for a one-hour conference each week for three weeks. The psychiatric nurse and the instructor shared the leadership. Those faculty members who were not participating at the time

with the psychiatric nurse were free to structure their conferences as they saw fit.

3. In the fourth week the psychiatric nurse had an individual conference with each of the instructors who had participated with her. During this conference they evaluated the clinical discussions in terms of the significance of the topic chosen, the amount and mode of participation by the students, the quality of group leadership exercised by the instructor, the method by which the psychiatric nurse fostered or hindered the desired outcomes, and the identification of the psychiatric concepts inherent in the problem. Tape recordings of the group meetings were played back and discussed.

This alteration of the focus and structure of the psychiatric nurse's conferences also represented a qualitative change in the goal of the conferences. The original goal, which had been in terms of student learning, had been broadened to include the goal of faculty growth.

Dealing with Confidential Material. The other area of change consisted of the psychiatric nurse employing a method for dealing with students' problems that were exposed in the conferences in a way that preserved the confidential nature of her unstructured discussions without alienating the faculty. The method as devised and used by the psychiatric nurse consisted of one or another of the following three approaches.

1. As students divulged problems in the group conferences, the psychiatric nurse encouraged them to go directly to the instructor who was most actively involved in the problem or who they felt might be the most helpful to them. After the problem had been explored in the group, a volunteer committee of two or three students then would go to the instructor to discuss the problem and to suggest the way or ways of dealing with it that had been identified by the group.

2. At the end of the discussion of a problem, the psychiatric nurse told the students what she thought needed to be communicated to an instructor or the total faculty. She then shared the material with the faculty, but she did not identify the individual students who had raised the issues.

3. After a student had explored a problem with the psychiatric nurse, she and the psychiatric nurse might invite the faculty member most directly concerned with the problem to attend the next student group conference for the purpose of discussing the problem with the students and helping them to come to some resolution. In these conferences, the psychiatric nurse was the leader of the discussion, and the other instructor functioned as a resource person.

These three approaches in communicating the emotionally disturbing experiences of students to the faculty were employed with about equal frequency by the psychiatric nurse. Their use helped to clarify the purpose of the unstructured conferences for both students and faculty, to penetrate the aura of mystery that had enshrouded the conferences, to dilute the faculty's fear of being under attack by students, to increase effective communication between the students and the faculty and between the faculty and the psychiatric nurse, and to bring about greater closeness between the students and their instructors.

Counseling in Individual Conferences

For the purpose of affording the student the opportunity to come to grips with some of the problems that impinged on her professional performance but that were either too threatening to her or too personal for discussion in the student group and because there were no unstructured group conferences for the junior students, the psychiatric nurse and the psychiatrist had individual conferences with students in the sophomore and junior classes. Although many of the problems that were brought to the team members significantly interfered with a student's academic or clinical performance, there also were numerous cases when this intrusion of problems did not occur.

Over the five years of the integration project, the psychiatric nurse had individual conferences with approximately 135 students from the sophomore and junior classes, and she spent between two and ten hours of conference time per student. A total of thirty-five of these same students were also referred to the psychiatrist.

The Structure for Referral. The students were free to seek conferences with the psychiatric nurse and the psychiatrist on their own. During the first three years of the project, the majority of such conferences with the psychiatric nurse were initiated by the student. In the fourth year about 75 per cent of the students who were seen by her were referred by other faculty members. In the fifth year, during which the psychiatric team was on partial leave, all the students who were seen by the team members were referred by other instructors. In the case of the psychiatrist's conferences, with few exceptions, the students were referred to him by the psychiatric nurse, the other faculty members, or the nurse or the physician in charge of the student health service.

In the process of their work with students in individual conferences, the psychiatric team learned that those students who first had been seen by the psychiatric nurse before being referred to the psychatrist were much more amenable to seeing the psychiatrist. During their conference with him they also were less anxious, freer in their responses, and more open and spontaneous in revealing themselves than those students who had been referred directly to him. These qualitative differences in students' responses were due partly to the fact that, in regard to their fear of "being psyched," the psychiatric nurse posed less of a threat to students than did the psychiatrist. The differences were due more, however, to the fact that as the psychiatric nurse worked with a student in uncovering pertinent information and in clarifying her problem, the student generally experienced the psychiatric nurse in a highly personal way. This personalized experience helped to alter the student's distortions and reduce her fear of psychiatric matters. When the necessary groundwork for psychiatric consultation had been laid by the psychiatric nurse, most of the students had a satisfying experience with the psychiatrist and much of his time and effort were saved.

In view of these positive outcomes of the psychiatric nurse's conferences with students, the structure for referring students to the psychiatric team was modified; all students who were to be seen by the psychiatrist were to be seen first by the psychiatric nurse. After as many conferences as were necessary to clarify the student's problem, the psychiatric nurse, sometimes in consultation with the psychiatrist, determined whether referral to the psychiatrist was indicated.

One criterion by which the psychiatric nurse determined the advisability of referring a student to the psychiatrist was the extent to which she was able to appraise a student's strengths and limitations and to estimate her potential for change in those areas that were pertinent to her professional role. Another criterion, of course, was the seriousness of the student's problem. Generally she referred those students whose problems were significantly interfering with their performance all along the way in the program, those whose inherent capacities could not be evaluated by the psychiatric nurse because they were obscured by a heavy layer of anxiety, and those whose limitations in the emotional area were such that the potential for change seemed dubious to the psychiatric nurse.

Topics Discussed. Students raised and discussed a wide range of problems in the individual conferences. Some of these were:

Questioning one's motivation for nursing and experiencing difficulty in making a decision of whether to remain in the program or to withdraw from it.

Failing in the program; setting up the situation to be failed out of the program.

Difficulty in organizing study assignments and anxiety in taking examinations.

Fear of an instructor.

Anxiety about not having boy friends.

Problems related to sexual relationships before marriage, the pros and cons of premarital intercourse, and the basis of making a choice regarding one's behavior.

Pregnancy outside of wedlock and the alternatives for handling the situation that were open to the student.

The impact of a parent's alcoholism, chronic physical and mental illness, divorce, or death.

Insufficient financial resources to pay for psychotherapy or to pay for continuing in the educational program.

Referral for Psychotherapy. Of the thirty-five students referred to the psychiatrist, six were referred elsewhere for psychodiagnostic evaluation, and eighteen entered individual psychotherapy.

The students for whom psychotherapy was recommended were expected to take the responsibility for informing their parents of the recommendation. Except for two cases in which the chairman of the department informed the parents because the student had refused to do so, all the students initiated the discussion of psychotherapy with their parents. In most instances when the student accepted the recommendation for psychotherapy, the parents also accepted it. In the case of a student who did not want it, her parents went along with her decision. At the request of a student or of her parents, one or both team members had a joint conference with the student and her parents for the purpose of clarifying the student's problems with her parents and of interpreting to them her need for psychotherapy. The opportunity for such a conference was made known to each student for whom psychotherapy was recommended.

The following student comments in response to the psychiatric nurse's question "How do you feel about psychotherapy and have you ever considered it for yourself?" reveal attitudes of acceptance, curiosity, ambivalence, and fear of dependency toward psychotherapy.

> At one time I thought about therapy, but because I shared the problem with you [the psychiatric nurse], I was able to iron it out.

> I recognized I needed therapy. In the beginning I felt uneasy and didn't want to talk about it. Gradually I got more comfortable because people recognized a change in me. The faculty and the students supported me in a very positive way. I began to feel that to be in therapy is not so bad.

> It was good for me to see how therapy helped my friend. She has problems, but that doesn't mean she is abnormal or crazy. This made me realize that psychotherapy is not such a stigma after all.

> Once I thought about psychotherapy but I felt I should be able to solve my own problems or that other people would think so.

> I never thought of therapy for myself—only in terms of interest and curiosity.

From these comments, which were typical, it can be seen that the students themselves were not unduly resistant to the idea of psychotherapy.

On the other hand, several faculty members (both younger and older) were somewhat less than enthusiastic about psychotherapy for students. The students who were undergoing psychotherapy required the instructor's assistance to enable them to keep their appointments. Such assistance consisted of changes in class or clinical practice schedules and in the provision of makeup work in those areas in which students had had to miss certain specific learning experiences.

In the early stages of psychotherapy many students also went through temporary periods of negative acting out against patients and authority figures, which resulted in their ineffective performance. During such times the instructors were called upon by the psychiatric team to give added support to these students. The following comment by a faculty member, solicited by the psychiatric nurse, identifies some of the difficulties engendered by students who were in psychotherapy.

> Sometimes we expect too much from students in terms of their ability to undergo psychotherapy and to carry the nursing program. It is a grueling experience for students. I feel we are put at a disadvantage when the number of disturbed students who need our support is such that the instructors have no time left to help the so-called normal student. Would we take a student with this much physical disability and keep her in the program?

As this instructor's comment reflects, some of the faculty members felt that because of the heavy demands of the nursing curriculum, students should not enter psychotherapy during the two-year clinical period of the nursing program. The essential point which was overlooked by this restricted view, however, was that for some students, the demands of the nursing program created a burden in addition to those with which they already were saddled.

The fact of the instructors' mixed reactions about students undergoing psychotherapy during the clinical part of their program raises several important questions. As is the case with several of the issues raised in this book, these questions are essentially a product of hindsight; the psychiatric team did not consider them, at least on a conscious level, during the time of their collaborative work. These questions follow.

What were the faculty's expectations of the outcomes of psychotherapy?

Did knowledge of the fact that a student was in intensive psychotherapy significantly influence an instructor's perception of her, and if so, was such a view likely to operate for or against the student?

How did the faculty members perceive their role in relation to the student in psychiatric treatment?

Were there occasions when the psychiatric nurse and the psychiatrist unwittingly set the therapeutic goals for the student in therapy above the educational goals, and as a consequence, made unreasonable demands of the other faculty members with respect to the kind and degree of support to be given to students?

Further investigation of the issues posed by these questions could have serious implications for the psychiatric integration program.

During the fifth year of the integration project, a student had a psychiatric emergency over the weekend. The psychiatric nurse was called by another student, who urgently requested psychiatric help for her classmate. In the absence of a policy for handling such emergencies (acute panic, suicidal intent, depression, and psychotic episode) during hours when the department of nursing was not in session, the psychiatrist and the psychiatric nurse, under his guidance, took the necessary therapeutic action. Their therapeutic action was correct and effective, but they neglected to communicate with the chairman of the department before taking it.

This episode was discussed with all the faculty members in one of the group meetings with the psychiatric team. As a consequence, policies and procedures were developed for guiding the members of the psychiatric team and the other faculty members when called on for help in a psychiatric emergency.

Dealing with Confidential Material. In the beginning of the second year of the project, some of the younger and older faculty members were extremely wary of the psychiatric nurse's interviews with students. Because the psychiatric nurse had not shared with other faculty members the problems that students revealed to her, some of which were interfering with a student's performance, several instructors regarded the psychiatric nurse's interviewing activities with intense suspicion (see Chapter 8, July 16 and July 21, 1959). As with the unstructured group discussions, the psychiatric nurse soon recognized that to the degree she continued to have a confidential relationship with some students, she inevitably would alienate some instructors. This situation was a slippery one for the psychiatric nurse to handle, especially because she had been trained to regard as privileged communications problems brought to her in private. She and the rest of the faculty members had to learn together that a wide margin exists between betraying a student's confidence and selectively sharing pertinent information with other faculty members who might be in a strategic position to help the student.

As a result of the faculty's reactions to the conferences, the psychiatric nurse and the psychiatrist devised a method for sharing with the faculty pertinent information brought to them by students without jeopardizing the student's trust and confidence in them. The method of communicating confidential material to the faculty consisted of the following steps: At the beginning of every individual conference with a student, or sometimes during it, the psychiatric nurse or the psychiatrist would tell the student that to be able to help her as much as possible she or he might find it necessary to share with some faculty members certain general aspects of her problem but that the specific details would be withheld. Then the team member would tell the student that before the conference was over she or he would convey to the student those aspects of the problem that she or he felt needed to be shared with the faculty. This knowledge gave the student the opportunity to raise questions about or take issue with the psychiatric nurse or the psychiatrist about whatever was to be communicated to the faculty.

In most instances this method of dealing with students' privileged communications was successful in eliminating any lurking mistrust of the psychiatric nurse or the psychiatrist on the part of the students. It also helped to develop their trust that all the instructors were deeply concerned with their welfare and were involved in the corporate endeavor of trying to help them.

As for the faculty members, this method penetrated their distrust of the conferences and of the psychiatric nurse. They began to appreciate the importance of holding certain communications in confidence. They developed respect for those colleagues who kept certain information confidential, and they increased their skill in holding confidential material themselves.

The following situation illustrates that this method also was successful in engaging the students and the faculty members in joint endeavors to resolve problems.

> Whenever Florence Hurley was assigned to the care of a woman patient she became so tense, anxious, tongue-tied, and helpless that she was unable to complete the nursing care without receiving a great deal of help from her instructor. After the student, at her own request, had had several individual conferences with the psychiatric nurse in which she talked about her discomfort with all women authority figures, the psychiatric nurse and the instructor worked closely together on the problem. The student responded positively. Just as she had begun to noticeably improve, she was to be transferred to another service consisting of only men patients. The psychiatric nurse suggested to the current instructor that it might be helpful if the student could remain on her service for an additional week. After consultation with the instructor on the men's service, it was agreed to follow through with the suggestion.

It can be hypothesized that the student's growth was as much a result of the two instructors' and the psychiatric nurse's sincere interest in the student as it was a result of the additional experience provided for her to work out her problems in relation to caring for women patients.

REFERENCES

1. Neal, Mary V. *Disaster Nursing Preparation: Report of a Pilot Project Conducted in Four Schools of Nursing and One Hospital Nursing Service.* New York: National League for Nursing, 1963, pp. 33, 34.

2. Norris, Catherine M. "Greetings from the Lonely Crowd," *Nursing Forum,* 1 (1), 72–82 (Winter, 1961–1962).

Chapter Seven

THE WORK WITH THE
INDIVIDUAL INSTRUCTOR IN
CLINICAL CONFERENCES

The effect, if not the prime office, of criticism is to make our absorption and our enjoyment of the things that feed the mind as aware of itself as possible, since that awareness quickens the mental demand which thus in turn wanders further and further for pasture.

HENRY JAMES, *The New Novel*

In the belief that the nurse teacher is the chief resource for achieving the goals of psychiatric integration, the psychiatric team, during the second year of the project, began to help the individual instructors to improve their skills in teaching the students how to effectively handle the problematic behavior of patients. The fifty-minute clinical conference which every instructor held with her group of sophomore students each week was used to provide the assistance. Such a utilization of these conferences required that the focus of the discussions be shifted to clinical situations that had created interpersonal difficulties for the students.

These conferences were directed toward assisting the students to learn methods of helping patients who exhibit disturbed behavior and to learn more about the processes which facilitate recovery and how to prevent interferences with these processes. Problems that the students had encountered in the clinical situation with patients and with medical and nursing personnel were explored. These explorations focused on the students' interpersonal tensions arising from confusion about their roles as nurses and learners, problems involving unresolved attitudes toward authority, stereotyped responses to illness and death, and unrealistic expectations of themselves and others.

The psychiatric team worked with the instructor by attending the student conference and, immediately following each conference, reviewing and evaluating it with the instructor.

The Participating Instructors

The arrangements for the participation of instructors took into consideration whether or not the evaluation session following each student conference could be fitted into the instructor's schedule. In the second year of the project, when the activity was initiated, four younger instructors—Miss Drew, Miss Harris, Miss Jensen, and Miss Hunt—participated in this activity. In the third year the psychiatric team worked with three older instructors—Miss Reed, Miss Thomas, and Miss Vance—and in the fourth year, with three younger instructors—Miss Foster (for the first time), Miss Drew, and Miss Jensen (for the second time).* Miss Scott's teaching schedule made it impossible for her to participate in this experience. At her request, however, at the end of the second year the psychiatric nurse collaborated with her in all her student seminars.

During the first year of the activity, the psychiatric team worked with each of the four instructors during a series of three consecutive student conferences. This period of time proved inadequate for uncovering whatever difficulties the instructor had in leading this type of seminar and for establishing a working relationship in which the psychiatric team members and the instructor were sufficiently comfortable with each other to pave the way for change and growth. Consequently, during the next year (the third year of the project) this experience was extended to include a series of six clinical conferences with each of the participating instructors. In the third year of this experience no changes were made in the number or structure of the conferences.

Goals and Methods

The specific objectives of the psychiatric team's participation were to help each instructor:

1. To explore behavioral problems on an emotional rather than a purely intellectual level.

* For the convenience of the reader, the members of the younger group have been given names beginning with letters in the A–N section of the alphabet, and those in the older group with letters in the R–W section. Thus, Miss Vance, for example, is immediately identifiable as a member of the older group, and Miss Harris as one of the younger group.

2. To increase her skill in identifying the problems of immediate concern to students.

3. To clarify her role as leader of the clinical conferences.

4. To allow herself to be experienced by students on a personal level. (Such a personal teacher-student relationship does not imply a social relationship, but rather a professional one in which the teacher reveals her own feelings and attitudes about matters of concern to the student.)

5. To develop an operational framework for the conferences.

The psychiatric nurse and the psychiatrist did not know in advance the best way to proceed in the student conferences. Initially they sat back and waited for the instructor to bring them into the discussion. This approach did not work out successfully. The students had certain preconceived notions about psychiatric matters and psychiatric personnel; for example, they harbored the stereotype of a psychiatrist and a psychiatric nurse who could read their minds and make them act against their wills. Their anxiety about the role and function of the psychiatrist was particularly intense because they had not had the contacts with him that they had had with the psychiatric nurse in individual and small group conferences. The passivity of the psychiatrist and the psychiatric nurse did nothing to dispel their notions. Uncertain about the reasons for the presence of these two people, they became uncomfortable and communication was inhibited.

In an attempt to handle this problem the psychiatric nurse and the psychiatrist tried a second approach. One or both of them participated actively in the discussions and at times assumed the leadership. This participation made the students feel more comfortable, but in several instances the instructor reacted unfavorably because she felt that the members of the team were usurping her role with the students.

Gradually the psychiatric team began to combine both techniques. In some conferences the instructor served as leader and the psychiatric nurse and psychiatrist remained inactive unless the instructor called on them as resource persons. In other conferences the members of the psychiatric team took the leadership while the instructor observed them, and when she resumed the leadership, tried to utilize some of the principles and techniques that they had demonstrated.

For a time this combined technique was used in work with all the instructors. Progressively, however, the members of the psychiatric team shifted from this framework to one in which they recognized each individual instructor's needs, desires, and goals, and were relatively passive or assertive according to the instructor's seeming needs at the moment.

In line with the psychiatric team's efforts to tailor the conferences and their roles in them to fit each instructor's particular needs, an orientation period was arranged for each instructor individually. The briefing consisted of the members of the psychiatric team identifying the goals of the conferences, discussing the general structure, exploring how the instructor would be most comfortable in functioning and what role she wanted the psychiatric team to take in the beginning sessions, and clarifying how the students would be oriented to the experience.

During the one-hour evaluation session that followed each seminar the members of the psychiatric team and the instructor evaluated the seminar with respect to the significance of the topic chosen, the amount and mode of participation by the students, the quality of leadership exerted by the instructor, the way in which the psychiatric nurse and the psychiatrist had functioned and their effect on the discussion, and the psychodynamics underlying the subject matter of the discussion. To assist the instructor and the psychiatric team in recalling the details of the student seminars, all seminars were tape-recorded.

Often more professional problems were opened up in the evaluation period than could be handled during the allotted six weeks. Accordingly, several instructors sought and were given continued help on an individual basis by the psychiatric nurse.

Problems Engendered by the Double Focus

In contrast to the usual teaching-learning situation, in which there is one learner or group of learners with one set of objectives, the clinical conferences in which the psychiatric team participated were utilized for helping two separate groups of learners—the instructor and the students—each of which had its unique set of goals. This duality posed problems for each of the participating individuals or groups over and beyond those that are characteristic of the normal single-focused teaching situation.

THE STUDENTS' PROBLEMS

The students, of course, were accustomed to situations in which all the resources of both personnel and equipment had been introduced for use in their instruction and quite naturally viewed the presence of any such resources in the conference room as in some way related to their performance. When such a relationship was not obvious, they endowed the resource person with a mysterious and somewhat frightening purpose. As has been pointed out, until the members of the psychiatric team participated in their learning situation, they felt uneasy about their presence.

The tape recorder also was a subject of the students' concern. As was the case in the psychiatric nurse's unstructured group conferences with them, the students were also apprehensive about how the taped material would be used and about whether their discussions would be available to the rest of the faculty. Sometimes such preoccupations interfered with their spontaneity, and communication was inhibited. The orientation of the students, therefore, had to include a clarification that the tapes were being used to help the instructor and the psychiatric team. In one situation in which students continued to be inhibited, the team voluntarily removed the tape recorder.

THE PSYCHIATRIC TEAM'S PROBLEMS

The psychiatric nurse and the psychiatrist were confronted by problems that were inherent in their dual teaching role. Because as far as they were concerned the emphasis of the conferences was on the faculty members' professional growth, it was sometimes necessary for them to ignore temporarily the immediate needs of the students so as to meet those of the instructor. Sometimes it was difficult for them to postpone the satisfaction that is derived from giving help to students when they need it. Often it required a high level of frustration tolerance to wait and not move in. However, their staunch belief that in the long haul the students would profit most from the growth of their instructors enabled the psychiatric nurse and the psychiatrist to climb over most of the hurdles with relatively minimal difficulty. The value of the support each received through the other's physical presence, empathy, and example cannot be overestimated.

THE INSTRUCTOR'S PROBLEMS

Of the three individuals or groups participating in the clinical conferences, the instructor was most affected by the dual focus, because it forced her to assume two roles. Whereas throughout the experience the students remained students and the members of the psychiatric team continued to be teachers, the instructor was expected to function simultaneously as a teacher and as a student. Furthermore, one of these roles (that of student) constituted a role reversal for her with respect to her relationship with the largest number of participants in the experience—the students; she had to undertake the task of learning in front of an audience before which she was appearing as an authority. The fear of loss of status with her students as well as with the members of the psychiatric team was therefore an omnipresent threat.

Further compounding the difficulty of role and status was the fact that the instructor was expected to learn and teach new content, utilizing new methods. Moreover, unlike the situation in the faculty discussions with the psychiatric team, where she was also a learner, in the clinical conferences the instructor was the lone student participating in the experience; she could not resort to camouflage or to hiding among a group of fellow students. Also the goals of the experience were more specific and clearly defined than were those of the faculty discussions, so that her attainment or nonattainment of them was likely to be more obvious.

Small wonder that some of the instructors approached the clinical conference experience with indifference or even open rejection. The extreme instance of this approach was the instructor who defied all the psychiatric team's efforts to secure her cooperation and managed to avoid the experience until the last possible moment, when she participated in a somewhat less than enthusiastic manner. Other instructors displayed a surface acceptance which hid authoritarian and controlling attitudes. For example, one instructor, who in her need for approval volunteered early for the experience, was obviously resistant to it despite her surface compliance.

On the other hand, some of the instructors exhibited potential readiness for the new experience by their willingness to participate and experiment and seek help. One instructor in particular showed genuine interest and receptivity; she was flexible, accepted suggestions, and tried new ways of approaching the material.

The Content

The content of the clinical conference experiences, as far as the instructor learner was concerned, consisted of the knowledge and skills involved in leading students through five steps that were identified as essential to the seminar process, namely,

1. Eliciting an appropriate topic for discussion.
2. Securing the students' participation in the discussion.
3. Uncovering the students' feelings and reactions.
4. Summarizing the data and conceptualizing the problem.
5. Exploring appropriate and alternative possibilities for handling the interpersonal problems associated with the topic.

ELICITING AN APPROPRIATE TOPIC FOR DISCUSSION

This step was found to be more complicated and to require greater skill than might appear at first glance. Unless all the students were stimulated to participate in the selection of the topic, at least insofar as they committed themselves to an acceptance or a rejection of it, it was exceedingly difficult, if not impossible, to engage them in the exploration. If premature closure was to be avoided, it was necessary for the instructor to be certain that the topic chosen was of concern to the majority of the students and that consensus was reached before it was finally decided upon.

The first requirement, therefore, was that the instructor allow sufficient time for eliciting problems for discussion. It was also important that she lead the students from the selection of a problem that in actuality was masking another problem around which the students were experiencing a notable degree of anxiety. For this task the instructor had to be sensitive to the meaning of both verbal and nonverbal communication, including silences that attended a suggestion. When principal sources of concern were withheld but the instructor had some hunches about what might be bothering the students, it was incumbent on her to raise the issue herself. At other times it was important that the resistance to bringing problems into the open be discussed.

SECURING THE STUDENTS' PARTICIPATION

In addition to participating in the selection of a topic for discussion, it was important that all the students be actively involved in the discussion of the topic. Various techniques for promoting participation were suggested to the instructor, including making such comments as, "We haven't heard from everyone, yet"; "how about some other suggestions?"; and "what is your choice?" Calling on individual students directly was also suggested.

When the first two steps of the seminar were unsuccessfully negotiated, the conference turned into a stereotyped experience in which the students talked around the problem. In such instances direct intervention became necessary. During the early stages of the work with an instructor, the responsibility for intervening usually fell to either the psychiatric nurse or the psychiatrist. As some instructors grew more secure and skillful, they were able to intervene on their own.

UNCOVERING THE STUDENTS' FEELINGS

This step, which was perhaps the most critical one of all, was a necessary prerequisite to the identification of the realistic and the unrealistic components of the problems presented by the students and the students' rational and irrational responses to these problems. Such attitudes, reactions, and responses formed the matrix of the psychiatric concepts to be integrated.

Uncovering the students' feelings generally took longer than did any of the other steps. Experience demonstrated that if sufficient time were spent in eliciting the students' reactions, ways of handling the problem effectively usually emerged. If, on the contrary, the group was hurried through this step and the primary emphasis was put on finding a solution to the problem, the problem usually remained unresolved.

As might be expected, this step was one of the most formidable for the instructor, and a large part of the guidance activities of the psychiatric team was concentrated on helping the instructors learn to negotiate it.

SUMMARIZING THE DATA AND CONCEPTUALIZING THE PROBLEM

Conceptualization is the process by which all the concrete data that have been gathered about a situation are put into useful order and then explained in terms of their interrelationships. It further involves putting one's speculation about the explanation into precise terms from which generalizations may be formulated. These generalizations can then be used to uncover the meaning and significance of similar situations.

The data on the problems presented by the students were not limited to the objective facts under discussion; they also encompassed the entire gamut of the students' and the instructor's subjective responses. Thus, the instructor was faced with the task of helping the students to formulate concepts about their own reactions to a situation as well as about the behavior of the patient or other person involved in the situation.

Exploring Alternatives for Handling the Problem

In instances in which the preceding steps had been carefully engineered, this particular step often involved the least time and effort. Once the students' feelings and attitudes had been brought to the surface, it was possible to differentiate between realistic and unrealistic aspects of the problem. It was found that when such differences were clarified, more effective ways of handling the situation evolved almost automatically.

Problem Areas

As the members of the psychiatric team observed the instructor's performance with respect to the five steps involved in leading the clinical conferences, they were able to identify the areas that were causing the most difficulty. Two of these problem areas—the lack of understanding about how to deal with psychiatric content and the instructor's underlying attitudes toward the leader-student relationship—were fundamental. In addition, certain specific problems stemming from these two basic ones seemed to call for special attention.

Dealing with Psychiatric Content. Some of the instructor's problems in leading the clinical conferences arose from the unique nature of the content under discussion. In contrast to content associated with the integration of other specialties, the content involved in psychiatric integration is derived from an individual's attitudes, feelings, reactions, modes of communication, and behavior. Inevitably, such content is not as safe, easily codified, easily recognizable, or accepted as the content the instructor was accustomed to teach. Thus her view that, "We already teach psychiatric concepts" was very different from the process of focusing on and exploring nurse-patient relationships in action.

Underlying Attitudes. Perhaps the greatest factor in the instructor's progress in this experience was her underlying attitude toward the functions of a teacher leader and the relationships that should exist between such a leader and her students. These underlying attitudes were usually uncovered after the second or third seminar with the psychiatric team. In the case of some instructors, friction was created as deeper attitudes of control and manipulation, which interfered with growth, came to the surface. In the case of others, negative attitudes decreased and potential readiness for growth emerged.

The greatest growth, perhaps, was observed in the two instructors with whom the psychiatric team worked in a second series of clinical conferences. The interval of one year between the first and second series provided opportunity for these instructors to assimilate their first experiences and to experiment with different ways of handling problems. It also enabled them, during the second series, to approach the experience on the basis of greater familiarity with the members of the psychiatric team. In one instance the instructor's authoritarian and controlling attitudes had modified to a considerable degree. In the other, positive attitudes emerged that had previously been hidden behind surface rigidities. Both instructors were much more comfortable with the members of the psychiatric team and were able to function on a collaborative level. They had grown in their ability to elicit students' feelings about the problem under discussion and demonstrated greater awareness of the psychiatric concepts involved.

Conceptualization. A more specific problem was the inability of the instructors to formulate concepts from the data obtained in specific situations. This weakness was understandable in view of the deficiencies of all graduate education in the United States. The majority of these programs provide their students with facts and opinions rather than with an understanding of processes, and the programs in which the Skidmore nursing instructors had been prepared apparently belonged to this majority. Although there were wide variations among these instructors in their knowledge of psychodynamics, there was a uniformly meager application of abstract concepts to nurse-patient relationships. Similarly, there was little attempt to abstract from the nurse-patient interactions any general concepts. Few if any of the instructors were able in their first experience to conceptualize the problem under discussion. This inability was in sharp contrast to the persistent reaffirmation by some that they did not need help in the area of psychiatric concepts. Both instructors who completed a second series of conferences with the psychiatric team achieved substantial growth in this area.

Uncovering Students' Feelings. Even more obvious perhaps was the tendency to disregard the fact that the students' feelings were an important, if not the most important, element in every problem that was discussed. The instructor tended to jump from a superficial exploration of the problem under discussion to an equally superficial answer. She paid lip service to the necessity for students to express feelings. Nevertheless, in practically every case the instructor experienced difficulty in eliciting subjective responses from the students. Her attitudes about the appropriateness of the students' openly discussing negative feelings about patients and authority figures and her anxiety about her role as a teacher, which had been generated by her own conflict about authority and dependency, tended to limit her effectiveness in dealing with behavior on an emotionl rather than solely intellectual level.

Personalizing Relationships. An inherent aspect of handling affect-laden material was the instructor's fear of personalizing her relationship with students by revealing her own feelings. Instead, some instructors tended to display a façade of closeness and warmth and to strive toward a pseudo-personalized relationship characterized by benevolently autocratic mothering or camaraderie. Their behavior toward students contained common elements, such as lack of explicitly defined expectations, insufficient limit setting, and avoidance of direct confrontation of the student regarding problematic behavior at the time of its occurrence.

Under such conditions, the students were apt to become confused about the instructor's role and where they stood in relation to her and to the program. Periodically, they were caught in a double bind of conflicting messages; a faculty member would gloss over her expectations, perhaps in the effort "to be understanding" and, at the same time would convey the idea that the student had better measure up to her abstruse expectations.* Nevertheless, some of the students' thinking and energy were dissipated in trying to guess the content of the hidden agenda and to conjure up ways to try to deal with it. Such student comments as, "We feel pressured to conform to the Skidmore mold"; "I'm just waiting for the ax to fall"; "I was told about my limitations too late to try to improve them"; and "Failure comes as a bolt out of the blue," revealed how some students were experiencing the double bind imposed on them by some faculty members.

This double bind in faculty-student relationships was, of course, an echo of what was occurring from time to time in intrafaculty relationships. The root problem in both situations was the same—many of the intrafaculty problems arose from the faculty members' fear of being direct about their feelings and attitudes. Therefore much of the psychiatric team's work with faculty members in both group and individual conferences was aimed at penetrating their indirectness and establishing a higher order of explicit communication, with students and with the psychiatric team. A potent force in achieving this goal was the ability of the psychiatric nurse and the psychiatrist to establish a personalized relationship with the instructor in the clinical conference activity.

---

* The double bind, according to Gregory Bateson's concept, occurs when messages containing diametrically opposed expectations are given (1). In the attempt to fulfill one of these expectations, the individual inevitably fails in living up to the other. Thus, he finds himself in an untenable situation in which it becomes impossible to secure the approval of the significant person.

An example in faculty interaction may clarify the concept. When an important school event occurs, some members of the older group may state that the faculty members should make their own decisions about attendance. If some younger members decide not to go, some members in the older group disapprove.

Some Learning Experiences

Possibly the best method of describing the way in which the psychiatric team worked with the instructors in the clinical conferences and the evaluation sessions is through excerpts from some of these experiences. The six experiences thus summarized here illustrate the following four ways in which the instructor's leadership of the conferences was deficient.

1. Inadequate leadership in the selection of a topic.
2. Elusiveness and insufficient guidance.
3. Overprotection and premature closure.
4. Alienation of students.

The reader may find it advantageous to compare the instructor's interaction in these four clinical and evaluation conferences with her functioning in the faculty meetings.

INADEQUATE LEADERSHIP IN THE SELECTION OF A TOPIC

October 14, 1959

The psychiatric team first participated in one of Miss Vance's clinical conferences one week ago. This conference had also been the first one that Miss Vance had had with this group of students. The students had been apprehensive about the use of the tape recorder, and the psychiatric team had explained that it was being used to help evaluate the discussion and to identify useful techniques in leading such groups, but not to evaluate the students' performance. One student stated, "It will take time to get used to this kind of conference, and you can't expect us to open up about all our problems at once."

During this second conference the students are enthusiastic, spontaneous, and attentive. They smile and giggle. They seem to have forgotten about the presence of the tape recorder. Participation is general and contributions flow. Faces are animated and eyes glisten. A student sitting next to the psychiatric nurse peeks at what she is recording. She grins sheepishly when the psychiatric nurse looks up, smiles, and winks at her. Cigarettes are passed and lit. Several students offer one to the psychiatrist and the psychiatric nurse. The students seem more comfortable than the instructor. They sense her insecurity and keep looking to the psychiatric nurse for direction. The conference takes some time to "get off the ground."

MISS VANCE. What problems do you have that would be helpful to discuss? [*She adjusts her glasses.*]

AMY WILSON. How do you get a patient to do what he is supposed to do when he constantly goes against the doctor's orders?

MISS VANCE. Yes, I know whom you're referring to, and he can be difficult. There are a lot of problems in that situation. How are the rest of you handling it?

BETTY KINSMAN. I just sort of kid him along.

PSYCHIATRIC NURSE. Perhaps before we get into the details of this particular problem we should find out if there are any more that are causing difficulty.

ALICE KANE. There is one nurse on the staff who does things in her nursing care that we have been told not to do. This raises all kinds of trouble.

LUCY TILTON. These patients treat us as if we were children. We have one patient who tries to keep the nurse for himself and he objects when we pay any attention to other patients.

LILLIAN GARY. I am bothered by immodest male patients who expose themselves in front of us.

MISS VANCE. Any other problems?

SONDRA STERN. A patient told me I was just right for his son. Is it right not to be too friendly with patients?

MISS VANCE. I don't know how to answer that because we first have to find out what kind of a relationship is going on. [*She gives a philosophical discourse on nurse-patient relationships in general, all the while fiddling with a lock of her long auburn hair.*]

[*The group looks to the psychiatric nurse for a decision to be made on the choice of a topic.*]

PSYCHIATRIC NURSE. How come you are looking to me?

GROUP. Because you write down everything that we say.

MISS VANCE. Now we have identified several interesting problems for discussion. Let's decide which one we'll concentrate on.

ALICE KANE. Let's discuss the relationship that Amy presented. Lucy and Sondra mentioned him also and most of us have taken care of him or, if we haven't, we've heard of him.

[*Burst of laughter.*]

EVELYN SAUNDERS. The patient himself determines what kind of a relationship with the nurse will take place.

PSYCHIATRIC NURSE. It sounds as if you are talking about the problem of how you can be a realistic authority and establish a professional relationship with an adult patient, particularly when he is trying to set up another kind of relationship that is antagonistic to your goals as a nurse.

GROUP. Yes! [*All of the students are turned toward the psychiatric nurse.*]

MISS VANCE. The feeling I get about this patient is that he is a very mobile person who at this time has very little physical discomfort.

EVELYN SAUNDERS. The patient is fifty-eight years old. He has had a history of hematuria and he had a prostatectomy. Both he and his wife were very worried before his surgery. They have one child, a nineteen-year-old son. He constantly interferes in the conversation between the students and the other patients.

MISS VANCE. Let's look at what you do and evaluate it.

FAYE HILL. He's not too sick and so he wants to be the cheerer-upper of the whole ward. He talks all the time.

LUCY TILTON. When I was giving a backrub to a bed patient, he asked me when I was going to do the same for him.

SONDRA STERN. He tells me how wonderful all of us are, how he loves the nurses, and how I am just the right girl for his son.

GLADYS JACKSON. I've been trying to give him more attention, such as talking to him without his asking for it. When he started on the business of his son for one of us, I told him that we were just interested in helping him to get well. And ever since then he's let up on all this sweet talk with me and I'm more comfortable with him.

FAYE HILL. I don't feel he acts like this with the head nurse or any other person in authority. It seems to be just with us students.

MISS VANCE. Dr. Ullman, could you tie some of this together for us?

PSYCHIATRIST. The students did pretty well in the situation, so that there are no real problems on that score.

PSYCHIATRIC NURSE. Gladys' response to the patient was most appropriate because she clarified her role to the patient and her purpose for being there in the first place. The patient's reaction indicates that this is partially what he has been looking for. Once he became certain that Gladys was interested in him as a patient and that she wanted to take care of him, he no longer had to resort to his seductive manipulations as a way of making sure he would get what he needed.

PSYCHIATRIST. Yes, you [*Gladys Jackson*] accomplished your goal of arresting the patient's behavior but without hurting him.

MISS VANCE. It's really more important to treat the patient as an adult.

PSYCHIATRIST. When the patient got out of hand, you handled it, and when he acted out the role of the father by suggesting his son for you, you didn't take him up on this.

LUCY TILTON. Do men always go through a second childhood?

[*The group looks at the psychiatrist and titters.*]

PSYCHIATRIST [*laughs*]. In this culture, sexual prowess is important. The aging process therefore can be quite painful. This patient's illness involves his penis, so that he doesn't separate his genito-urinary problems from the sexual area. Any illness involving the genitals always involves anxiety. Then, he has a young, nineteen-year-old son who is taking over the male role. The patient is acting out his own fantasies. He can't say to you "I'll prove I'm a male by seducing you." Instead, he handles the situation indirectly and covers over his preoccupations with humor and wise-cracking. He is trying to prove "I am as good as a man of nineteen years of age." When he was asking for the back-rub, he was being the father, but also inviting bodily contact.

The students unconsciously had got the patient's real message. You were able to trust your intuitive responses. When students don't get involved or caught up with the patient's problem, as Jane pointed out, the patient is more comfortable because he doesn't have to prove himself, which is accompanied by the fear that he can't make the grade.

The nature of the problems these students presented indicated that they understood the purpose of the seminars and the role of the psychiatric team. Miss Vance was apt to discourse philosophically, with a kind of ecclesiastical precision, and to focus on solutions instead of dealing with what was bothering the students. The students looked to the psychiatric nurse for direction. The psychiatrist was still a stranger to them. Miss Vance quickly picked up the cue for giving more direction. The students were alert to the core of their problem—the feeling of helplessness in taking their rightful role as an authority with adult patients—which in this situation was further complicated by sexual overtones.

This conference demonstrated a situation in which it was unnecessary, and moreover would have been poor tactics, for the instructor to suggest concrete ways of handling the problem. The student had discovered what to do on her own, and her approach had been useful to the patient. What the students needed was the opportunity to validate the appropriateness of their approach to the problem, some help in clarifying their own reactions to the situation, and an explanation of the psychodynamics of the patient's behavior, which provided them with the principles underlying their intuitive handling of the problem.

After the students leave the conference, the psychiatric nurse, the psychiatrist, and Miss Vance discuss it. They move their chairs to get closer to each other. The psychiatrist sits between Miss Vance and the psychiatric nurse. After a slight pause, during which Miss Vance tries to get settled by crossing and uncrossing her short legs and pushing her auburn hair behind her ears, she opens the discussion.

Miss Vance. The students found it very difficult to accept the validity of how they handled the problem themselves. I had some qualms about cutting into their discussion. I wanted to get one item completely discussed before moving on to the next.

Psychiatric Nurse. This was an excellent conference, Esther. The task of choosing a subject is not easy. The criteria for choosing a topic in this kind of conference are different from other nursing care conferences. You were inclined to choose a topic without getting choices from other students. It is necessary to have a topic that engages the entire group. Today the agreement went right around the room. We made the correct choice, which can't be pushed.

Miss Vance [*to the psychiatrist*]. Is it helpful to use the students' reactions and responses to the situation, or focus on the way they handled it?

Psychiatrist. It is important to elicit the feelings of those students who are not participating. Some tended to sit back.

Psychiatric Nurse. I felt there was some cutting off of their own feelings when the focus was on handling the situation.

Psychiatrist. That's true, but it's more difficult to get to these in this situation because of the sexual area. The important issue is that their handling of the problem was excellent and wasn't just an accident.

Psychiatric Nurse [*to Miss Vance*]. How do you feel about the way we operated?

Miss Vance. I did wonder whether I should ask Dr. Ullman to comment. At what point should I turn for help?

PSYCHIATRIST. Our aim is to leave it up to the instructor to discover what the students want to discuss. The instructor gets the facts out on the table—the feelings, attitudes, and various experiences in relation to the problem. This part of the conference will take the longest. The last part is to synthesize all the material The instructor can try doing this by herself or ask us to do it.

MISS VANCE. All three of us are conferring, so I don't think you and Jane should just sit here without contributing.

PSYCHIATRIST. We really aren't conferring. Our purpose is not to help by discussing the patient. Our purpose is to gradually eliminate ourselves. The initiative of the instructor helps us to do this.

MISS VANCE. But I consider myself as a specialist in my own area and you and Jane in yours.

PSYCHIATRIC NURSE. Your area certainly is the baseline from which you operate, but we hope something will be gleaned from these conferences that will be useful to you in your own area. Every instructor can use psychiatric principles to deal with common problems that involve the psychodynamics of the patient's presenting difficulties.

In her opening reference about wanting to finish the discussion of one item before moving on to another, Miss Vance was demonstrating her tendency to go off on tangential aspects of a subject. This difficulty was underscored in her attempts to identify what was important to the students. During the evaluation conference it was made clear that she was responsible for taking the leadership in the clinical conferences.

Miss Vance, who was somewhat resistant to psychiatry, showed that she believed that a dichotomy existed between the content of her own specialty and the understanding of and skill in handling problematic behavior. Such a view is not unusual for nursing instructors. It probably stems from an aggregate of causes, including insufficient psychiatric knowledge and experience, stereotyped notions about and fear of psychiatry, and resistance to change. Both the psychiatric nurse and the psychiatrist dealt with Miss Vance's opposition by suggesting that regardless of the clinical area, behavior problems occur and have to be handled.

Miss Vance seemed fairly comfortable in raising questions. She focused most of her attention on the psychiatrist. This behavior was understandable and to be expected, especially because this experience was the first opportunity that she had had to relate with him on a personalized level. Because it was also an untraditional approach for a nurse to work with a physician for the explicit purpose of increasing her skill in handling a teaching situation, such an experience was bound to raise anxiety beyond that normally present when one's own practice is being observed and evaluated.

In this situation the psychiatric nurse was faced with role conflict. On the one hand, she wanted the good will of the instructor, with whom she had a strong professional identification, but on the other hand, she had a legitimate authority role with her. These attitudes, plus her own reactions toward authority, aroused anxiety which early in this experience was expressed in her uncertainty about what to do. Moreover, her situation was similar to that of the instructor—it was more difficult for her to hide or to camouflage her reactions in these conferences than it was in the faculty discussions.

Elusiveness and Insufficient Guidance

In spite of all the attempts of the psychiatric team to secure Miss Foster's cooperation in working with them in this experience, she defied their efforts until the psychiatric nurse took the initiative and gave her a written schedule of the dates on which the psychiatric team planned to work with her. This resistance made it especially difficult for the team to help Miss Foster overcome her difficulties in assuming leadership with students.

June 28, 1961

This is Miss Foster's sixth and final experience in her series of clinical conferences with the psychiatric team. The students appear restless and uneasy, and their facial expressions add to the feeling of gloom. When Miss Foster asks them to choose a topic for discussion, they remain silent. Heads are bent. Occasionally, a head bobs up as a student searches the psychiatric nurse's face. Except for Miss Foster who is smoking, cigarettes remain untouched. The incessant clicking of a ball-point pen is the only sound. As the psychiatric nurse glances around the room, her eyes fall on Miss Foster, who peers at her over her rimless glasses as she pokes a hairpin into her blonde braids. They hold each other's glance as they seem to ask each other what is wrong.

Sue Eddy breaks the silence with a seemingly irrelevant comment that betrays her anxiety.

Miss Foster. What are you going to discuss today?

[*There is a long silence; the students look at the psychiatric nurse.*]

Sue Eddy. A patient who has ulcerative colitis made out his will today.

[*Silence. The students shift in their chairs.*]

Psychiatric Nurse. How does this happen to come up?

Sue Eddy. It was just a side line. [*Long pause.*] Larry died!

Natalie Phelps. The reactions of the other children to his death were something. How does a child know that he will die?

Miss Foster. The parents' reactions may reveal this.

Eleanor Neal. Larry had open-heart surgery and. . . .

Miss Foster. The mother was very concerned and brought the patient a present every day and he looked for this. Does the mother have too high expectations of what doctors and nurses can do? How does the nurse handle this?

Cynthia Bolton. Larry's father has been in a mental hospital. How do I find out more about this? How far should I go?

Eleanor Neal. How do you handle a situation in which the patient dies as an outcome of serious surgery?

SUE EDDY. The patient's father seems to have his feet on the ground.

MISS FOSTER. Larry's mother is unrealistic. You couldn't sit her down and tell her her son had a fifty-fifty chance for survival. No matter how you talk to her, she avoids facing problems. Let's go back to the patient.

NATALIE PHELPS. I was stunned by Larry's death.

JEAN UNGER. It's tragic. He got so much attention from everyone.

ELEANOR NEAL. Looking back on his condition, I think maybe it's better he died. [*Long silence.*]

MISS FOSTER. Besides having had open-heart surgery, the patient also developed a tumor in the trachea, and a tracheotomy was done. He couldn't eat. He aspirated and got pneumonia. He had a full course of radiation therapy. [*Long silence. Some eyes are lowered; others look up at the psychiatric nurse.*]

MARY HULL. Maybe in the long run it's better he died. I felt badly that his mother wasn't present.

SUE EDDY. It's the way he died that disturbs me. I heard that the tracheotomy tube came out and when the nurse ran to get the doctor, the patient suffocated. It's all so senseless! It was an error that could have been avoided. It's just plain negligence!

CYNTHIA BOLTON. What do you tell parents in a case like this?

MISS FOSTER. Natalie, is this what is bothering you too?

NATALIE PHELPS. I've heard at least five or six stories on how Larry died and they all indicate that his death seemed avoidable.

CYNTHIA BOLTON. The doctor said the patient was frothing at the mouth and should have been suctioned. There was nothing to suction.

MISS FOSTER. We will never know what happened, but how would you handle this situation with the parents?

PSYCHIATRIC NURSE. Is it realistic to expect that the patient would not have died if this incident had not occurred?

JEAN UNGER. The parents placed a lot of hope in his getting well.

MISS FOSTER. And who else did also?

NATALIE PHELPS. All the nurses hoped so too. Larry was the pet of the clinical unit.

MISS FOSTER. How do you feel about a child dying?

NATALIE PHELPS. It's hard to take. It's as though a child is just snuffed out. Adults at least have had a chance to live.

MARY HULL. It hurts me more to see a child like Patty Lucas who is so paralyzed that she will never get well. It's when a patient dies suddenly that it is so difficult.

PSYCHIATRIST. We are talking about unexpected death. People do die suddenly. This is not necessarily due to negligence. With sudden death, we are stunned, surprised, shocked. These reactions may be expressed by scapegoating somebody, as if a person is responsible for the patient's death.

PSYCHIATRIC NURSE. I hate to do this, but we have already run over our time. [*Like freed prisoners, the students grab their belongings and rush to leave.*]

PSYCHIATRIST. What was wrong with this class today?

SUE EDDY. The sun is out and it's hot.

PSYCHIATRIST. Why weren't we able to get with the problem?

MARY HULL. Sometimes we are just way out and off the beam.

PSYCHIATRIST [*looks at Miss Foster and the psychiatric nurse*]. Well, shall we release the prisoners?

[*The students get up, but instead of leaving for their next class, for which they are already late, the majority gather around the instructor.*]

In this session the students seemed to know the situation that they wanted to discuss, but they did not discuss it perhaps because of their fear of how they thought the instructor might respond. It is to be expected that the situation of the dying patient will arouse varying degrees of anxiety in the instructor, but by diverting the students from expressing their feelings about the death of the patient to a discussion of his parents, Miss Foster side-stepped the real problem concerning the patient and the nurse's role. Her avoidance of the problem may have confirmed the students' feeling that there was a realistic basis for being afraid to express themselves. One result was that they continued to blame the nursing staff because the opportunity for either validating or invalidating the rumor had been eliminated.

This conference also demonstrates how an instructor's own feelings of blame can intrude on her evaluation of a problem presented by students. Miss Foster's anger, which included blaming the nurse who was caring for the patient, may have been a reason for not expressing her feelings to the students. Her tendency to avoid expressing her own reactions and feelings placed the burden of the discussion on the students.

During the six conference experiences that the psychiatric team had with her, it became apparent that Miss Foster withheld her feelings and reactions from the students and consistently threw the leadership back to them. Her chief technique consisted of remaining detached about the topic under discussion. Even if she had reacted negatively, the students would at least have had something concrete and specific to relate and react to, and they would have been enabled to fight back, rebel, accept or reject, or compromise. In these conferences, however, the students had trouble in getting hold of anything substantial in their relationship with Miss Foster. Because it was difficult for them to experience her as a person, they did not always know where they stood with her. Their anxiety was expressed in their effort to be her "pet," because it is probable that from their viewpoint the only alternatives were to be a pet or to be rejected. In this meeting, although apparently in a hurry to leave, the students nevertheless remained and hovered around Miss Foster.

For several moments Miss Foster and the students talk among themselves. Their chitchat is punctuated by laughter. The psychiatric nurse and the psychiatrist wait. Then the students leave for class.

The moment the psychiatric team and Miss Foster are alone a feeling of uneasiness and discomfort settles in like a fog. The three of them try to get set-

tled. They move chairs. One closes the door. Another opens the window only to close it again. The psychiatric nurse adjusts the tape recorder. Miss Foster lights a cigarette and exhales with a sigh. She is the only one smoking. Then she takes off her glasses, energetically wipes them, and then rubs her blue eyes.

MISS FOSTER. I knew the death of Larry was disturbing the students. The doctor was fond of the child. Some of the staff feel he blamed his death on lack of nursing care.

PSYCHIATRIST. Why didn't you let these feelings come out? What is important here is to let the rumors come out in the open so we can find out whether they relate just to Sue Eddy's feeling or if her feelings are shared by the group.

This clinical conference required much more active leadership on your part. Such discussions won't filter back to department heads. The students left here feeling that rumors will be evaded and authorities will pass the buck. It is important to point out that the students may have a realistic basis for resentment.

This kind of conference requires two things of the instructor: She must not dominate the scene, but she must learn how to break through students' conventions and get at their feelings. They don't have courage to get these out themselves.

MISS FOSTER. The nurse who was caring for the child was not equipped to do so. I have such strong feelings about it that maybe I was overcompensating to keep them from coming out. I was afraid I'd slip!

PSYCHIATRIST. I don't feel it's appropriate, Claire, for these specific feelings about the staff to come out, since your reactions are on a different level from the students' because you have more information about the problem. But if you sit on your own feelings concerning the patient's death, the students will sit on theirs.

PSYCHIATRIC NURSE. Giving your own reactions is a way of eliciting feelings from students. Also, it would have been useful if, for example, you had asked Natalie Phelps to tell specifically what rumors she had heard.

PSYCHIATRIST. Because I felt we weren't getting anywhere, I thought that if I threw this point to the students they might get some insight as to whether they were putting the lid on their feelings.

MISS FOSTER. I was afraid if I let the problem of the rumor of negligence come out, I would be on a spot and have to tell what I know.

One goal that the psychiatric team had set in their work with Miss Foster was to help her to resolve some of her negative attitudes toward the psychiatric integration program and themselves. They agreed that for the most part the psychiatric nurse would remain in the background during the evaluation sessions, in the hope that she could establish a beginning basis for Miss Foster's trust and freer communication. The psychiatrist, on the other hand, became more and more direct in his comments to Miss Foster as the series of conferences proceeded.

During this conference, the psychiatrist acted out his negative feelings toward Miss Foster's elusive behavior. Perhaps his feelings were a carryover from the faculty discussions, where, up until this time, the issue of Miss Foster's evasiveness and withdrawal had never been dealt with or resolved (see Chapter 11, faculty discussion, April 6, 1962).

The psychiatrist indicated that the student conference had required more leadership by Miss Foster. He identified Miss Foster's difficulty in revealing herself to the students as the chief stumbling block to her effective leadership of the conferences. He spelled out one aspect of the instructor's role and functions when he made an important distinction between the inappropriateness of an instructor divulging her own negative attitudes about the nursing care given in a specific situation, because these attitudes might or might not have a realistic basis, and her responsibility to give the facts and communicate the impact of the patient's death on herself.

There was little spontaneity and enthusiasm in this evaluation session. For the most part Miss Foster handled her anxiety by lighting one cigarette after another, only to put each one out after one puff. However, she did reveal some of her own feelings about the situation, and her anger began to seep through.

As previously planned, the psychiatric nurse remained in the background. She observed the psychiatrist closely and was attentive to how he was dealing with Miss Foster's elusiveness. She gingerly made a suggestion to Miss Foster at the end of the conference. Although the verbal exchange was limited almost exclusively to Miss Foster and the psychiatrist, Miss Foster occasionally looked at the psychiatric nurse throughout the conference.

OVERPROTECTION AND PREMATURE CLOSURE

Many of the instructors tended to overprotect students from their fears and thereby to stifle the expression of their feelings, especially in situations in which the instructor felt anxious. Three examples of this type of behavior on the part of an instructor are presented here.

Whitewashing Authority Figures. When nursing students reveal to the teacher their negative feelings about other authority figures with whom they are working, the nurse teacher's own unresolved attitudes toward authority are apt to lead her either to close off prematurely the students' expression of such attitudes, or conversely, to feed into the students' negative feelings by joining sides with them against the authority figure under discussion. It was fear of the latter reaction that made the psychiatric nurse's unstructured student group conferences so threatening to the other faculty members. In spite of their intellectual knowledge that the dissociation of negative feelings is likely to prolong and exacerbate the conflict, most of the faculty members continued to operate on the false premise that feelings that are disregarded cease to exist. Miss Harris was confronted with this problem in one of the conferences in which the psychiatric team was participating.

February 8, 1959
This conference is the fifth and last in the series with Miss Harris. At the suggestion of the psychiatric team the tape recorder, which has been an inhibiting factor, has been removed. Participation is limited primarily to two students. The rest withdraw, although some listen. Others are preoccupied and have a far-away expression. No one acknowledges the presence of the psychiatric team.

Miss Harris. What do you want to talk about? The differences between taking care of babies and older children?

Julia Ferris. I like talking to older children.

Connie Vahn. I prefer older children too.

Mercedes Claridge. Miss Harris, you've told us you like older children better too. Why do you?

Miss Harris. I find the growth and development of the child after infancy more interesting. [*She pauses.*] What do you want to talk about today? How about you, Judy [*Whitby*]?
[*Judy Whitby is silent. The other members of the group are silent; their eyes are lowered and there is a general tone of uneasiness.*]

Miss Harris. What do you want to talk about?
[*Silence.*]

Psychiatrist. Am I the inhibiting factor?

Miss Harris. We are working on a play for Lincoln's birthday. Children like to participate in writing a play.

Stephanie Masters. But Miss Harris, we've only been with the older children for two days. We have very few post-op patients who are able to be up and around. Everything is against us.

Miss Harris. After the first time you do a play, it will be easier.
[*Silence.*]

Miss Harris. You don't necessarily have to have a play to entertain the children. You can sing to them [*She sings a song in a soft and dulcet tone.*]
[*Silence. Some shifting in chairs and squirming.*]

Miss Harris. You are not being graded on whether or not you can put on a play.
[*Silence.*]

Julia Ferris. We still haven't decided what we're going to talk about.

Mercedes Claridge. Does Mrs. Wayne have anything to do with our grades?

Miss Harris. No. What makes you ask?

Mercedes Claridge. In front of another supervisor she criticized a student for leaving a dirty pillow case on the chair. And the student didn't do it.

Stephanie Masters. It's a case of being either on the good or bad side of her, so I just avoid her.
[*Dolores Novick is withdrawn and preoccupied as she files her fingernails.*]

Mercedes Claridge. She criticizes students in front of others. I'm afraid of her. She. . . .

Miss Harris [*interrupting*]. You have to remember that Mrs. Wayne is responsible for knowing everything about the total situation, but this is impossible. She really doesn't mean it when she is critical. She just sounds critical. Her bark is worse than her bite. As a matter of fact, she has a wonderful sense of humor, once you get to know her.

MERCEDES CLARIDGE. Maybe so. But she criticizes students in front of others.

[*The psychiatric nurse and psychiatrist exchange glances.*]

MISS HARRIS. We aren't looking for mistakes. We appreciate that you are just learning.

PSYCHIATRIC NURSE. Sometimes humor acts as a mask for hostility and derogation. I wonder if it isn't this that the students are picking up and reacting to.

PSYCHIATRIST. What we are talking about is the element of disrespect. Isabelle [*Harris*] doesn't convey to students that they are inferior because she knows more than they do. The problem is not merely a matter of Mrs. Wayne's irritability and annoyance, but the fact that she equates students with inferiority. She makes people lose face in front of others. Under stress, this underlying attitude of disrespect and being critical may be brought into the open. As students, you already feel somewhat insecure about your own values and strengths in a new clinical experience, which in turn makes you even more vulnerable to being treated as an inferior.

It took a long time to uncover what was bothering the students. Protracted silences were frequent. Miss Harris reacted by trying to reassure the students. They responded with more silence and withdrawal. Anxiety was expressed about meeting Miss Harris' and the nursing staff's expectations.

Miss Harris allowed her own style and spontaneity to come to the fore. She seemed less hampered than some of the other instructors by the presence of the psychiatric team, but she did not use them. The psychiatrist and the psychiatric nurse, who were sitting apart, exchanged occasional glances. The students finally blurted out what was disturbing them. As they struggled to express their feelings, Miss Harris cut them off by trying to present a positive picture.

The students leave in silence. Miss Harris appears preoccupied as she adjusts the comb in her gray chignon. She retreats. An expression of sadness crosses her pale face and she slumps in her chair. There is a long silence. Each one waits for one of the others to speak first.

[*The psychiatric team and Miss Harris are silent.*]

PSYCHIATRIC NURSE. Well, how do you think the conference went?

MISS HARRIS. I do so want the students to enjoy this clinical experience. It upsets me that they don't like Mrs. Wayne.

PSYCHIATRIC NURSE. Hm hm. I know. [*Pause.*] It's not easy. In this conference you were primarily concerned with putting Mrs. Wayne in a good light. You seemed to be defending her to the students.

PSYCHIATRIST. It would be much easier to sum up and see situations such as these in a less personal way. The real reason the students' feelings took a downturn in the first place is that they were cut off before there was opportunity to identify what their feelings were.

PSYCHIATRIC NURSE [*gets up and walks over to the blackboard and draws a diagram*].

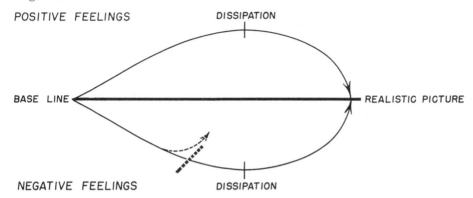

POSITIVE FEELINGS   DISSIPATION

BASE LINE   REALISTIC PICTURE

NEGATIVE FEELINGS   DISSIPATION

This baseline represents equilibrium, the goal of which is to have students view the total picture, to see the reality with a minimum of distortion. Isabelle, you brought the discussion of Mrs. Wayne to the baseline before trying to find out what the negative feelings were about her. Your goal was not to explore Mercedes' [*Claridge*] feelings, but rather to humanize Mrs. Wayne. When the student herself begins to move toward the baseline, then we can help her to look at the positive side of the picture. But if in the attempt to get at the baseline we cut off the negative feelings prematurely, they will continue to simmer underground, as will the unrealistic picture of the person involved. Similarly, a realistic picture cannot be attained as long as an idealized view of the situation and the potentialities are held. [*She sits down.*]

[*Miss Harris listens attentively.*]

PSYCHIATRIST [*gets up and walks to the blackboard*]. In Jane's diagram the point didn't ever evolve at which the students started to move toward the baseline. This is because their negative feelings were interrupted before all of them had been ventilated.

MISS HARRIS. I'm so annoyed with Mercedes [*Claridge*] anyway. She seems to act out all her negative feelings in the clinical situation. Maybe this is one of the reasons I shut her up.

[*Long pause.*]

PSYCHIATRIC NURSE. This is our final session together. It would be helpful to us if you would indicate what you got from these sessions and what wasn't very useful, and also make some suggestions for improvement.

MISS HARRIS. At the conferences in which I was leader I was so involved that I can't remember much. When you and Dr. Ullman were more active, I had a chance to observe. Dr. Ullman's summary today was very helpful. I would like more analysis of my own interaction with students. How do you get at students' deeper feelings?

PSYCHIATRIST. Well, for one thing, you are careful not to insert your own views. You try to get as complete a picture as possible of how, for example, the students see Mrs. Wayne. Eliciting students' feelings is a matter of different emphasis.

MISS HARRIS. There are a lot of other problems going on. There is tension aroused because of a conflict in philosophy between another clinical instructor and myself. Then, too, several in this student group have serious personal problems that spill over into the clinical and teaching setting.

PSYCHIATRIC NURSE. This isn't an easy area to teach in, especially since the student is torn about being a child herself. [*Pause.*] Do you have any suggestions for us that might help our work with the other faculty members?

MISS HARRIS. I think that it would help if you and Dr. Ullman would function as leaders for the first few sessions while the instructor observes, so she can get some pointers. After that, she could step in as leader and try to apply some of what she has learned.

In the beginning of this evaluation period the psychiatric nurse looked to the psychiatrist to initiate the discussion. When his leadership was not forthcoming, she moved in. The mood shifted to one of interest when she drew the diagram on the blackboard.

The members of the psychiatric team were in harmony with each other. All their efforts were directed toward trying to help Miss Harris to use her warmth and sensitivity on a more productive level.

The conference closed on a positive note, with Miss Harris making valuable suggestions for the future. Her suggestions disclosed that the psychiatric team had expected the instructors to perform skillfully before giving them any tangible help.

Exhortation. There are few situations in nursing practice and education that arouse as much anxiety, stir as many feelings of helplessness and hopelessness, and result in as many problems of withdrawal as does the situation presented by a dying patient. Throughout the period of the project this problem came up over and over again in the psychiatric team's work with faculty members and students. On several occasions, some faculty members expressed surprise that even though the topic had been explored repeatedly, the problem continued to exist. There always was the expectation of a final resolution.

The way in which the psychiatric team tried to help an instructor learn to help students meet the problem is illustrated in the following experience.

May 4, 1960

This is Miss Thomas' fourth session in the first series of clinical conferences in which the psychiatric team participated. The students have been having clinical experiences with cancer patients. They appear overwhelmed by these experiences. One student completely withdraws. Others sit back and passively observe. Miss Thomas speaks in a very low voice, which at times is almost inaudible. She keeps brushing aside a strand of her black hair from her forehead.

MISS THOMAS. What do you want to discuss today?

[*Silence.*]

MISS THOMAS. Why don't each of you tell us the kind of patients you are taking care of and how you feel about them. How about you, Alice [*Kane*]?

EVE DERRICK. I feel like I have cancer on the brain.

ALICE KANE. At this hospital, all the patients have cancer. It scares me.

EVELYN SAUNDERS. It is so difficult to be reassuring, and I'm unable to do anything that really helps.

SELMA KRUTHERS. I'm scared for myself. I don't know how I'll take care of patients, because I don't feel confident.

ALICE KANE. I'm afraid they will ask questions about whether they have cancer. I feel on edge! I am afraid I'll say something wrong and that I won't be able to get out of the middle.

ARLENE PRESTON. What makes me leery is the patient's depression. I don't know how to give him something to live for.

MISS THOMAS. Is the problem you want to discuss today—how to nurse a patient who won't get well?

SELMA KRUTHERS. I came into nursing feeling that I wanted to help patients get well. I learned that we can help patients feel less alone, but I'm not so sure about our ability to do this. I feel uncertain about what we can talk about and how far we can go. When a patient accepts dying, is this easier for him than when he has something else to blame dying on?

MISS THOMAS. Alice [*Kane*], maybe it would help to give a specific patient situation.

ALICE KANE. I took care of Mr. Warner.

MISS HUNT. Was the patient satisfied afterwards? Did you feel satisfied?

ALICE KANE. The patient died the following day.

PSYCHIATRIC NURSE. How did this make you feel?

ALICE KANE. I felt sad. Later, I realized that considering his condition, death was best for him.

EVELYN SAUNDERS. I'm not as concerned when a patient can't talk. Then I can do all the giving. I don't have to worry about being on the spot.

MISS THOMAS. Could you expand on that? What were you afraid of?

EVELYN SAUNDERS. I didn't realize death could occur so rapidly. And to someone so young.

MISS THOMAS. Having cancer doesn't automatically mean a person is going to die. What would you say when a patient asks you, "Am I going to die?"

PSYCHIATRIC NURSE. Linda [*Thomas*], could you speak louder?

SELMA KRUTHERS. I would say, "You mean because you have leukemia you think you are dying?"

SHARON TEELEY. I'd say something like, "With any blood dyscrasia, you are bound to feel fatigued."

ALICE KANE. I'd tend to leave it alone. I'm scared of it.

MISS THOMAS. An important aspect of nursing patients who have cancer is to share everything with the doctor, especially what you told the patient. It also is necessary to find out from him what and how much he has told the patient about his condition and the patient's response. All of this information should be put on the Kardex so the nursing staff will know what to do. [*Her tapered fingernails tap her arm rest.*] We also can help the patient by fostering whatever religious beliefs he has. All of this helps. It is essential for all of us to work together.

PSYCHIATRIC NURSE. The time is just about up, Linda.

MISS THOMAS. Do you think this discussion has helped you at all?

[*Silence.*]

MISS THOMAS. We have to try to see how we can be the most helpful to the patient.

ALICE KANE. I feel better because now I know I'm not alone. Everyone has the same problem.

The key issue in this conference was how the nurse can give hope to the dying patient. Neither Miss Thomas nor the students were able to pinpoint a specific situation. No one looked to either member of the psychiatric team for help.

Miss Thomas was in tune with the students' sense of helplessness in responding to patients who are dying of cancer. She dealt with the essential aspect of the students' fear of what to say. However, in her desire to reassure the students she did not pursue this aspect deeply enough, but instead, exhorted them to help, to communicate, and to utilize religious beliefs. The students left the conference in much the same mood in which they came to it.

> *After the students leave the room, there is a long silence. The atmosphere is oppressive. Several minutes are spent in trying to adjust the ventilation. As the psychiatric nurse lights a cigarette, the psychiatrist, with a sheepish grin, asks her for one, too. She teases him about not smoking. Miss Thomas watches the psychiatric nurse's face intently. She sighs as she tugs at an earring in her pierced ear. Finally, the three get settled.*

[*Silence. The psychiatric nurse lights a cigarette.*]

PSYCHIATRIST. How about my bumming one from you. [*He grins.*]

PSYCHIATRIC NURSE. Monte! I thought you had quit smoking.

[*Long silence.*]

PSYCHIATRIC NURSE. How do you think the conference went today, Linda?

MISS THOMAS [*sighs deeply*]. I want so much to help the students.

PSYCHIATRIC NURSE. Hmmmm. I know. [*Pause.*] Eve Derrick, who first raised the problem of patients with cancer, went mute. She was very much involved; however, Linda [*Thomas*], you didn't seem clear about what to do about her.

PSYCHIATRIST. Linda, you raised the essential question. The point is, did you emphasize it enough? The key question here is—"What does the patient want?" He wants hope. Hope that he doesn't have cancer or hope that he won't die. The only valid guideline in working with these patients is to put into practice the idea of instilling hope.

PSYCHIATRIC NURSE. You know, there was one point that was not clarified. Although Linda gave the students some of the guiding principles through which to screen their responses, we did not get to what holds them back in responding to cancer patients.

PSYCHIATRIST. The students' fear of lying, deceit, indirection. This has to be explored with them. There is a difference between lying on a personal level and lying to help the patient struggle more effectively.

MISS THOMAS. Dr. Stone does this with all his patients. I don't approve of lying to patients. I never have had to be defensive with patients. You don't have to be if you can justify your own conscience.

PSYCHIATRIST. You can lie by leaving things out.

MISS THOMAS. But then you aren't stating the truth.

PSYCHIATRIC NURSE. Students think of a lie in terms of black and white. We need to help them use truth in a rather indirect and evasive way.

MISS THOMAS. I don't agree.

PSYCHIATRIST. The physician has only two choices in situations such as these. The first is to help the patient face the issue. The second is to help him evade death. This involves conscious espousal of the patient's denial.

PSYCHIATRIC NURSE. Because we teach students to be conscientious and forthright, espousing the denial is apt to be equated with lying.

PSYCHIATRIST. The problem is not fear of death but, rather, living with the knowledge of impending death. The human being is the only animal exposed to this kind of fear. One can live with this knowledge if one has lived a full life.

PSYCHIATRIC NURSE. When a person cannot live with the knowledge of death, this is where the nurse comes in. She is the one person who is the closest to the patient in terms of time and physical proximity. In taking care of him, she participates with him in the physical activities of living. In this way the nurse can help the patient experience hope in living by supporting his denial.

PSYCHIATRIST. It's also important to mobilize the patient's religious feeling. But neither can you make such feeling exist when it doesn't.

[*Miss Thomas listens attentively, with hands folded and nods.*]

PSYCHIATRIC NURSE. We have to help students understand that fear of death is based on emotional separation rather than physical death. Generally, the danger of death happens only once to a patient. Once the patient has died, he is not there to know about it.

PSYCHIATRIST. Yes, and then he doesn't know the course that is to follow. He will confront the nurse to get a negation, a denial. Our evasion of the patient means affirmation of death to him. The choice for the patient is to give up or to struggle. If the patient has intuitive awareness that the struggle still ends up in death, he may want a way out of the struggle. He may ask the nurse's permission to give up. Giving up results in depression and apathy, which are emotional suicide.

The dying patient is concerned with a problem in living—his finiteness. He doesn't have the liberty of indulging in the fantasies about the future as do other patients.

MISS THOMAS [*attentive*]. Hm, hm.

PSYCHIATRIC NURSE. It sounds as if you are talking about the dying patient experiencing time in a way that is different from the person who is well.

PSYCHIATRIST [*gets up and goes over to the blackboard*]. Try to imagine that each of us has a built-in hourglass. I'll put three on the blackboard. The first represents time as it is experienced by the well person. The second, by the dying patient who does not have cancer, and the third, by the dying patient who does have cancer. Because the well person is involved in all the various activities of living, he is unaware that the sand of time is running. He therefore doesn't have to see that his built-in hourglass is slowly emptying.

In the case of the patient who has an illness which eventually will terminate with his death, his living activities may be somewhat limited. Hence, he becomes more aware that the sand is moving. But just so long as there still is sand left in his hourglass, the patient does not see the hourglass itself. To the degree that this patient is able to be involved in other activities, the hourglass becomes obscured, if not invisible.

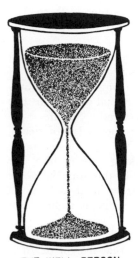 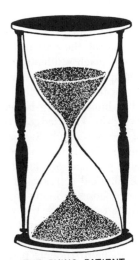 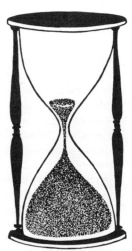

THE WELL PERSON   THE DYING PATIENT WITHOUT CANCER   THE DYING PATIENT WITH CANCER

With the patient who has cancer, the physically destructive aspects of the disease decrease the possibility for him to participate in activities of living. He becomes aware that the sand has almost run out. As his hourglass becomes empty, it becomes more visible to him. On some level, he becomes aware that for him time is almost at an end. He sees nothing but imminent physical destruction. He then can either face death or deny it. The degree to which the patient has lived a full life in the past will influence his reaction to the reality of time running out. It will directly affect the degree of recognition or denial utilized by him.

[*Miss Thomas and the psychiatric nurse, pensive and interested, nod to each other in agreement. Miss Thomas looks to the psychiatric nurse as if asking her for something.*]

PSYCHIATRIC NURSE. In regard to the patient who is dying from cancer, then the task of the nurse is to provide a framework for the patient in which the hopelessness is reduced and from which some hope can spring.

PSYCHIATRIST. Exactly.

[*Miss Thomas nods in agreement.*]

PSYCHIATRIC NURSE. This is more or less difficult depending on the nurse's own conscious and unconscious feelings about death, which would hinge on how full a life she herself has lived in the past and is living today.

MISS THOMAS. One of the ways we can build a framework of hope for the dying patient is to utilize his religious beliefs.

PSYCHIATRIC NURSE. Very true. But it also is easy to get boxed in by one's religious beliefs.

What strikes me most about our conference today is that the nurse can be the key figure in the life of the dying patient.

PSYCHIATRIST. This is the reality. When a patient dies, the family, because of their somatic preoccupations, tend to fade into the background. The doctor, who may see the patient several times a day, isn't of much help because he can't alter the course of disease. So it is the nurse who becomes the single, most important person in the patient's life. Regardless of the pain in dying, the patient experiences less pain to the degree that he can share it with this one person—the nurse.

In this evaluation conference the members of the psychiatric team were chiefly concerned with helping Miss Thomas to create an operational framework of realistic hope for the dying patient. Their emphasis was on the issue of how to shift from a moralistic appraisal of what the dying patient's needs should be (which, in essence, are merely an echo of the nurse's needs) to what the patient himself wants and needs. The psychiatrist identifies some of the psychodynamics underlying the experience of dying. The psychiatric nurse translated these into the nursing role. The psychiatric nurse and the psychiatrist demonstrated different roles and functions which complemented each other. Together they exerted an influence that neither could have accomplished alone.

Many emotions were experienced—resignation, self-righteous indignation, hopelessness, sadness, tenderness, and, finally, hope. Among this threesome, the drama of caring for the dying patient was partially re-enacted.

"Reassurance" and Missing the Problem. The tendency to overprotect students, particularly in discussions of anxiety-laden topics, was so persistent among the instructors that the members of the psychiatric team often found it desirable to intervene in the student conferences even after the instructor was supposedly ready to assume the leadership without help. The second series of conferences with Miss Jensen furnishes a case in point.

Miss Jensen had volunteered early to have this experience with the psychiatric team. She put great emphasis on wanting help from the psychiatric team and repeatedly stated that she was eager for constructive criticism. She seemed to be seeking the approval of both the psychiatric team members and the total faculty by being among the first to have this experience. During her first series of conferences with the team she sought an individual conference with the psychiatrist to discuss her progress. (However, after one occasion in which the psychiatrist pointed up some areas for improvement, she directly attacked the psychiatrist in a faculty group meeting [see Chapter 8, July 14, 1959]).

Shortly before the conference that is being presented the members of the psychiatric team had a briefing session with Miss Jensen in which they reiterated the goals of the conference, reclarified their own roles and stressed how important it was for her to orient the students. All three agreed that Miss Jensen would take the leadership and call on the psychiatric team when she felt need of their contributions.

October 12, 1960
This is the first session in the second series of conferences with Miss Jensen. It is also the first time that these students have had contact with the psychiatrist. No explanation is given regarding the purposes of the conferences, the reasons for the psychiatric team's presence, or the use of the tape recorder.

Miss Jensen shifts in her chair, as her blonde ponytail swings from side to side. Although the surface atmosphere is one of friendliness and spontaneity, there is an undercurrent of tense guardedness.

MISS JENSEN. For the next six sessions, Dr. Ullman and Miss Schmahl will be with us. You've all had Miss Schmahl before, so you know what these classes are all about, don't you?
[*Members of the group nod in agreement.*]
MISS JENSEN. You all know Dr. Ullman?
GROUP. We've seen him around.
PSYCHIATRIST. Hi!
MISS JENSEN. Okay. Very good! You can discuss whatever you want to. What would you like to talk about today?
JO NISTROM. I had a lot of reactions to a patient I was taking care of. But I'm not taking care of him any longer. How friendly should you be with patients?
ROSE MORRIS. I wonder about our relationships with personnel. Everything is so disorganized.
MISS JENSEN. Any other problems?
[*Natalie Phelps raises her hand.*]
MISS JENSEN. Yes, Natalie, honey.
NATALIE PHELPS. Maybe we could talk about the organization of the clinical unit.
PSYCHIATRIC NURSE. I'm not exactly clear. How is this a problem?
NATALIE PHELPS. You feel helpless up there. Everything is so disorganized that there's no place to go.
[*Silence.*]
[*Miss Jensen's green eyes meet those of the psychiatric nurse.*]
PSYCHIATRIC NURSE. Why not talk about the most embarrassing and humiliating experience you have had this week?
VERA BOND. I have a patient who is dying. What do you do with a patient when so many modifications of care have to be made? What's wrong with me that I'm having so much trouble? His stomach is distended. His teeth aren't in.

He's grotesque looking. I'm afraid of hurting him and of pushing him toward death sooner.

Jo Nistrom. You have to ask for help in turning him. What about his eating if his teeth aren't in? I don't see why we put the patient through so much suffering when there's no hope.

Rose Morris. Our goal in nursing is to preserve life. We are so green.

Miss Jensen. This patient needs a lot of physical care. If the nurses don't take care of him, who will?

Psychiatrist. Vera, was it your patient's appearance or the fact that he is dying that makes you afraid?

Vera Bond. His appearance.

Psychiatric Nurse. Before you ever saw the patient, how did you feel about being assigned to take care of him?

Vera Bond. I had heard about him. I dreaded it.

Rose Morris. His appearance is much worse than it was one week ago.

Polly Hadley. How can he still be alive and look like this? I find myself referring to him as "it" instead of "he."

Beatrice Kaplan. He looks sick. But I expected to see something else—to look like he was in pain or frightened.

Natalie Phelps. The sight of him didn't bother me so much. It's more the thought of death itself.

Psychiatrist. Don't you expect a person who is dying to be human?

Natalie Phelps. I expect that dying patients won't be able to talk or to relate with me.

[*Miss Jensen squirms in her chair and peels her nail polish.*]

Psychiatrist. A dying patient can die in a moment or two months later. You tend to assume that the dying patient is on his last leg.

Psychiatric Nurse. If your own anxiety gets in the way, you will become more timid in handling the patient. Why assume that taking care of the patient is "pushing"? And therefore, death will come, now?

Vera Bond. I was all shook up after taking care of him.

Rose Morris. This throws me.

Polly Hadley. It's such a shock.

[*Silence.*]

Psychiatric Nurse. Try to describe what it is that shocks you and throws you.

Natalie Phelps. It's being taken off guard.

Vera Bond. I cried.

Psychiatric Nurse. How come?

Vera Bond. I got something out of my system.

Psychiatric Nurse. Like what?

Vera Bond. Fear of contributing to his death.

Jo Nistrom. Aren't there times we should leave the patient alone?

Miss Jensen. You have to modify the care so you don't create more physical exertion for the patient.

Jo Nistrom. What's the sense of beating my head against the wall? I think he should be left alone.

Psychiatrist. Are you asking, "Does a patient who has multiple fractures and pain, for example, have to have nursing care? Are you setting up the dying patient as a special case? Are you assuming that when a patient is in distress he doesn't want to be bothered?

Jo Nistrom. With the dying patient, the care is without any purpose. It won't get him well. With the patient with fractures, pain has a purpose.

Psychiatric Nurse. I get a feeling of a difference between the technical use of the word *dying* and the process of dying, which is part of living.

Psychiatrist. We can't know sometimes at the moment when someone is dying. There are people on the street who are dying. Another kind of dying is where a person is dying, in a more literal and immediate sense. Should medical and nursing procedures be modified only because the patient is labeled as "dying"?

Psychiatric Nurse. What are your feelings about dying?

Jo Nistrom. I think of it in terms of the patient—his spirit. If the patient has given up the struggle and is apathetic, shouldn't the nurse go along with this?

Psychiatrist. How can you give hope to the patient?

Jo Nistrom. By comforting him—by being neither positive nor negative.

Psychiatrist. The question before the nurse is, what do you expect to give the dying patient? Lasting life?

Psychiatric Nurse. The basic question here seems to be: Whose judgment is the basis for giving nursing care, the patient's or the nurse's? The nurse's role is to help the patient change his feelings of futility. By not accepting the patient's feelings of hopelessness, she gives hope.

Vera Bond. You are saying that with improvement in our own attitudes the patient may get better physically?

Psychiatric Nurse. No. The nurse has to have realistic goals. Part of the nursing responsibility is to help the patient cope with dying. This is the problem.

Jo Nistrom. Then we should impose our attitudes on the patient, regardless.

Miss Jensen. Okay, kids. We have to stop now.

[*Students stay behind and ask Miss Jensen questions regarding clinical assignments and what to do about things they don't know how to do.*]

At the beginning of this conference the students pulled topics out of the air. With the help of the psychiatric nurse they finally chose the topic of the dying patient.

The anxiety was so high that both Miss Jensen and the students attempted to block out feelings about the dying patient by looking for hope in the specifics of what to do. Miss Jensen and the psychiatric team were working at cross-purposes. Because of the longer-than-usual association between Miss Jensen and the psychiatric team, Miss Jensen's difficulty in leading this particular conference, and the intensity of the students' feelings, the psychiatric team took a more active part than the plans had called for.

The student Jo Nistrom became engaged in a contest with the psychiatrist. As the student's anger increased, Miss Jensen continued to recede into the background until finally she completely abdicated her role as leader. The final note of the conference was a challenge to the psychiatrist by the student.

After the students leave, Miss Jensen plunks down in the chair next to the psychiatric nurse. As the psychiatrist begins to talk, she starts again to pick at her nail polish. She looks at him and appears to be listening attentively. She nods in agreement. Her deep sighs are punctuated by murmurs of "hm," "hm."

PSYCHIATRIC NURSE. Dot [*Jensen*], you need to be more explicit about the purpose of these conferences to students and about what Monte's and my roles are. As soon as I asked them what had been embarrassing, they got the point. It was necessary to deflect Jo Nistrom who wanted to get into physical care, which got away from the students' reactions.

MISS JENSEN. But when do you discuss the problem of nursing care?

PSYCHIATRIC NURSE. At this point it was more important to pursue the students' reactions and their concept of dying. These were getting in the way of their giving the nursing care the patient needs.

MISS JENSEN. I'm inclined to jump the gun too soon. I have a feeling of what is bothering the students and I want to move on. I don't see any point in beating a dead horse.

PSYCHIATRIST. Jo Nistrom's statement about routinely impersonalizing a nurse-patient relationship is irrelevant. The problem was not under what conditions care should be modified. Jo was saying, "I have a gripe." She was only interested in the position of how care should be modified.

PSYCHIATRIC NURSE. She was all involved in a tangential aspect of the problem. It was not central.

PSYCHIATRIST. The problem here and now is the students' feelings and reactions to dying. What is your reaction to this?

PSYCHIATRIC NURSE. I wonder what the point is of our eliciting students' feelings and how it all adds up if the instructor cuts the feelings off. How about it, Dot?

MISS JENSEN. Feelings, yes. But it is also important to give them reassurance. They all realized that they felt helpless.

PSYCHIATRIST. But they do not recognize the underlying feeling of helplessness. They rationalize it. Jo [*Nistrom*] was offering a program of action which was a way of covering up her own feelings of helplessness. . . .

PSYCHIATRIC NURSE. They used the terms *shocked, surprised, thrown* to label the dying patient.

PSYCHIATRIST. The patient's appearance, because of elements of strangeness such as the ascites, makes the nurse feel helpless. The label *critical* that we attach to the dying patient, as well as "Last Rites," influences the nurse's feelings of helplessness.

PSYCHIATRIC NURSE. The instructor's task is to link the student's feelings of helplessness to what she can do, rather than doing nothing.

By jumping the gun, Dot, you end up reading into a situation what isn't there, as in this case when you assumed the students recognized their feelings of helplessness. At the same time you also miss what exists in the situation, because you aren't listening to it or looking for it. You know, when the three of us worked together the first time two years ago, one of the things to come out was your tendency to overprotect students.

MISS JENSEN. I think what happened today is some of the same thing.

During this evaluation conference Miss Jensen became defensive about eliciting students' feelings, because she believed she knew what they were feeling without any exploration. She stressed the desirability of reassuring the students. She agreed that she might tend to overprotect students. The meeting closed with surface agreement.

The overall quality and direction of Miss Jensen's functioning in this kind of conference revealed her tendency to overprotect students from their fears and thereby to cut off their feelings. Her surface acceptance of the students' feelings continued to cover authoritarian and controlling attitudes toward them.

Such attitudes posed several disquieting questions which had broad implications for the integration project as a whole. What was a faculty member's investment in acquiring psychiatric knowledge and techniques? Was the wish to emulate the psychiatric team tied to helping students grow? Were some faculty members seeking to use psychiatric knowledge primarily as a mechanistic gimmick for self-aggrandizement and for the achievement of power? These were some of the questions about which the psychiatric nurse developed misgivings as the project progressed.

ALIENATION OF STUDENTS

April 15, 1959
This is Miss Drew's fifth conference in the first series.

MISS DREW. What would you like to discuss today?
[*Silence.*]
MISS DREW. How about Mrs. Seward? She has been causing a lot of concern to everyone.
[*Silence.*]
MISS DREW. Well, if not Mrs. Seward, how about Mrs. Hallery?
[*The members of the group shake their heads in the negative.*]
MISS DREW. I don't know then.
NANCY SPIEGEL. Well, here I go with both feet. It isn't patients that are bothering us. It's the atmosphere on the clinical unit.
MISS DREW [*begins to squirm in chair*]. Jane, is it all right if we discuss this here?
[*All turn and face the psychiatric nurse.*]
PSYCHIATRIC NURSE. It probably is a good idea, Eileen [*Drew*], especially since this is what seems to be on the students' minds.
ANN CLIFFORD. I get the feeling that the nursing staff feels we are in the way. It's an intangible kind of thing. All I know is I give a great deal of myself.
MISS DREW. How about you, Nancy? You brought up the problem.
NANCY SPIEGEL. I feel ill at ease, as though I'm only a nuisance.
JUNE TRAVIS. I didn't like it, Miss Drew, when you told the juniors who are team leaders that we aren't adequate.
MISS DREW. I was referring to the fact that the junior students, instead of working with the total staff, work almost exclusively with the sophomore students.

NANCY SPIEGEL. You were talking about the juniors being inadequate as team leaders?

MISS DREW. That's right.

NANCY SPIEGEL. This kind of reputation can spread to other clinical areas. We were told by another student group that we are snobs. Are we being aggressive?

ANN CLIFFORD. We aren't allowed to assist the doctors with treatments, like taking blood or helping with bone marrows. Sophomores aren't given enough responsibility. . . .

MISS DREW [interrupts]. Is this also a problem in assignments?

ANN CLIFFORD. I feel there is no point in wanting to learn if you can't use it on the unit.

JUNE TRAVIS. There was more physical care in other experiences.

MISS DREW. Does nursing only consist of the physical?

NANCY SPIEGEL. We're insecure with the emotional aspects.

ANN CLIFFORD. We keep telling the head nurse we want to assist. We feel defensive when we sit in the nurses' station with nothing to do.

LOUISE ATKINS. We want to be busy, but don't know how to go about it.

MISS DREW. Why hasn't all of this come up earlier? If Nancy [Spiegel] hadn't brought it up, it probably wouldn't have come up at all.

JUNE TRAVIS. We don't want to jump to conclusions. We've been trying to work it out ourselves.

MISS DREW. What can we do?

NANCY SPIEGEL. I don't know, because I don't know how we are accepted by the staff.

EDITH HALL. Is it just us who aren't accepted, or the whole department?

JUNE TRAVIS. Other students have gotten along.

MISS DREW. How do each of you feel you are accepted? Any concrete illustrations that we aren't? Have you ever felt this way in your other clinical experiences? Some of you have worked on this unit before. What is the difference now?

LOUISE ATKINS. It was better before. We've tried so hard to do well.

ANN CLIFFORD. I have worked well with individual staff members but not with them as a group.

MISS DREW. You are liked by the staff. They do look forward to seeing you. At times they get annoyed as I did this morning when you just stand around. We have attempted to give you more responsibility. On the whole, your organizational skills are good. Some not so good, but this can be expected. Yesterday, I walked into the utility room which was like "The Wreck of the Hesperus." Yet all of you were sitting around looking pretty, as though there was nothing to do. Should your assignments be heavier?

NANCY SPIEGEL. It's mostly on us.

PSYCHIATRIC NURSE. I'm puzzled about what is happening here. The group is uncomfortable, but we don't know why. Is the inability or difficulty in finding what to do the real problem? There is an irritant. What is it? I don't think we've put our finger on the real problem.

MISS DREW. I don't think we have either.

[Janet Smoler, a student, joins the conference and sits down.]

PSYCHIATRIST. Are there any particular members of the staff that you feel have a "chip on their shoulders"?

JUNE TRAVIS. I don't even know the head nurse. I haven't seen her function as a nurse.

NANCY SPIEGEL. I like her better than the rest of the staff.

ANN CLIFFORD. The head nurse studies our faces every time she asks us to do something, as though she expects us not to want to do it.

MISS DREW. Have you always been willing?

GROUP [in unison]. Yes.

ANN CLIFFORD. Miss Yeager isn't liked.

NANCY SPIEGEL. She seeks power. She's always directing.

MISS DREW. What does this do to you? We have to know!

[Long silence.]

JUNE TRAVIS. There's another aspect we haven't gotten to. This is the clinical experience where students get sorted out. This is the real place a student is tested.

MISS DREW [Her brown eyes look pleadingly at the psychiatric nurse]. Jane! Will you please help me?

PSYCHIATRIC NURSE. I think we ought to get down to what the rumors are. What have you been hearing?

MISS DREW. This is exactly why I mentioned staff. This is what I've been trying to get at. You have mentioned everyone except one person—me. I'm the problem. Can we shift to this now?

NANCY SPIEGEL. I'll kill you kids.

JUNE TRAVIS. Okay. I'll start. We don't know where we stand with you.

PSYCHIATRIST. I'm clearer now. What the students are asking is quite simple. They want more direct and concrete evaluation all along the way—good and bad. When the student is vague about where she stands, her own anxieties and distortions take over.

PSYCHIATRIC NURSE. We saw this kind of distortion in the students' fear of dismissal.

JUNE TRAVIS. We need to be guided as things are happening. In our nursing care conference, I felt I needed more guidance.

MISS DREW. But, June, you functioned very well.

The students had tremendous difficulty in choosing a topic for discussion. They rejected Miss Drew's suggestions. After choosing a topic, they talked around it. There seemed to be some friction on the surface. The students were bright, interested, and eager, and they endeavored to get out what was gnawing at them. Something kept holding them back. Miss Drew was putting them on the defensive. In her annoyance, she became aloof and cold and pushed the students away. Her pent-up anger had alienated the students, who responded by "waiting to be bounced."

With some support from the psychiatric team, the students did not retreat; they struggled to get closer to Miss Drew and to tell her what was wrong. Miss Drew became uneasy and cried out to the psychiatric nurse for help.

The problem finally erupted into the open. For the students and their instructor, new possibilities for change and growth were born.

From the students' reactions to their clinical experience, it appeared that in her withdrawal from the students, Miss Drew may also have abdicated some of her authority and responsibility for selecting and guiding student assignments in the clinical setting, in favor of the head nurse. One of the most significant aspects of this meeting was Miss Drew's willingness to seek help directly from the psychiatric nurse. However, the psychiatric nurse, in her myopic view of the disruptive process that was going on in the faculty group, temporarily overlooked Miss Drew's change and growth (see Chapter 8, July 19, 1960).

The psychiatric nurse, the psychiatrist, and the instructor are alone. Miss Drew is deep in thought, her short legs extended before her and her blonde head resting on her hand. She stares at the psychiatric nurse with a sad smile. She glances at the psychiatrist, and he glances at the psychiatric nurse. Miss Drew sighs and lights a cigarette. Despite the pensive silence, there is an air of expectancy.

PSYCHIATRIST. I'll tell you what I think has happened. In your exploration of the problem you put the students on the defensive.

MISS DREW. I could kick myself for not having had a conference about what went on in the clinical setting.

PSYCHIATRIC NURSE. This really isn't the problem.

PSYCHIATRIST. There seems to be something in your attitude that is a little aloof and standoffish. You stand back and tell the students what's wrong with them after the incident is all over. Now they are waiting for this. Your insecurities as a teacher make you defensive. The students have picked up both the aloofness and insecurity.

The students aren't asking you to be Pollyanna-ish. It is better to get angry at the time than to allow the anger to build up and then get annoyed at the students. You put the initiative on the students such as when you asked them why they don't bring the problem up in a conference with you. This really is a matter for your initiative.

MISS DREW. Why has this happened with this group and not others?

PSYCHIATRIC NURSE. This is a pretty eager and sharp group, Eileen. They want more from you. You don't step in early enough and tell them what's wrong so new ways of learning can be opened up. Because these students are bright, they will run into different kinds of problems. Their standing around doesn't mean lack of interest or initiative, but rather fear of incurring your ill will by making a mistake.

PSYCHIATRIST. Since the students have been described as "instructor-oriented," this needs to be taken up with them directly.

MISS DREW. I feel the students keep busy as long as I am around, but that they avoid working when I am not.

PSYCHIATRIC NURSE. It is quite possible that the students feel you and the staff have joined sides against them, in which case they would fear the staff also.

MISS DREW. Where do I go from here?

[*Long silence.*]

PSYCHIATRIC NURSE. A giant step has been taken in helping the problem by the students' talking about the feelings that alienate them from you.

PSYCHIATRIST. The students want you to be direct. When you are annoyed, you can't be positive. Annoyance involves aloofness, coldness, and judgment. Annoyance is associated with the removal of the instructor. A good teacher is one who can call a spade a spade; get angry when it is called for in response to the actual situation. When you aren't direct, your responses to the students are out of context. The immediate critical situation no longer is the real situation. All situations become generalized with feelings of anger, annoyance, impatience, and so on.

[*Thoughtful pause.*]

PSYCHIATRIC NURSE. Do you overestimate the students' own initiative? I think that all of us are guilty of expecting students to be able to do certain things without our ever having taught them. They need some spelling out.

PSYCHIATRIST. When students pick up your feelings of annoyance, the question arises in their minds, "When will I get bounced?" As humans, we are not indoctrinated toward being direct with critical feelings. You need to shift your orientation of "What bad is going to come out in these clinical conferences and how will Jane, the students, and Monte put me on the defensive?" to "How can I use these conferences in a way that will help me achieve more satisfaction from my relationships with students?"

Understandably, Miss Drew responded to the team's directness with some defensiveness. When, however, it was pointed out that the students were expressing the desire to be close to her and were asking her to give more of herself, a new dimension was added to the picture. There were moments of self-blame, of anger, of hurt, of disappointment, of shame, of trust, of hope. The three participated in the painful and moving discovery of the self.

The essence of Miss Drew's problem was her insecurity as a teacher. This difficulty was not unique to her, although her willingness to face the problem and to work on it with the psychiatric team was by no means usual.

This particular group of students had integrated many of the principles of effective communication into their own behavior. Their struggle to deal with the difficulties in their relationship with authority figures was a demonstration of one of the objectives of psychiatric integration—the development of the ability to communicate with authority figures.

Up until this time, Miss Drew had had an on-the-fence attitude toward the integration program. From this point on, however, she was very responsive to the suggestions of the psychiatric team and demonstrated numerous sources of potential and growth. Because the psychiatric nurse and the psychiatrist were able to overlook her surface rigidities and to focus on the positive aspects of her behavior, they were successful in helping her to work on a very productive level.

The benefits realized by an instructor were related more to her attitudes toward the experience and her capacity for change than to the amount of information and knowledge that she acquired. In the beginning of this experience it was not possible for the psychiatric team to ascertain which instructors would be most likely to be helped by it. If the team had been able to pick up clues about this matter, priority should have been given to those instructors who gave the greatest promise of growth.

REFERENCE

1. Bateson, Gregory, et al. "Toward a Theory of Schizophrenia," *Behavioral Sciences*, Vol. 1, pp. 251–264, 1956.

Chapter Eight

THE WORK WITH THE FACULTY
GROUP: THE STAGE OF IMPACT

Great ideas, it has been said, come into the world as gently as
doves. Perhaps then, if we listen attentively, we shall hear, amid
the uproar of empires and nations, a faint flutter of wings, the
gentle stirring of life and hope. Some will say that this hope lies
in a nation; others, in a man. I believe rather that it is awakened,
revived, nourished by millions of solitary individuals whose
deeds and works every day negate frontiers and the crudest
implications of history. As a result, there shines forth fleetingly
the ever threatened truth that each and every man, on the foundation of his own sufferings and joys, builds for all.

ALBERT CAMUS, *Resistance, Rebellion and Death*

Unless the faculty member is free to communicate with her
colleagues on a rational basis—in light of the professional problems under
discussion—not much integration can occur. As has been pointed out, during
the first year of the project the psychiatric nurse recognized that the faculty
members felt they were not sufficiently free to communicate with each other,
and the individual was inclined to be subservient to group values and pressures. Frequently, decisions were made not on the basis of a rational course
of action for the problem at hand, but rather, in regard to what the younger
or older group advocated or seemed to advocate. It was in consideration of
the problems of communication within the faculty group that the original
conception of psychiatric integration as primarily a curriculum study was
broadened to a participant-observational study of faculty and faculty-student
interaction.

Because a considerable emphasis was put on the faculty in the integration
program and this emphasis continued throughout the project, the process of

psychiatric integration will be described and analyzed largely in relation to the faculty group discussions. The uniqueness of this approach is another reason for emphasizing the faculty discussions in this book. As the eight reports of other integration projects reveal, this book is the only one that identifies the process in step-by-step sequence by which the faculty and the project staff became integrated with each other.

The psychiatric nurse's and the psychiatrist's work with the faculty in the group discussions associated with the project was characterized by a three-stage dialectical process.* These may be summed up under the headings of:

1. *Stage of Impact: Initial Presenting Attitudes* (the second year), or the period in which the faculty members felt the initial effect of the introduction of an integration program, the shift of the psychiatric nurse's role from peer to leader, and what these changes might mean to them.

2. *Stage of Recoil: Reactive Phase* (the third year), or the period in which the faculty members, as they became aware of the necessity for their own involvement and commitment to the work of the project, rejected it.

3. *Stage of Synthesis: Resolution Through Change and Growth* (the fourth and fifth years), or the period in which a higher order of explicit communication among the faculty members and the psychiatric team was achieved, and a time in which the psychiatrist and the psychiatric nurse became synthesized into an interdisciplinary team.

The general pattern in which the three-stage process evolved in the project will be considered within the context of the faculty group discussions.

Initiation of the Faculty Discussions

In accordance with the plan drafted by the psychiatric team at the end of the first year and accepted by the faculty, arrangements were made for weekly one-hour meetings of the entire faculty and the psychiatric team. Attendance at these meetings was required of each faculty member.

When these meetings were started, at the beginning of the second year of the project, there were eleven full-time faculty members in addition to the psychiatric nurse. Since the end of the first year, one member had resigned and had been replaced. Five of them were members of the older group, and six of them, including one new member who was assuming the clinical teaching responsibilities formerly carried by the psychiatric nurse, belonged to the younger group.

The purposes of these discussions were to provide the participants with an opportunity:

* At the end of the five-year period of the first grant, these stages of faculty group interactional process were identified by the psychiatrist.

1. To explore, with the help of experts in psychiatry and psychiatric nursing, the interpersonal problems as they emerged in the professional experience of the nurse as a student, as a nurse, as a teacher of nurses, and as a colleague, and to learn to handle these effectively through the application of psychiatric concepts to the teaching-learning process.

2. To explore together the interaction process among colleagues in a live situation and to become aware of how the group was functioning, so that there would be greater participation on the part of all the members and that the group would function more effectively.

STRUCTURE AND SUBJECT MATTER

Although the psychiatric team at times prepared suggestions to be taken up at the meetings, there generally was no agenda. Frequently they were unstructured, with the goal of a given meeting evolving out of the discussion. No preparation for them was required and the discussion was spontaneous. The expression of attitudes and feelings was sanctioned and facilitated through gradually exposing and exploring problematic behavior *at the time of its occurrence*. This approach fostered personal involvement. At the same time, a participant could achieve anonymity through passivity, withholding, or withdrawal.

The topics around which the discuissions revolved were related to common interests—the curriculum, teaching and clinical supervision, evaluation of students, administrative policies and practices, and evaluation of the psychiatric integration project. Because each of these subjects had facets that had a direct bearing on self-concept, the individual faculty member was involved from the outset with affect-laden material associated with approval and disapproval. Thus, in addition to problems connected with the educational program, the subjects of exploration included intrafaculty tensions arising out of status and authority differences, problems pertaining to democratic process, decision making, and emotionally based alignments.

ROLES

The "line" hierarchy characteristic of meetings of an organizational group did not apply to these meetings. All the participants were expected to take the learner's role. Because such a role involves a change in thinking and attitudes, assignment to it was at cross-purposes with the faculty member's need to preserve or elevate her status. Fear of losing status frequently was the primary source of resistance to change and thus was a major impediment to the attainment of the goals of the meetings and of the integration project.

Because there were no clearly defined guidelines for the meetings, the members of the psychiatric team were looked to for direction. The team responded by providing leadership and by functioning as a catalyst in facilitating group interaction. Thus, the status of the psychiatric nurse was shifted from her status in regular faculty meetings, where she was an inside member of the group. Her leadership status in this group arose primarily from her rational authority as an expert in psychiatric nursing. The psychiatrist, as a man, a physician, and a consultant, was perceived essentially as an authority and an outside member of the group.

Unresolved Attitudes toward Authority

The faculty members' fear of each other gradually came into the open in the second year of the project. Up to that time any direct expression of feelings or attitudes had been assiduously avoided. The fear of disapproval generally was related to the individual's preconceived attitudes and expectations about authority figures and to the attitudes and responses of the group with whom she was working, as well as those of the students.

The following vignettes are composites of the discussions that took place at three meetings that occurred in sequence. They illustrate the faculty members' fear of disapproval by and retaliation from each other and the way in which these concerns led to techniques of evasion, avoidance, and scapegoating.

The Faculty Schism

In the faculty discussions that preceded these three meetings, the participants had manifested difficulty in communicating with directness and specificity. Regardless of the topic under discussion, the meeting eventually broke down. Issues that were brought up for discussion were too deep and too contentious to be faced with equanimity. The status of some faculty members was threatened, and the usual faculty grouping—according to status —was conspicuous. Acknowledgment of this grouping first occurred at the following meeting.*

April 7, 1959

Last week, in the course of a regular faculty meeting, centering on the evaluation of students, communication was once again short-circuited, so that the faculty was unable to proceed with its business. At the beginning of this meeting, therefore, there is a great deal of tension and a somber mood prevails.

PSYCHIATRIST. It appears we are having difficulty in communicating with each other. Before we can continue with the evaluation of students, we better try to get our own house in order. Do we have problems in being direct with each other?

* As a reminder, the members of the younger group have been given names beginning with the letters in the A–N section of the alphabet, and those in the older group with letters in the R–W section. Thus, Miss Scott, for example, is immediately identifiable as a member of the older group, and Miss Jensen as one of the younger group.

Miss Scott. Yes we do. I think the age difference between faculty creates some difficulties.

Miss Vance. I think that younger faculty feel older faculty have special information that they withhold from the younger group.

Miss Reed. Students have a good deal of trouble with authority and I need help with this.

Miss Jensen. I don't know what we are talking about or where we are supposed to be going.

Psychiatric Nurse. This is an example of how we tend to skirt intrafaculty issues by shifting our attention to students. Could we pin down this discussion to concrete examples of our communication difficulties? I think it is important to evaluate how we interact with each other.

Miss Reed. I wasn't shifting the topic. [*She smooths her white upswept hair.*]

Miss Foster. I've been observing that not one younger faculty member has spoken today. Where do you draw the line between being direct and being disrespectful?

Psychiatric Nurse. You mean you are concerned that faculty will get angry if you express how you feel? Do you have feelings that you are reluctant to express?

Several Members. Yes.

[*Silence; aimless doodling; exchange of nervous smiles.*]

Miss Willis [*Her brown eyes sweep over the group*]. I wonder why faculty seem to discuss their problems with everyone but me.

Miss Jensen. Often we are led to believe that we have a choice to make, when in reality there is none. It is like a case of "Hidden Persuaders." I was asked if I was going to attend a particular event. I was asked in a way that communicated the expectation that I was supposed to attend, but at the same time it was presented to me as if I had a choice.

Psychiatric Nurse. Perhaps one of our problems pertains to insufficient clarification when certain situations require a command performance.

Psychiatrist. An essential aspect of any democracy is the command performance. There are times when it is perfectly legitimate not to permit a choice.

Miss Graf. A good example of the discrepancy between what faculty verbalize and what we really expect of others is in relation to time. I feel there is much emphasis and value placed on time. Although never directly stated, I feel that we are expected to enter and leave the situation at a specific time and that we are checked up on. We talk about this among ourselves but never get it out in the open.

Miss Drew. I feel guilty about leaving before a certain time even if my work is completed. I find myself tip-toeing around.

Miss Hunt. Older faculty are usually in the situation by a certain time. This makes me feel we are expected to do the same.

Miss Willis. I am uncomfortable when younger faculty may have to work beyond a certain hour or to attend functions that occasionally occur on weekends. [*She runs her fingers through her gray hair.*] This doesn't concern me as much about the older faculty, perhaps because they are used to the tradition of hours.

Miss Vance. Are we apprehensive about being free agents? Am I a free agent with an appointed position, or do I have a job in which I work on an hourly basis?

Miss Willis. Maybe we ought to look at our own departmental policies in relation to the college. Perhaps we need to be clearer about the channels of communication.

Miss Scott. I am in conflict as to whether I should conform to the clock and thereby reduce my guilt or to use my own judgment and go on feeling guilty.

Psychiatrist. It is the ability to allow conflict to develop and be resolved by the individual in her own way that helps to create a professional environment.

An examination of the process of the meeting reveals that four members (two in the older and two in the younger group) stayed outside of the discussion, either remaining silent or occasionally responding to such less-charged topics as policies, curriculum, and teaching loads. However, these four were not necessarily uninvolved; some of them engaged in forming a separate group of their own. They whispered and wrote comments to each other, exchanged glances, doodled, nodded, smiled, and mumbled.

A study of the discussion gives some indication of the degree of anxiety that was present. In an attempt to assuage their anxiety, the faculty members tended to become sidetracked by discussions of "right" and "wrong" behavior and thereby to become involved in setting new policies or discussing students instead of expressing their feelings about the current policies.

Nonetheless, for the first time the faculty began to deal with the concrete issues that were barriers to effective communication. Three problems were identified.

The identification of the first problem was precipitated when Miss Foster, with astringent candor, pointed out that as yet not one younger faculty member had spoken. With the help of the psychiatric nurse, some younger faculty members identified one problem in intrafaculty relations as fear of openly expressing themselves.

The atmosphere became charged with anger as members of the younger group identified the second problem—the difficulty of knowing what was expected of them and of determining when and whether they had a legitimate choice. Members of the younger group had difficulty in accepting certain responsibilities; at the same time they resisted anything that appeared to be rules or regulations. The members of the older group were apprehensive about stating their expectations directly and setting the necessary limits, although they expressed disappointment and annoyance when they were not fulfilled. Consequently, the members of the younger group often found themselves caught in a double bind. Miss Jensen gave an example of this dilemma.

The third problem related to the emphasis and value placed on time, particularly as this emphasis pertained to entering and leaving the work situation at a specific hour. Attitudes and responses included feelings of being "checked on" and conflict between feelings of guilt and disapproval on the one hand and anger and self-righteousness on the other.

Role of the Psychiatric Team. At this meeting, the psychiatric nurse and the psychiatrist were in tune in their roles and approach to the faculty. It was the task of one or both of them to intervene by referring to the faculty's avoidance of a problem. The psychiatric nurse moved in quickly and picked up Miss Reed's and Miss Jensen's comments, which were only sidetracking the key issue and leading the meeting astray.

When one faculty member alluded to her concern about speaking openly because of fear of arousing the anger of others, the psychiatric nurse and the psychiatrist stimulated group participation by eliciting other members' feelings. At that point more members began to contribute to the discussion and verbalize some of their attitudes. The psychiatric team did not deal with the problem of how to involve other members of the group, perhaps because the degree of blame aroused some anxiety in themselves.

The psychiatric nurse and the psychiatrist both clarified the faculty's tendency to equate democratic process and free choice with the absence of any requirements or expectations.

SCAPEGOATING, COUNTERSCAPEGOATING, AND SCAPEGOATABILITY

A predominant feature of the next two meetings was the pattern of placing blame on others.

April 14, 1959

PSYCHIATRIC NURSE. In the emphasis to work together as a group, I have the feeling that there may be insufficient appreciation and recognition of the individual instructor.

MISS SCOTT. I'd like to know how we feel restricted or made to conform?

MISSES VANCE, JENSEN, AND DREW. We are controlled by our own class schedules.

MISS VANCE. How can we possibly keep our own imagination and creativity going? [*She peers over her glasses.*] The problem of the teaching load has been continuous.

PSYCHIATRIC NURSE. Perhaps we use schedules as a way of closing off possibilities for having to change.

MISS REED. We already have chopped off too many hours from the curriculum.

MISS WILLIS. This is primarily a curriculum problem. It is important to identify functions of each member and decide about teaching loads.

PSYCHIATRIST. In some ways we have gone astray, and yet we really haven't. The principle of personal responsibility applies to everything we have said.

MISS WILLIS. On campus, faculty members are not required to attend special events such as concerts. Maybe we have been pretty rigid in expecting new faculty to attend classes taught by other faculty members. But we do expect attendance at traditional events.

PSYCHIATRIST. The major issue is not these special events, but the everyday ones. It is interesting that even though we discussed the problem of time last week, we have hit the crucial point, namely, what gets in the way of our work? There are many facets of the problem that can't be changed. Part is the curriculum, and some is with faculty's teaching loads. These cannot be worked out here. Our concern should be in the area of atmosphere—that which stymies creativity. Is there anything in the philosophy of teaching that limits instead of strengthens the use of self?

MISS JENSEN. Having to do work that rightfully is the job of the secretary interferes with my own growth. Is this the responsibility of professional people?

MISS GRAF. I understand that this is because the secretaries are loaded down and also that they have to be paid time-and-a-half for overtime.

MISS FOSTER. I don't have enough time to plan for my teaching, let alone to take four hours to type students' evaluations.

MISS WILLIS. We have faculty meetings to discuss these problems. Why wasn't this brought up then?

PSYCHIATRIST. Obviously there is a great deal of feeling about this so that for one reason or another it couldn't be brought up. What was made as a suggestion was transformed into a rigid institution of drudgery. Where and how did this happen?

MISS WILLIS. The secretaries are overloaded with work.

PSYCHIATRIST. This is not the issue.

MISS SCOTT. He's saying the group does this to themselves. Let him finish. [*Her gray eyes snap.*]

MISS HARRIS. It is the manner in which the suggestion was presented.

PSYCHIATRIST. But why wasn't this discussed?

MISS JENSEN [*yanks her blonde ponytail*]. Because I was sputtering inside.

PSYCHIATRIC NURSE. Dot, it might have helped all of us to settle the problem if you could have sputtered outside.

MISS REED. I haven't any feelings about this. I don't see any problem.

MISS JENSEN. I do, because we have more students than some of you and therefore we have more recopying of evaluations to do.

MISS FOSTER. I don't want to shift the blame, but the secretaries' attitudes are some of the problem. They treat us deplorably. They don't even try to understand our handwriting.

PSYCHIATRIC NURSE. We seem to be blaming others rather than looking at why we didn't bring this problem into the open instead of allowing it to fester.

PSYCHIATRIST. All of us have unresolved feelings about authority, and then we blame them rather than looking at our own feelings. In the Service, this is known as "griping." Are there alternative ways of dealing with these feelings that will get away from anger, guilt, and annoyance?

MISS HARRIS. I think the secretary business is a real problem.

PSYCHIATRIST. Nevertheless, our own background and feelings toward authority get in here.

PSYCHIATRIC NURSE. It seems that these situations become a trigger for feelings that haven't been resolved and that one of us is made a scapegoat for problems that are never talked about within the group.

PSYCHIATRIST. Can this situation be worked on with the idea of making a compromise?

In this meeting members of the younger group blamed the older group. Feeling attacked, some members of the older group became defensive and helpless and ignored or cut off the members of the psychiatric team.

Most of the discussion was carried on by four members of the older group, three members of the younger group, and the psychiatric team. The members tended to withdraw from facing problems openly—the same pattern of behavior that had been creating many of the difficulties in which the faculty members currently found themselves. Although the psychiatric nurse and the psychiatrist clearly stated the problem as one of placing blame on others, they did not pursue a discussion of it when the rest of the faculty did not pick it up. They felt that the group was not ready to deal with it.

The day after this faculty discussion, the psychiatric team, as planned, participated with Miss Drew and her student group in a clinical conference and evaluation session. In this session, Miss Drew voiced some problems and concerns about her relationship to the students in the clinical setting (see Chapter 7). This experience had great impact on Miss Drew, and it became an important milestone in her own growth and maturity.

At the next meeting the pattern of blaming was continued, with the discussion centering on the "Kay Fried Incident." This incident, which had occurred several months before, involved the failure in the clinical area of one of Miss Jensen's students. Unfortunately for everyone concerned, Miss Jensen neither explicitly warned the student about her poor work before final evaluation nor alerted the appropriate persons in administration so that they might communicate with the student's parents. Intrafaculty relationships were seriously disrupted, and the faculty meeting at which Kay Fried was evaluated drifted and deteriorated into the alignment of faculty members into pro and con camps. From that day on, the forbidden subject had never been brought into the open, and as a result, further seeds of fear and resentment had been sown.

April 21, 1959

The scapegoating during last week's faculty discussion stir up and revive the painful memories of the "Kay Fried Incident." Inhibitions cause a generalized lockjaw. The silence is punctuated by the click of ball point pens. Cigarettes are gaspingly puffed on and conversation rises in a smoky cloud to separate the faculty members from each other. One older faculty member clears her throat in open annoyance. Miss Harris and Miss Jensen, with nervous insolence, look over each other's shoulder to see what the other has written, and snicker and exchange insinuating smiles and garble "Uh, uh's."

PSYCHIATRIST. Would you like to give your reactions to the meeting of last week? [*Silence.*]

PSYCHIATRIST. Or would you want me to do it?
[*Silence.*]
PSYCHIATRIST. Two weeks ago we got down to brass tacks about faculty relationships. Last week we began to discuss what gets in the way of our potential leadership. Some of the feelings that were expressed included being enslaved to
schedule needs and resistiveness in coping with this. We heard expression of
feelings without being very critical of their rationality. Concern was external-
ized by griping. Griping includes feelings of protest which, when expressed,
provide relief, but very little can be done about the situation. If there are such
feelings present, accompanied by the freedom to express them, then we can
look at them and explore what possibilities there are for a change. Now, would
the rest of you react to last week's meeting?
[*Silence.*]
[*Miss Harris and Miss Jensen talk to each other but cannot be heard by the
group; they knowingly smile at each other. As one writes something, the other
glances over her shoulder and then nods in agreement.*]
PSYCHIATRIST. What is the difficulty?
MISS JENSEN. It is a tense and uneasy situation.
MISS VANCE. Faculty have been uneasy since last week's meeting.
PSYCHIATRIC NURSE. I felt that faculty were worlds apart from each other during
the faculty meeting that preceded this one.
MISS HARRIS. I feel we have made some movement in the right direction. I thought
the members felt some satisfaction that the issues were beginning to be explored.
PSYCHIATRIST. Why are we having trouble getting off the ground?
MISS HUNT. In other meetings the focus is on students. Here it is on us. [*She
scratches her ash blonde head.*]
MISS JENSEN. Some members feel they were used as a scapegoat.
PSYCHIATRIC NURSE. Did this happen?
MISS JENSEN. Yes. [*She picks at her nail polish.*]
MISS SCOTT. I have a grave feeling of a deep chasm between the two age groups,
and that as a group we are farther apart than ever. [*She smooths the chestnut
knot on top of her head.*] But I think this phase is transitional.
MISS DREW. I didn't think about it until I was involved in this scapegoating my-
self.
PSYCHIATRIST. Could you share with us what you mean?
MISS DREW. Not yet. [*She lowers her brown eyes.*] I have to think about
it.
MISS WILLIS. I felt like a scapegoat. Why don't faculty come to me?
PSYCHIATRIST. Sometimes issues are apt to get tied up with a person, especially
with a person who has authority, and then the group behavior takes on the
quality of directing an attack.
MISS WILLIS. I want to be one of thirteen rather than looked to for decisions.
MISSES VANCE, HARRIS, AND JENSEN [*in unison*]. But this isn't possible.
MISS HARRIS. I don't think we were scapegoating, but Miss Willis seemed to take
it this way. Should we discuss what we want and expect from those in authority
positions? Also, I feel that authority does have certain responsibilities for decisions that are not up to the group.

MISS THOMAS. May I please speak now? I'm also a member of this group. [*She pats her black bangs.*] I also felt just as resentful about having to make out the final evaluation records instead of the secretaries doing it.

MISS SCOTT. Now we are doing what we did last week—griping!

MISS HUNT. [*Her hand shakes as she lights a cigarette.*] Faculty keeps discussing hours and then blames authority. We seem to emphasize understanding of students, but not of each other.

PSYCHIATRIC NURSE. What impedes communication? We need to stick with more concrete problems. What are our tensions connected with?

MISS JENSEN. I felt I was used as a scapegoat in the case of the dismissal of my student Kay Fried. Even though this was a faculty decision and I had made up my own mind about what to do, I would never dismiss a student again after what happened.

MISS VANCE. The fact that you didn't tell the student ahead of time is the issue that made you a scapegoat. We got involved in tension rather than issues.

MISS SCOTT. I felt just as guilty in not questioning our decision to dismiss the student.

MISS WILLIS. Out of all this, we learned something good, such as policies. The important thing is what does faculty want to do?

MISS THOMAS. If only Miss Jensen could have shared her feelings of guilt. We were in a real mess.

MISS SCOTT. One of our difficulties is dealing with group versus individual decision.

MISS HARRIS. Is this not a place in which a policy was involved and we were allowed to make a decision contrary to policy? Shouldn't this have been the decision of the administrative group? [*She runs her hand under her gray chignon.*]

MISS SCOTT. We want the administration to be a big stick.

PSYCHIATRIST. Griping is for the purpose of putting things into a hopper, not that this is necessarily a realistic appraisal of what really exists. Griping can be constructive only when it is brought out in the open and tied to concrete action.

We have gotten into the problem of scapegoating, counterscapegoating, and scapegoatability. It takes at least two people to allow this to happen regardless of the negative behavior on the part of one person. When a decision such as the dismissal of a student falls more heavily on one instructor, she has greater responsibility to deal with the feelings that come out of the situation. Dot Jensen didn't have sufficient data to back up her decision. Faculty did not back her up nor did anyone consider the possibile results of the decision. So in reality, this was not a group decision. To say that the group could not back up Dot Jensen because they did not know the student is a rationalization. A group decision exists only when there is total group participation. The feeling of urgency led to making an immediate decision without thinking it through. Our chief concern here is with leadership, democracy, and individual responsibility.

The participants' difficulty in coming to grips with central issues might well have been due to their fear of exposure and fear of being assaulted by each other. Miss Willis felt she had been made a scapegoat by younger faculty, while Miss Jensen felt she had been scapegoated by older faculty. Miss Drew declined to share what she meant by being involved in scapegoating. Miss Thomas, bristling with anger, caustically implied that the group had kept her from participating.

The pattern of placing blame became more apparent as such self-righteous attitudes as exoneration of one's self in order to avoid personal responsibility began to color the meetings. Scapegoating became a case of "the best defense is an offense": attacking each other was a defense maneuver against exposing oneself. Under such conditions, it is extremely difficult for one person to intrude on the scapegoating process because of one's fear of being attacked himself. Thus, the scapegoating process developed and was perpetuated. One of the most destructive and demoralizing aspects of placing blame is that once it gets into operation, it almost inevitably results in a split in the group.

Group participation was more general, although two members in the younger group had little to say.

Role of the Psychiatric Team. During this meeting it became apparent that the psychiatrist was more and more inclined to assume the role of sole authority. The psychiatric nurse contributed in the beginning, but as the meeting progressed her unresolved attitudes and feelings toward the rest of the faculty members became a barrier to her direct intervention. She shared some of the younger group's anger toward the older members, but at the same time was angry with some younger members. She did not want to take sides. When threatened by the danger of becoming entangled, she retreated, and the psychiatrist took over the leadership.

Because these discussions occurred early in the project, the nature and definition of the psychiatric nurse's role had not yet unfolded, and the members had apparently felt less need than formerly to define it for her. The faculty members' basic conflict about her remained. She had not yet gained their trust and acceptance, partly because she had let them down by relinquishing her responsibility as a rational authority. Had she been functioning alone in this situation at this time, she probably would have had to deal with the problems on a more didactic and superficial level. In other words, in a situation like this, in which the emphasis is on interactional process, something of value is derived from the presence of an outside and unbiased expert—in this case, the psychiatrist.

The psychiatrist repeatedly focused on uncovering and exploring the existing tensions, and he dealt with the resistances in the context in which they were occurring. He pointed out the function of "griping" and differentiated feelings about a situation from a realistic appraisal of it. As he dealt with the problem of placing blame by clarifying that it involves at least two people, he avoided placing blame himself. He helped the faculty members to deal with reality when he identified the evasion of individual responsibility as one of the chief stumbling blocks to effective communication.

Breakdown in Intrafaculty Communication

The focus in these meetings on some of the barriers to effective communication, such as emphasis on time, decision making, leadership, personal responsibility, and the democratic process, gradually paved the way for the faculty to become embroiled in the evaluation of each aspect of the psychiatric integration program.

This evaluation was going on near the end of the quarter. At this time, in addition to a separate examination for each nursing course, the sophomore students were given a general examination covering some areas of medical-surgical, pediatric and emergency nursing, including the content in the thirty-six-hour course on psychiatric concepts taught by the psychiatric nurse and the twenty-hour course in social science concepts taught by the psychiatrist. As has been noted, these two courses were to be represented by a question prepared by the psychiatric nurse and the psychiatrist which was to be weighed as 10 per cent of the general examination. Neither of these courses carried separate course credit, and in neither of them were graded assignments or a separate course grade given. Thus, the only evaluation in which the psychiatric team was involved was the construction and scoring of this question. The psychiatric nurse was to correct and grade the responses.

In constructing this question the psychiatric team drew on a student's actual experience with a patient and attempted to recapture all the anxiety inherent in it (see Chapter 6, pp. 132–33). Since the other faculty members were not expected to discuss their examination questions or to get clearance for them, the psychiatric nurse and the psychiatrist assumed they were to use their own judgment in preparing their item on the examination; it did not occur to either of them to discuss the item with the rest of the faculty before giving it to the students.

In the process of collating the questions submitted by the various faculty members, a younger member discovered the one submitted by the psychiatric team. The nature of it was almost immediately transmitted to various faculty members. Snide remarks and side comments from members of the younger group indicated their disapproval and fomented further discord. This incident alerted the psychiatric nurse to another source of friction and altercation between the two faculty groups and further emphasized the extent to which the faculty schism was operating as a block to effective communication.

Barriers to Communication

May 19, 1959

Psychiatrist. In any group there are many lines of cleavage that create difficulties. Separations are natural and necessary. We have been exploring some
of the emotional overcast that is involved in difference. Should we spend another session or sessions in this area, or should we move into other areas, such
as personal reactions and feelings toward the work of psychiatric integration?
Revamping of the integration program should come from the group.

Miss Thomas. I think there are some mixed feelings about Jane's exam question.

Patient Situation. Robert S., a twenty-eight-year-old single man, was
admitted to the hospital with the diagnosis of spontaneous pneumothorax. His four-week hospitalization was relatively uneventful. He
was on complete bed rest until four days prior to discharge, when he
was allowed up.

You are assigned to care for this patient. He is able to take his own
bath; you give him back care and make his bed. While you are making his bed, the patient stands a short distance away, watching you
work. As you look up, you observe that the patient has had an erection
and is openly masturbating.

1. What are your initial and spontaneous reactions to the patient's
behavior?

2. What physical manifestations specific to you would be apt to accompany your reactions?

3. On impulse, how would you automatically handle the situation?

4. On further reflection and analysis, evaluate the above. In what
respects was your handling of the situation appropriate, and in what
ways was it inappropriate? Why?

5. If you found yourself in a similar situation again, what would you
see as an effective way of handling the patient's behavior?

6. How do you feel about this nurse-patient situation as an exam
question?

The Examination Questions. (See Appendix C for students' responses. Subsequent to the first use of this question, only items 4 and 5 were graded.)

Miss Foster [*adjusts a hairpin in her blonde braids*]. How do you intend to
grade this?

Psychiatric Nurse. Not on how the students handle the situation, but rather
their ability to face their feelings and anxiety about what is happening.

Miss Foster. In other words, you will punish a student for being hostile. [*Her
blue eyes narrow.*]

PSYCHIATRIST. We are concerned with the extent that a student is aware of the various facets of a situation, that she understands to be frozen is part of anxiety.

MISS HARRIS. Should this kind of a question be in an examination? Won't the student's tendency to freeze be increased by the examination situation itself?

MISS DREW. It doesn't belong here. I don't like the question.

MISS THOMAS. It seems that the psychiatric team should be trusted to know what students can handle.

MISS HUNT. This question counts for 10 per cent of the overall exam. What if the students can't express their feelings?

MISS SCOTT. Students have written about this problem in normal growth and development.

PSYCHIATRIC NURSE. Since this question raises so much controversy, I can't help wondering why no one came directly to me to ask about it.

MISS FOSTER [peers over her rimless glasses]. It's just that you weren't around, and besides, there wasn't time.

MISS JENSEN. It is useless to discuss the matter at all. Nothing will be done about it anyway.

MISS REED. I guess there is need for some background to the question. [She places both hands on her slim hips.] It just so happens that the exam question is taken from the exact same situation that happened to one of my own students.

PSYCHIATRIST. Each of you has the responsibility to decide what the basis is for your dislike and whether it is realistic, and how our purposes might be achieved in a better way.

MISS DREW. I still don't like the question, but now that I know this incident really happened. . . .

MISS REED. A faculty member has the right to give the kind of question she thinks is suitable.

PSYCHIATRIST. It is not enough merely not to like a question.

MISS VANCE. Is the problem because this is a sexual situation and that it is not chosen on the basis of frequency, but because of the shock it creates? [She twists a strand of her auburn hair.]

MISS JENSEN. Students don't see this kind of behavior in my clinical situation.

PSYCHIATRIST. We are getting away from the central point. We are not introducing the question because the situation occurs every day.

MISS HARRIS. How will parents or lay groups view the question? Students will talk about it outside.

PSYCHIATRIST. I would withdraw the question if, on the basis of nursing experience, it is not realistic, but not because it is a sexual question.

MISS WILLIS. Dr. Ullman, Jane, and Miss Scott know what students have had and need. We should trust them. I wish I had had this background. I wouldn't know what to do in such a case. The decision is left up in the air, and Jane and Dr. Ullman need to know now.

PSYCHIATRIST. There is no need to have the question if the majority don't go along with it.

[Silence.]

PSYCHIATRIST. The majority seem to want it.

MISS DREW. I still don't like it, but I'm willing to try it out.

MISS HARRIS. How will parents and the public see this? The social stigma continues to exist. This is the problem.

Contrary to what one might expect, the older faculty members seemed to be the least threatened by the content of the examination question. (Or it is possible that the older members did not take a stand on the issue since the younger group could be depended on to do so?) Periodically, some older members referred to their own experience with male patients who had had erections while they were taking care of them.

However, the question brought forth an uproar from the younger members. Tenaciously they denied the existence of such a problem and reinforced their armor of self-righteousness as they united in vehemently opposing the question on moral grounds. Some faculty members had obviously been threatened by the kind of behavior described in the examination question, so that it was difficult for them to discuss it even in the abstract. It is logical to ponder whether they could have allowed themselves to notice the occurrence of such an event in the clinical setting, and also how they might have handled it with students.

Miss Thomas, who was aware of the younger group's anger about the question, brought the problem into the open. In so doing, she referred to it as "Jane's question," when in reality the question had evolved from the psychiatrist's clinical conference with a group of junior students and their instructor, who was a member of the older group. This assumption on Miss Thomas' part illustrates that during the early stages of the project the rest of the faculty was confused about the collaborative roles of the psychiatric nurse and the psychiatrist.

In reality the content of the examination question was not the only issue. The genuine issue was the arbitrary way in which the psychiatric team had gone about handling the examination question without first discussing the matter with other faculty members. Such assumption of independence on the part of newcomers to the program further exacerbated the existing authority-dependency conflict. Further fuel was added to the conflagration when the older members reminded the younger members of the psychiatric nurse's and the psychiatrist's special knowledge and importuned them to trust the judgment of this team. Miss Jensen scornfully communicated the younger group's attitude that in the eyes of the older group the psychiatric team could do no wrong. Out of this discontent of the younger group was bred open rebellion.

There was some breakthrough in the opposition when the younger group became aware that the examination question was based on a situation which had confronted one of the students. Miss Drew was the first to evidence some sign of reconsideration. When the psychiatrist stated that there was no need to have the question if the majority did not go along with it, instead of coming to a decision the group responded with silence. The silence was not simply a matter of the faculty not wanting to make decisions; rather, because the psychiatric team had taken the authority for decision-making, the participants did not perceive themselves as a decision-making group.

Role of the Psychiatric Team. In this meeting, there were beginning signs that the psychiatric nurse was being made a scapegoat. She responded by becoming angry, defensive, and less active. Because of her abdication of her legitimate authority and because the psychiatrist had taken over the authority role, the psychiatric nurse was more vulnerable to being scapegoated. It was also more difficult for the faculty members to deal rationally with whatever hostility they may have had toward the psychiatrist for his having ascended to the authority position in the group. It was possible, therefore, that some of the members' attitudes toward the psychiatric nurse were a displacement of negative reactions to the psychiatrist.

SOME INTERVENTION ON THE FACULTY CLEAVAGE

In the interim between this session and the one to follow, the general examination, with the psychiatric team's question included, was given to the sophomore students. The psychiatric nurse graded the team's portion of the examination, after which each instructor discussed the total examination, including the psychiatric team's question, with her own group of students. There was a rumble among the faculty members about how the team's question downgraded some students on their entire examination.

The week after the students took the examination, the members of the psychiatric team, at their own request, had a one-hour session with the total sophomore class to discuss the examination question. The other faculty members had agreed to this meeting and were invited to attend. They turned out en masse. The psychiatrist led the class. The students were most responsive and participated eagerly. They were open and free regarding their immediate reactions to the question and in their discussion of it (see Appendix C).

In spite of the students' favorable responses, there was little change in the attitudes of some of the younger faculty members. The examination question became a *cause célèbre* for two possible reasons. On one level, it may have been used to justify a backlog of pent-up feelings that included feeling victimized by a series of injustices they felt had been perpetrated by the older group. On another level, it could have been a symbol of the psychiatric team's assumption of an independent status that they thought had not been accorded to them. It might be noted that although the examination question was used for the remaining period of the first grant, no objection was raised to it in subsequent years. It is a moot question whether this abatement of discord signified faculty growth or whether it was due to a displacement of conflict with the psychiatric team on to other activities in the integration program.

The examination question continued to be discussed in the faculty meetings for several weeks. Finally, the psychiatric team attempted to utilize these discussions to move toward one of the interim goals of the integration program—the healing of the faculty schism.

June 30, 1959

PSYCHIATRIST. The basic goals of a psychiatric integration program are partly related to the goals the psychiatrist has for a patient. These include not to magically wave away anxiety or to eliminate stress, but rather to shift anxiety from self-defeating modes of coping with it so that the individual has more mastery over problems and so that his life is not led by his problems. Techniques here have to be changed as our situation changes. In a group such as this, we don't have the time to work this through as in therapy.

Essentially, this is what we are doing with the student via the exam question. We take advantage of one stressful situation and exploit it to understand it. This will not eliminate the situation, but will help to modify it. We asked ourselves how to design a question which would produce a stressful situation.

PSYCHIATRIC NURSE. In terms of evaluation, if this was considered a sexual question, then there is no basis for evaluation. If, however, it is regarded as a question in which the sexual aspects are not being tested, but rather the question, "To what extent is the nurse aware of the patient's inappropriate response and of her own inappropriate response, and how do these get in the way?" then there is a legitimate basis for evaluation.

Let's take the case of a medical or surgical patient who is incontinent or has a fecal impaction. Even though the situation is unpleasant, there is no question whatever about taking care of the patient. Should a student's own attitudes hinder her in cleaning up the patient or removing the fecal impaction, the instructor has no alternative about how to handle the situation. Nor does she have any conflict about the role of the student's personality in the evaluation of clinical performance.

The exam question attempts to get at how the student's attitudes facilitate or impede her taking care of the patient. In every other area of medical practice, with the exception of psychiatry, there is no question about allowing personal feelings to interfere with medical treatment or nursing care. We are not unique in putting psychiatry under a cloud.

PSYCHIATRIST. I don't want to belabor last week, but some faculty were focusing on the sexual aspects of the question. I had the uneasy feeling that some faculty were in disagreement and were not going to discuss it. This makes for poor communication, which has been going on right along. I feel some aspects of the problem need further exploration.

MISS HARRIS. From the way you are talking, it is as though you and Jane are primarily focusing on the student. I thought the focus of the integration program was supposed to be on faculty.

PSYCHIATRIST. The primary goal of psychiatric integration is the learning of the student; the faculty is merely an intermediate point and the way of achieving the goal.

[*The younger members of the group whisper, pass notes, and smile at each other.*]

PSYCHIATRIST. We have been primarily interested in looking at the exam question from one point of view. And a breakdown in communication has occurred.

PSYCHIATRIC NURSE. I am not concerned only with the reaction to the question, but with our relationships as a whole.

PSYCHIATRIST. We need to focus on the concrete incidents that create problems and specify what these problems are, such as focusing on the exam question. We need to be unified in this.

MISS DREW. Why do we need to be unified?

PSYCHIATRIST. The issue before us is whether the exam question helped to move the integration process ahead or backward. I was excited about the students' response to the question and their discussion of it, but I felt your lack of enthusiasm and that the class felt flat.

MISS THOMAS. I get the feeling that those who don't agree with the question feel that a respectable school wouldn't give this kind of question.

MISS JENSEN. The group didn't object to the question being given, written about, or discussed in class. It is the fact of grading it that causes disagreement.

MISS DREW. But this kind of situation doesn't happen very often.

PSYCHIATRIST. But now you are focusing on the sexual aspects.

MISS FOSTER. Sex only produces more stress in the student.

[*Miss Harris and Miss Foster whisper to each other, nod, and exchange notes.*]

PSYCHIATRIST. Is there something you want to say? If so, it should be addressed to the whole group rather than a private communication.

MISS JENSEN. I can understand what you are saying, but it is difficult to divorce what the grade does to the student.

MISS DREW. Younger faculty are the ones who are disagreeing.

MISS JENSEN. We are completely split right down the middle.

PSYCHIATRIST. Would you agree that the issue is: This was a legitimate question, but there was need to have explored the method of grading and what results this would bring?

MISS WILLIS. There is a need to identify what is to be evaluated in a narrative question. Maybe this is where psychiatric integration fell down. I still feel that you and Jane knew how to evaluate the responses. I feel faculty ought to concede.

[*Miss Jensen and Miss Harris discuss how the question had too much influence on the overall grade of the total exam, which tested all areas.*]

PSYCHIATRIC NURSE. Monte and I should have discussed the basis for evaluation with the faculty group. You seem troubled by the fact that we lower the grade when the student does not express any reactions.

MISS THOMAS. Lower your voice, Jane.

MISS SCOTT. The statement that Eileen [*Drew*] made about a faculty cleavage intrigues me. It seems to come up in other areas.

PSYCHIATRIST. This problem of cleavage, or a split, has come up in other intra-faculty situations, and now it is related to our exam question.

MISS HUNT. Nevertheless, I feel the opinions expressed by Miss Jensen and Miss Foster represent a fresh point of view.

PSYCHIATRIST. In which direction are we going to move? Toward the evaluation of the integration program or discussion of the cleavage? I would prefer to move in the former.

MISS JENSEN. We've regressed ever since the "question." We don't even hear each other. We continually cut each other off.

PSYCHIATRIST. I take exception to this when our poor communication is used as an example of moving backward. The faculty cleavage has always been here. Only now it is in the open.

MISS SCOTT. Not only do we not listen to or hear each other, but there is continual note-writing and side glances. [*She holds her hefty body rigidly.*]

PSYCHIATRIC NURSE. Such behavior is rude and discourteous and it makes me terribly uncomfortable.

MISS WILLIS. There is a need for more knowledge on the part of faculty. We don't know what the students know.

PSYCHIATRIST. Your point is well taken, but it is not really related. We might have analyzed with faculty the principles that are involved in each question.

MISS THOMAS. I suggest that we get back to the evaluation of the integration program and discuss the clinical conferences with the individual instructor and Dr. Ullman and Jane.

At this meeting anger and resentment abounded. Once again blaming and counterblaming occurred. Members of the older group were noticeably passive during this meeting; one of them did not participate at all.

The younger faculty members were unified in their opposition to the examination question, but differed in their reasons for it. Miss Harris felt that the psychiatric team was more concerned with students than with faculty. This perception of the team further aggravated the feeling of the younger faculty members that interest in and appreciation and recognition of them as individuals were lacking. The complete bypassing of both Miss Scott's and the psychiatric nurse's direct references to the acting-out behavior of some younger members indicated a high degree of anxiety in the group.

By helping to increase the psychiatrist's ascendancy to power, the older members relinquished their realistic authority and, on the surface, their authoritarian approach to decision making. However, they maintained the authoritarian framework by taking the side of the authority figure, who was the psychiatrist, as when Miss Willis exhorted the younger members to concede to the psychiatric team.

During this period, because of their feelings of frustration and need for satisfaction, the members of the psychiatric team tended to equate the older members' lack of open disagreement with them as acceptance of the integration program. The younger members shared this interpretation. As a matter of fact, the older members had not aligned themselves with the psychiatric team, but had adopted a *laissez faire* attitude. However mistaken, the younger members' belief that the older group and the psychiatric team had joined forces against them aggravated their hostility. The psychiatric team, especially the psychiatric nurse, became the target for this hostility.

At the same time, there was some hope when Miss Drew, Miss Jensen, and Miss Scott confirmed the existence of a faculty schism. Facing this fact was the first step in resolving the problem. Several beginning steps in intervention on the faculty cleavage occurred.

Role of the Psychiatric Team. The task of the psychiatric team was to guide the discussion from its current focus on faculty members' personalities, whereby direct attack often was experienced, to a relating of the purposes of the examination question to the general purposes of the total curriculum as well as to the more specific ones of the integration program itself. The psychiatrist attempted to put the discussion in perspective by placing the points made within the broader framework of integration. He clarified that the primary goal of integration is the student's learning and pointed out that focus on the faculty was merely a way of achieving this goal. In a general sense, he related the broad goals of psychotherapy to a long-term goal of psychiatric integration, namely, to shift from self-defeating modes of coping with anxiety induced by professional problems to modes that result in increased mastery of such anxiety. The examination question was an illustration of how to exploit a stressful situation in the nurse-patient context in order to understand it.

The psychiatric nurse was active through most of the meeting. She and the psychiatrist were very much in tune with each other. She clarified the relationship of the students' feelings and attitudes to the quality of nursing care given by them by putting the whole issue within the framework of giving physical care to a medical or surgical patient. She thereby illuminated the existing prejudice toward psychiatry.

On several occasions she referred to the fractious conduct of some of the younger members, but to no avail. Finally, when the psychiatrist intervened, the disruptive behavior ceased. In spite of her determination not to withdraw from the group, the psychiatric nurse felt her resolutions founder.

In the effort to differentiate the roles of the psychiatric nurse and the psychiatrist in an integration project, the question that immediately comes to mind is how this situation might have been handled by the psychiatric nurse had she been functioning alone. This question takes on even greater significance in view of the psychiatric nurse's periodic feelings of helplessness. At best, one can only speculate about the answer.

It might be hypothesized that because of the intensity of negative feelings, degree of breakdown in communication, and resistance to change, the faculty members at this time would not have permitted one of their peers to deal with an intrafaculty problem on any level except a superficial and didactic one. As discussed in Chapter 5, the reluctance of the faculty members to use each other's specialized knowledge and skills was one of the causes of the difficulty in intrafaculty relationships. The ensuing difficulties encountered by the psychiatrist, an outside and unbiased expert, would seem to validate this point. If the psychiatric nurse had been functioning as the only expert in this particular field, she probably would have had to approach psychiatric integration from an entirely different vantage point.

Prelude to Disruption

Faculty Rivalry with the Psychiatric Nurse

As has been stated, hostility toward the psychiatric nurse was also engendered by the series of weekly unstructured discussions which she had with groups of sophomore students. The following meeting took place after the summaries of these discussions, which she had prepared at the end of the first year, had been distributed to the students and the faculty members (see Chapter 6).

July 14, 1959
Three members of the older group and one from the younger group are absent from this meeting.

Miss Foster. Even though Miss Thomas and Miss Harris aren't here, they have expressed the desire to participate in discussing Jane's unstructured group conferences with the sophomores as well as her individual conferences with students. [*She tucks some stray strands of blonde hair into her braids. Misses Vance, Jensen, and Drew all agree that discussion of the topic should proceed even though Misses Willis, Scott, Thomas, Harris are absent from the meeting.*]

Miss Foster. I can speak for Miss Harris.
Psychiatrist. Does the group agree to move in this direction?
[*All agree except Miss Foster.*]
Psychiatrist. Is this okay with you?
Miss Foster. Oh, sure. I was just stating feelings about the focus getting narrower. I don't care what we do.
[*Miss Vance asks the psychiatric nurse for clarification of the purpose of the class and for a description of how it is managed.*]
[*The psychiatric nurse starts to speak.*]
Miss Foster [*interrupts*]. Shouldn't we know when a faculty member is the problem so we can handle it?
Miss Vance. Counseling individual students and working with a group are very different.

MISS FOSTER. Miss Harris feels the same way. Students don't get as close to us now. They don't tell us about their problems with nursing service personnel. Whenver a problem arises and I ask them about it, the student responds, "Everything is all right now. We've told Miss Schmahl."

MISS DREW. I feel it's okay when students take personal problems to Jane. But when nursing personnel or faculty are involved, I feel the problem should go to the clinical instructor. I feel uncomfortable when a third person is involved.

MISS HUNT. I think it's a good idea for the students to have someone to go to; someone who is not involved in giving grades.

PSYCHIATRIST. I don't think there is any question that students can and have profited from these classes with Jane. They are eager for this kind of experience and have solved problems that otherwise may have gone by the board.

MISS REED. I feel that Jane's classes with the students have made it easier for me to know the students better.

MISS VANCE. We get to know students too well. That's one of our problems.

PSYCHIATRIST. Let's get back to the original question. There is much to hear from the other clinical instructors and we are not hearing from them. There is a problem, and we aren't getting at it.

MISS DREW. The students are one up on us. They can discuss us, only we don't know about it.

MISS VANCE. Aren't Jane's group conferences the same structurally as all the rest? The problem seems to be with faculty themselves. They are worried about what goes on that they don't know about.

MISS FOSTER [in an almost inaudible tone]. That's different.

PSYCHIATRIST. The only way we can get to the bottom of the problem is to stick with it.

[Miss Foster leaves the meeting twenty-five minutes before it finishes.]

PSYCHIATRIC NURSE. I think the fact that we are getting bogged down now is another indication of our lack of communication.

MISS JENSEN. I seriously question the advisability of using classes as gossip sessions about faculty. I question that the college would sanction this. Students discuss other faculty members with me and the rest of us. The suggestion that students discuss such matters only in these conferences is ridiculous. Students call them "gossip sessions."

PSYCHIATRIST. Perhaps Jane had better tell us about the discussions. She is the only one who really is in a position to know what happens.

PSYCHIATRIC NURSE. The goal of the conferences is to provide opportunity for students to discuss whatever problems arise in their relationships with patients, nursing personnel, faculty, and each other. The purpose is not to pass judgment on situations or the people under discussion, but rather to help students identify those feelings and attitudes that are unrealistic and irrational and therefore hinder their functioning as a student and a nurse. One of the goals is to help them arrive at a more realistic picture of those with whom they work. It is a way to help them work out some of their authority problems through me, so that, hopefully, they in turn can communicate better with all of you.

PSYCHIATRIST. I take strong exception to this experience being labeled a "gossip session."

Miss Jensen. Okay, okay! [*She nods vigorously.*] Perhaps we ought to discuss how the students all of a sudden have become so different and how this experience affects the whole nursing program.

Psychiatrist. Should we continue this next week?

[*Silence.*]

Miss Vance [*twirling her glasses*]. If all of this isn't ridiculous!

Miss Drew. We have to continue. We haven't finished yet.

Miss Jensen. We haven't even started.

Psychiatrist. That's not true. We have made a beginning.

Psychiatric Nurse. Another aspect is how faculty feels I handle any discussion with students that might involve them, for example, whose side am I on?

Psychiatrist. This is a problem on a different level that has to do with the particular qualifications and abilities of the person leading the conference. This will come out in the wash. We need to decide the initial issue first: "Are these conferences ethically right?" [*He turns to Miss Jensen.*] I don't know if you've changed your mind at all. . . .

[*No response.*]

Psychiatrist. Is this kind of a conference with students just too divisive for the goals of psychiatric integration? It is helpful to students, but is it too threatening to faculty? Should Jane's conferences continue, but perhaps with some change of focus to minimize the bad effects, or to maximize the possibility of the student going to her own clinical instructor? Or should the conference be eliminated altogether? Should the form be radically altered—such as having other faculty participating with Jane in these conferences?

The primary concern of the faculty members during this meeting was the fear that they themselves were the focus of discussion in the student conferences. Some of their responses indicated that they were feeling threatened regarding their status with students and each other. They were involved in the difficulty of identifying their own nursing and teaching roles, the respective and combined roles of the members of the psychiatric team, and the relationship of one to the other.

The entire meeting took on the moralistic tone that had characterized the discussion of the psychiatric team's examination question. This moralistic theme, which arose rather frequently, may have been used as a defense against handling affect-laden problems.

Miss Foster's penchant for anfractuous conduct was illustrated in the following pattern of behavior. At first she did not want to discuss the conferences without all the faculty members being present; then she said she could speak for the absent ones; then she was the one dissenting vote in the decision to go on with the discussion; then she left the meeting before it ended, not to return.

Throughout the meeting Miss Jensen responded to the psychiatrist in an openly hostile manner; she was the only member who did not greet him at the beginning of the meeting. The psychiatric nurse also was the target for much of her hostility.

Miss Vance was the only participant who did not yield to the temptation of scapegoating. She openly expressed her feeling that the problem was the faculty members themselves rather than the student conferences, but to no avail. The group was completely split off from the psychiatric team.

Instead of becoming an integrated group, the faculty began to disintegrate. In short, it was running amok. Before this disruptive process could be arrested, it was necessary to understand it. Why were the members of the younger group approaching every problem so belligerently? Some negative feelings about the possibility that the psychiatric nurse might infringe on faculty-student relationships were legitimate, but the degree of self-righteous indignation was not. Why were the younger faculty members so angry? What was going on in the current situation that caused them to be so resentful? Did they feel that some older faculty members might exploit them, even though they themselves allowed it? Were the faculty members really angry with the psychiatrist himself, or were they angry with him because they were viewing him as merely a shadow or extension of the psychiatric nurse?

Role of the Psychiatric Team. The central task of the psychiatric team was to cut through the diffuseness and to keep the faculty focused on the initial issue, namely, the academic soundness of the group conferences with the students. It was a tactical mistake to have focused on the ethical aspects of the conferences, for they were not the key issue. Rather, they provided a way for cutting down the psychiatric nurse.

The psychiatrist began to identify the unique role of the psychiatric nurse when he commented on the value of the group conferences to the students. Instead of allowing the discussion to continue with invalid assumptions, he called on the psychiatric nurse as a qualified specialist to clarify what was happening in the conferences. He left no doubt about the relationship between the way in which the conferences were being handled and her special qualifications and abilities.

Just as he had left the final acceptance or rejection of the examination question up to the faculty, so he left the decision about the conferences up to the group. He put the issue in the most realistic framework—what was best for students. In making it clear that the students were finding the experience useful, he put the burden of the problem back where it rightfully belonged—with the faculty members themselves. At the same time, he was definite about the willingness of the psychiatric team to revise the structure of the conferences.

The psychiatric nurse did not have much to say. On one occasion she commented on the poor communication. She was completely cut off and was not able to respond to Miss Vance's request for clarification of the student group conferences. Only when the psychiatrist suggested that the group needed clarification of the conferences from the psychiatric nurse did the faculty members hear or listen to her.

If in her explanation the psychiatric nurse had given some concrete examples, she would have provided a more vivid picture of the student experience. She might also have responded to Miss Drew's suggestion that she should limit her function to handling students' "personal" problems, by raising the question: "What constitutes a student's 'personal' problem?" She might have pointed out that generally any person's "personal" problems involve people, and in the students' case, these people would include their teachers. Also she could have explained that if she were to limit her functions to helping students with problems that occur outside the educational context, she would only reinforce the stereotyped image of herself as a therapist who "psychoanalyzes people" but who has little to do with the educational process or with the clinical practice of nursing. But because she felt under attack, she tried to withdraw from further incidents and to seek refuge in the impersonality of a theoretical presentation.

BEGINNING SIGNS OF ACCEPTANCE

Shortly after this meeting two episodes occurred which were significant because they represented a beginning attempt on the part of some individual faculty members and the psychiatric nurse to take constructive action about intrafaculty relationships.

The first of these incidents took place immediately following the meeting that has just been described. Miss Vance, a member of the older group, sought out the psychiatric nurse and asked, "Do you know what I was trying to accomplish in our meeting? Did it come through?" The psychiatric nurse remained noncommittal and asked Miss Vance to clarify her question. Miss Vance continued, "I was trying to push faculty into realizing that they talk about your conferences with students as if all that is discussed is themselves."

This remark may have been intended by Miss Vance as a way of supporting the psychiatric nurse as well as seeking approval from her. It placed the psychiatric nurse in a precarious position inasmuch as it provided the necessary stimulus for her to give in to the temptation of acting out her own anxiety by taking sides in the faculty schism.

In the second incident the psychiatric nurse attempted to learn something about the reasons for the younger group's deep resentment toward her. She resolved to confer with Miss Jensen, who had been quite vocal about her anger and resentment during the faculty discussions and had directed much of her hostility toward the psychiatric nurse. The following excerpt is an extract of the conference.*

* All this material was cleared with "Miss Jensen."

July 16, 1959

Miss Jensen and the psychiatric nurse are working together on an assigned curriculum problem. As has been the case in most of their previous collaborative efforts, their relationship is quite free and their communication marked by give and take. The psychiatric nurse is puzzled about why things seem to go fairly smoothly between them in individual contacts, whereas Miss Jensen is openly hostile to her in the faculty group discussions. The psychiatric nurse plans to bring the problem into the open after the business at hand.

PSYCHIATRIC NURSE. In the past, I think you and I have had a pretty good relationship, and I've always enjoyed working with you. I'm aware, however, that for some time now we've been estranged. I don't understand why, and I'm very concerned about it.

MISS JENSEN. I can see why you would feel this way, as I've continually cut you off in the faculty meetings.

PSYCHIATRIC NURSE. What do you think this is all about? Your reactions may help to shed some light on what is also bothering the other members of the younger group.

MISS JENSEN. Sure I can. [*Her blonde ponytail bobs up and down as she nods her head.*] First of all, the older faculty completely surround you with an aura. It's gotten to the place that we can't do anything "unless Jane is here." Also, I think some older faculty give lip service to mental health, but they don't listen to any of the rest of us. You have been put high up on a totem pole. Others including myself have had this happen, only to fall to the bottom. I keep wondering when this will happen to you.

Also, the younger faculty are just as angry at Dr. Ullman as they are with you. Yet, Jane, it's really not either of you we're angry at, but instead at the older faculty members. I'd hate to be in your position.

Supposedly, the emphasis of the integration program is on faculty. Yet how is the integration project helping the younger group?

PSYCHIATRIC NURSE. All of Dr. Ullman's time is spent in working with the faculty.

MISS JENSEN. Okay, but what about you working with us?

PSYCHIATRIC NURSE. I agree that I haven't worked closely with the younger faculty members, but I've also felt that they haven't allowed me to.

MISS JENSEN. It's true that we haven't worked with you, and sometimes it's gotten to the point that we have deliberately avoided you.

PSYCHIATRIC NURSE. I know. I've felt it. I wonder what I am doing that alienates me from the younger faculty?

MISS JENSEN. There is a lot of anger about your individual conferences with the students.

PSYCHIATRIC NURSE. Hm, hm. Are you aware that the students come on their own to discuss a whole variety of problems with me?

MISS JENSEN. I know this, and frankly, if I had had you around when I was a student, I'd have been parking myself at your door-step. I feel that the older faculty members really don't care about the younger members as people. The only time any concern about us is expressed is when one of us has a home or health problem.

PSYCHIATRIC NURSE. And yet the instructors are the very backbone of the faculty and the nursing program. Without them, there would be no program.

MISS JENSEN. I know, but I don't think the rest of faculty feel this way. Also, I become impatient with the older members' constant emphasis on the future because I feel such emphasis is accompanied by little regard for and understanding of the feelings and problems we have right now, today.

PSYCHIATRIC NURSE. I'm sorry we both have to stop now, Dot. All of this has been most helpful to me. Your comments give me a better idea about some of the underlying areas of friction. Before you leave, I'm curious to know what your reaction was when I raised this problem today?

MISS JENSEN. I had really expected you to discuss this with me, and I had even thought about bringing this up with you, myself.

In spite of her negative responses to the integration program and her ambivalence about the psychiatric nurse, it was obvious that Miss Jensen trusted the psychiatric nurse sufficiently to be quite open and free in expressing her feelings and attitudes toward her. Besides being courageously forthright and direct, Miss Jensen was remarkably perceptive about the faculty situation. She demonstrated unusual insight into the sources of the various difficulties. She corroborated the fact that the younger members were angry both with the psychiatrist for having usurped faculty's authority and with the psychiatric nurse. She recognized that the older group had vested the psychiatric team with superior status, but she erroneously concluded that this was synonymous with accepting them. She pinpointed that much of the faculty members' suspicion about the psychiatric nurse's group discussions and individual conferences with students was stimulated by the psychiatric team's duplication of the authoritarian pattern of interaction from which the younger members were trying to emancipate themselves.

INEFFECTIVE COMMUNICATION BY THE PSYCHIATRIC TEAM

July 21, 1959

One by one the faculty members straggle into the meeting. Younger and older members sit next to members in their own group. The psychiatrist and the psychiatric nurse separate as they sit and wait for everyone to assemble. The climate is strained. The younger members mumble among themselves. When someone utters a forced laugh, the psychiatric nurse jumps.

The team continues to wait. Finally, they are told that certain members will not be attending. Four are absent, three of the older group and one of the younger group. Some of them have missed the last three meetings. With one exception, there has been no notice or explanation of these absences.

PSYCHIATRIST. In continuing the discussion of Jane's group conferences with students, we need to ask,

1. How do the conferences get in the way of or dilute faculty-student relationships? The instructors are separated from this experience and students very well might by-pass the instructor in terms of clinical problems.

2. How can Jane handle the situation in which a particular instructor is being discussed by students without her being present?

3. Should there be this kind of group conference with the students?

Miss Thomas. I would like to get into the matter of individual conferences with students.

Psychiatrist. These are separate and apart from these group conferences.

Miss Thomas. There is noticeable absence of student discussion of problems they are having with nursing service personnel.

Psychiatric Nurse. Perhaps, some of this problem of the instructor not knowing what is happening would be alleviated if the instructors participated with me in the group conferences with their particular students.

Miss Jensen. Students do ask about personnel problems, but they stop at a certain point. There is the problem of one group of students who have discussed nursing staff in these conferences and then passed on their attitudes to another group of students.

Psychiatric Nurse. Exactly. One of the purposes of the conferences is to try to get at this very problem. It is by helping students to clarify their feelings and attitudes about nursing personnel that we can help students deal with the irrational elements and thereby achieve a more realistic picture of staff.

Miss Thomas. There is bound to be a great deal of anxiety in knowing you are going to be talked about. And when do students have opportunity to discuss Jane when she is not present?

Psychiatric Nurse and Psychiatrist [in unison]. In one of our clinical conferences with Miss Drew, she herself brought up the problem of her relationship with the students.

Miss Drew. I would have been even more uncomfortable and felt left out if I had not been there.

[The group unanimously agrees to the suggestion that the instructors participate with the psychiatric nurse in the unstructured group conferences with students.]

Miss Foster. I have the feeling that students are even more apt to come to us with their problems when they see us in this kind of role—and not to you. [Her blue eyes rest on the psychiatric nurse.]

Miss Thomas. I didn't know that Jane was seeing the student, Alice Carlson, or that anything was wrong.

Miss Jensen. I feel pretty foolish when, at the end of four weeks I discover a student had a problem.

Psychiatrist. Jane and I have a rule of thumb in our individual conferences with students. In the beginning of the conference we tell the student ahead of time that it may be necessary to share some general points with faculty, but that before we do, we will tell her exactly what will be shared. This gives her the opportunity to discuss any problems that may arise in connection with the material to be communicated to faculty. [See Chapter 6.]

Miss Thomas. Then there was the case of Cynthia Masters.

PSYCHIATRIC NURSE. Is the discussion of individual students the purpose of this meeting? We haven't finished evaluating the integration program.

MISS THOMAS. I don't have any other time to discuss students with Dr. Ullman. You do. If this meeting is going to be so structured that we can't talk about what we need to. . . .

MISS JENSEN. This is a sample of what happens after a student has had an individual conference with Dr. Ullman. We don't know what has happened and are left holding the bag.

PSYCHIATRIST. We can't finish the evaluation now, anyway, so why not move on to discussion of students? Okay?

[*Miss Thomas presents the problem of Cynthia Masters. Miss Foster leaves the meeting twenty-five minutes before it is finished.*]

The entire discussion at this meeting was carried by four faculty members and the members of the psychiatric team; three members (two in the younger and one in the older group) were completely silent. One younger member continued her pattern of leaving before the end of the meeting. Undoubtedly, from time to time certain responsibilities required some faculty members to be absent from a meeting or leave it early. However, the continuation of this pattern on the part of a significant number of faculty members might be construed as a withdrawal from the struggle of learning to work together because of fear of personal attack.

This meeting pinpointed some serious difficulties in communication between the rest of the faculty and the psychiatric team. The psychiatrist opened the meeting by providing a framework for continued evaluation of the integration program and problems around the psychiatric nurse's group discussions with students. The faculty participants avoided declaring their position in regard to the three questions posed by the psychiatrist.

Large reservoirs of fear and resentment about the possibility of the faculty members themselves being discussed by the students and the psychiatric nurse were tapped. Miss Thomas and Miss Jensen both referred directly to the problems created by differences in status between the psychiatric nurse and the other faculty members. Miss Thomas revealed some apprehension about the fact that the psychiatric nurse was the only faculty member to have an ongoing and collaborative relationship on an individual basis with a member from another discipline. This was the second occasion in which faculty members had expressed the desire for more direct help from and contact with the psychiatrist.

Both the psychiatric nurse and the psychiatrist referred to Miss Drew's positive experience when, in their conference with her and the students, she had raised the problem of her relationship with students. Competition to achieve and preserve status was revealed and illuminated as a deep-seated problem that was woven through the fabric of all intrafaculty relationships.

There was a noticeable shift in the interaction during this meeting. The younger members were more open. There were fewer side comments and undercurrents of innuendo. Miss Drew expressed her reactions quite freely. Th group reached a unanimous decision to participate with the psychiatric nurse in the conferences.

Role of the Psychiatric Team. The team's goals in this meeting consisted of trying to break through the faculty's avoidance of coming to a decision about the psychiatric nurse's student group conferences. This meeting was a remarkable demonstration of how the other faculty members either by-passed or openly rejected what the psychiatric nurse had to offer. When, for example, the psychiatrist spelled out three questions to serve as a springboard for further discussion and Miss Thomas digressed to a discussion of students and the individual conferences with them, she accepted his redirection that the individual conferences were separate from the group conferences. Later on, however, when the psychiatric nurse tried to get the group to continue evaluating the integration program, Miss Thomas responded querulously. When in the very beginning of the meeting the psychiatric nurse suggested that the instructors participate with her in the student group discussions, this overture was completely ignored.

It was on occasions such as these that the psychiatric nurse felt bogged down and seriously wondered if all the effort was worthwhile. Not infrequently she yearned for the tranquil days of teaching psychiatric nursing.

This discussion uncovered the tendency of the psychiatric team to withhold information about pertinent aspects of students' problems. Because of their psychiatric education and orientation, which stresses keeping confidences, this was an easy trap to fall into. Perhaps one reason for the psychiatric team members' poor communication and collaboration with the faculty was their own lack of communication with each other about the differences between those aspects of students' problems that should be shared with the faculty and those that should be treated as a privileged communication. It took the psychiatric nurse and the psychiatrist some time to learn that those experiences in the integration program in which the faculty had no opportunity to participate on some level were ones that eventually and inevitably came under fire.

Withdrawal seemed to be a defense operation which the faculty members used to handle fear of personal attack and retaliation from each other. At this time, neither the psychiatric nurse nor the psychiatrist made any move to intervene in faculty withdrawal from attendance at and participation in the meetings. The psychiatric nurse also was afraid of further attack if she did so. Considering her own anger with the faculty, it seems pertinent to speculate about whether her avoidance of intervention also may have grown out of her fear that she might counterattack. Waiting also became a way for her to establish equilibrium within herself. In this stage of the project the psychiatric nurse was dependent on the psychiatrist and from time to time sought refuge from the faculty's hostility by hiding behind him.

Summary

In the faculty group discussions the initial attitudes were primarily those of surface acceptance. On the part of some, this acceptance was accompanied by a potential and readiness for a deeper and more whole-hearted acceptance. In others, the surface acceptance was a cover for indifference and, in the case of some, covert negative rejecting attitudes. Receptive attitudes and the chameleonlike behavior of some faculty members may also have masked anxiety and may have stemmed in part from their inordinate need for approval.

The stage of impact consisted of the faculty testing their colleagues, particularly the psychiatric team, and exploring the limits of the specific roles of the two team members. The team's functions in the faculty group pertained to uncovering and exploring existing tensions, professional issues, and problems, and to dealing with them in a way that was both critical and constructive. The chief obstacle to uncovering problems on a group level was the fear of the faculty members that their personalities were under scrutiny and judgment and that they would lose face in front of their colleagues. The pattern of scapegoating which developed as the meetings progressed was a reflection of this fear.

By the end of the first year, there were the faint beginnings of a derailment of faculty relationships. At the same time some action had been taken to resolve some of the issues that estranged the faculty members, the psychiatric nurse, and the psychiatrist from each other.

Chapter Nine

THE WORK WITH THE FACULTY GROUP: THE STAGE OF RECOIL

From what source come these unmanly fears that prevail among us? These dark forebodings? This despairing impotence? What is it that has shaken the nerves of so many? . . . The particular projects which we debate so angrily are not so important. . . . It is not the facts of the crisis which we have to fear. They can be endured and dealt with. It is demoralization alone that is dangerous.

WALTER LIPPMANN, *Leadership and Opinion.*

The stage of recoil, or the reactive phase, was the second period of the integrative process among the faculty and the psychiatric team. It was a time in which individual responses to change were uncovered. It was the period during which the faculty members openly reacted to the integration project and to the psychiatric nurse and the psychiatrist.

The faculty discussions had been interrupted by one month of vacation. The length of time of the meetings had been extended from one hour to one and one-half hours per week. In the middle of March, 1960, the tape recorder was introduced for the first time, and it continued to be used in the meetings for the remainder of the third year and throughout the fourth year of the project. When the psychiatric nurse asked for the faculty's permission to tape-record the sessions, the members unanimously agreed.

In the third year of the project there was some change in the makeup of the faculty. A younger instructor was replaced by Miss Newcomer. An older instructor was on a sabbatical leave for three quarters and returned for the summer quarter. A younger instructor was on leave during the second and third quarters and returned for the summer quarter.

A Schism between the Faculty and Psychiatric Team

The past year's experience with the faculty meetings on integration demonstrated that spontaneous discussions tended to be diffuse and lacking in continuity. In an attempt to bring them from the general to the specific level and to encourage the utilization of concrete data, the psychiatric team endeavored to develop an operational structure for the meetings. Accordingly, the following alternative suggestions were presented to the faculty at the first meeting of the year 1959–1960 (the third year of the project).

1. Faculty members would raise problems which would be discussed serially by the group.
2. Each instructor would present a problem and, if she was able to, would clarify how the psychiatric team and group could help. The psychiatric team might function as a subcommittee in screening problems for presentation to the group by helping the instructor to identify the problem and by establishing priority of problems through determining those that were rich enough for ninety minutes of discussion.
3. The meetings would be utilized for the evaluation of student behavior. This alternative would preclude the discussion of other problems.

The second suggestion was accepted, and the faculty agreed to think about various problems and situations and have them ready to discuss with the psychiatric nurse two days before the next meeting.

The next three excerpts from meetings illustrate the faculty's response to the plan to operate within some kind of structure.

RESISTANCE TO DISCUSSING PROBLEMS

September 29, 1959

No faculty member has approached the psychiatric nurse about problems for discussion as planned, whereupon the psychiatric nurse has sought each member individually. Each faculty member has responded with surprise at her request for suggestions, and no one has had any suggestions for topics for discussion.

During the meeting many of the faculty members retreat into note taking and doodling or withdraw by hiding their faces in their hands, tightly folding their arms as though to protect themselves, or maintaining stubborn silence. Muttering, deep sighing, and pencil tapping by younger members punctuate the ponderous silence. Angry and furtive glances dart across the room.
[There is a long and resolute silence.]

PSYCHIATRIST. We are dealing with the concept of resistance. There is a reluctance to discuss problems. Last week we moved in by trying to set up a structure for the meetings. This is based on Jane's and my philosophy of interaction, that we don't just sit back and theoretically discuss how human beings interact.

We must get specific and concrete and identify problems so we can explore the application of psychiatric concepts. Problems cover a wide range and need not be always anxiety-laden, nor ones in which the whole group is involved.

The territory of problems is wide and complicated. Jane and I are not concerned with evaluating feelings and personal reactions, except as these get in the way of teaching. Our task is not to undermine the individual's sense of self-worth. If we can solve some of the problems, the pain in doing it is worth it.

The success of the recommended structure places a greater responsibility on the individual. It requires looking inward and how we are affected by others. I asked Jane to think about how she sees this.

PSYCHIATRIC NURSE. I am not wedded to a particular structure. Like all of us, I am primarily concerned that we begin to discuss some of the problems that arise in our work with students, nursing service personnel and each other. Last week I thought we had agreed to try out having one instructor present a situation, a topic or problem for discussion. I was excited by the numerous possibilities such a plan presented. I felt we had taken a constructive step toward working together.

MISS HUNT. Jane used the word *excited*. She uses it all the time. After all, we have our own favorite areas too. I feel that Jane thinks we should be as interested in mental health as she is.

PSYCHIATRIST. We need to look at the resistances. What are some of the rest of your reactions?

MISS VANCE. I haven't even thought about a topic since our last meeting. I thought we had to have a major problem.

MISS DREW. I thought that it was all settled that Jane would come to us and ask us if we had a topic for discussion. And I didn't mind. Yet when the time came and she did ask me, I objected.

MISS THOMAS. I thought it was all settled that Dot [Jensen] would present a problem.

MISS JENSEN. Jane came to me, and she had the impression I was going to present a situation for discussion. I did raise my hand last week in agreeing with the proposed structure.

MISS GRAF. Do we have to have such major problems? Are mine important enough for this august group? [She rolls her blue eyes.] And I feel like Audrey [Hunt]. I just can't get as excited about the whole thing as Jane does. I fear that we are expected to conform.

MISS NEWCOMER. I'm new here, but I'm selfish about sharing myself. [She runs her hands through her bright red feather cut.]

MISS FOSTER. It just slipped my mind that we were supposed to identify a problem. I thought someone else was going to present.

MISS WILLIS. Do we really want to support the team approach of working together with Jane and Dr. Ullman? Something seems to be going on in the group that I can't put my finger on.

PSYCHIATRIST. Obviously Dot [Jensen] got the responsibility, so the group didn't have to carry it out. What really happened is that Dot stated she had a problem and that some time, upon reflection, she might want to present it. The primary process here is one of wishful thinking.

How and why did this happen? First, there is the pressure of the work load. Then there is the expectation that everyone should be as excited and involved as Jane. But this attitude really has no basis. Neither Jane nor I are interested in proselytizing mental health. Such interest is very different from the desire to look at problem areas. It is not our expectation that you would be as preoccupied as we are.

Miss VANCE. This is a matter of a person's particular interest.

PSYCHIATRIST. It is a question of anxiety. We are asking you to bring in situations about which you have feelings. We do not bring in problems because of lack of interest, but because of anxiety.

Miss THOMAS. Why are we spending so much time in discussion of this? [*She impatiently flicks one long fingernail against another.*] I feel my own area is belittled. I'm here, but I won't play.

PSYCHIATRIST. The fear of conformity—fear that we are trying to make you think alike and lose your individuality—is present. This is like raising a red herring to a psychiatrist, who is concerned with helping individuals discover their uniqueness.

Uniqueness comes and unfolds only through sharing and social intercourse. If a problem is shared, we can arrive at an objective way of solving it. It is not an issue of conforming; but of conforming to the truth. Our goal is not to have you go against what you genuinely feel.

PSYCHIATRIC NURSE. There seems to be a tendency for us to feel that in working as a group, we lose our individual uniqueness. This is an occupational hazard.

PSYCHIATRIST. In asking you to share problems, we are not concerned with personal problems. We do get involved with the individual, but this is only to the degree of helping to improve the educational program. It does not mean sharing things that aren't the concern of faculty.

[*Miss Foster writes, and continues to do so throughout the meeting. Miss Newcomer looks over Miss Foster's shoulder. Miss Jensen looks at the psychiatric nurse as the psychiatrist is speaking and mouths,* Won-der-ful!!!]

Miss HUNT. I don't see why we have to see Jane about the problems we are going to discuss. [*She shakes her closely cropped blonde head back and forth.*]

PSYCHIATRIST. Jane's function is to help the faculty member increase her skill and deepen her level of dealing with these problems.

[*Protracted silence, deep sighing, energetic doodling.*]

Miss WILLIS. We don't have enough time. We feel under pressure to do this kind of problem solving. We have lost something as a group.

Miss VANCE. I would like to explore why we are so contagious to each other. We act like jugglers who are afraid that we are going to lose a ball. There is an underlying current of fear.

Miss REED. A topic I would like to discuss is whether I define limits too closely for students? Am I too rigid? Students are frightened of me at first.

PSYCHIATRIST. There is group resistance, and the faculty needs to form an opinion about this. Is there fear that we will lose our identity in this group? That we have to think in a certain way?

In this meeting there was a piling up of tensions. Hostility smoldered. The members evaded all responsibility for the meeting and struggled against becoming involved. They placed the burden for suggesting a topic on Miss Jensen. Each attempt to evolve some plan for getting at problems stimulated anger, rejection, and withdrawal. There was a powerful undercurrent of fear. Miss Vance and Miss Willis observed and commented on the group atmosphere.

A forward step was taken when some faculty members openly directed their hostility toward the psychiatric team. When the psychiatrist tried to impose his ideas, they responded with anger and rejection, as for example, when Miss Graf sarcastically questioned whether her problems were important enough to the group, especially to the psychiatric team, and when Miss Thomas stated that she felt her own area was belittled and that she would not play the game the psychiatric team was trying to force upon her.

At the end of the meeting Miss Reed demonstrated positive movement. She was the first participant to raise a problem that concerned her behavior with students. The psychiatrist completely ignored her suggestion. In response, were the faculty members beginning to feel that it was useless to talk about something personal, because the psychiatric team was not listening?

Role of the Psychiatric Team. In this meeting the psychiatrist became more authoritarian. All the suggestions for discussion were made by the psychiatric nurse and the psychiatrist, although they were unaware of this at the time. In addition to the controls that already had been placed on the faculty's authority for decision making, there now was an attempt to control the content to be discussed.

The psychiatric nurse abdicated her authority in favor of the psychiatrist, so consequently, the faculty members perceived her primarily as an extension of him. The contumely directed against her caused her to revert once more to passivity and withdrawal.

A COMPROMISE

Immediately prior to the next meeting, the psychiatric nurse and the psychiatrist conferred about how, and in which direction, to move in the meetings. The psychiatric nurse feared that if the current situation were allowed to continue, the meetings would have to be abolished. She anticipated two possible outcomes from such a crisis. If the faculty members were faced with the threat of terminating the meetings, they might be motivated to take some responsibility for them. On the other hand, the meetings might be terminated, in which case the faculty's contact with the psychiatrist would be cut off, and the integration program would thereby be placed in serious jeopardy.

The central problem in the group seemed to be the omnipresent struggle for power between the younger and older members, and between the faculty and the psychiatric team. Under such conditions the psychiatric team felt it was probably too much to expect the faculty to function as a total group and thought there might be greater freedom in communication if it was temporarily divided into two groups—younger and older—to work with the psychiatric team. Regrettably, the psychiatric nurse and the psychiatrist were unaware of how their own behavior operated as a disjunctive force.

October 6, 1959

PSYCHIATRIST. When we know the psychiatrist is losing ground and when resistance is overwhelming, we need to find out why. Some reasons include:

1. The current structure isn't working, and the reasons for this may be varied.
2. We may have expected the unreasonable in terms of the degree of freedom required to bring problems in the open.
3. Some of the resistance may be due to the many sore spots that were touched on last year and left unresolved.
4. Therefore, perhaps we have underestimated group differences. We have referred to these allegorically and euphemistically. If we could look at the differences, this might be helpful.
5. This year, there is a kind of inertia that I don't quite understand.

Because of these various points, Jane and I are suggesting another structure for your consideration. We suggest:

1. To divide the total faculty group into two groups according to the younger and older subgroups. Jane and I would meet with each group once a month. This would account for two of the four periods now given over to our meetings.
2. The third week would be left open for individual faculty conferences with me. These would be completely open in structure and faculty could discuss whatever is on their minds.
3. In the fourth week, the two groups would come together for a total group meeting. Jane and I would be responsible for choosing the topic.

There would be no pressure on the group to come up with a subject each week. It might be easier to explore problems without having to deal with the feelings of the other group. In reality, both groups have different problems. In principle, we are concerned with a unified group and the three proposals really are a preparation for this.

[*Miss Jensen maunders; shakes her head "no" when psychiatrist refers to a split in the faculty group. The rest of the group is silent.*]

MISS WILLIS. The older faculty who have tenure have different problems from the younger group. I don't know if the older members need help. I don't know what the problems are of the younger group.

MISS JENSEN. With this arrangement, we don't spend as much time. Are we running away from our problem?

PSYCHIATRIST. Yes, but strategically. Our goal is toward a total and unified group.

MISS JENSEN. I'm disappointed. We should be able to handle this in the large group.

MISS FOSTER. There is more resistance this year.

MISS DREW. I don't like this. It seems as if we can't move. Is it due to the structure that we have to go to Jane first? How about discussing our problems willy-nilly?

MISS FOSTER. We are more resistant. I'd like to try it this way.

MISS WILLIS. Why are we breaking the groups into younger and older?

PSYCHIATRIC NURSE. Last year we did scratch the surface and did get into some touchy areas. Freedom in this kind of situation is crucial for communication.

MISS THOMAS. I thought Jane only came to faculty for problems when none of us had approached her.

MISS REED. I didn't understand that she was supposed to come to me.

PSYCHIATRIC NURSE. Does anyone besides Eileen [Drew] want the group to remain as it is?

[Miss Drew and Miss Graf indicate they want to work in the large group without any structure.]

MISS THOMAS. Who says we aren't able to communicate? Just because we don't come to Jane and Dr. Ullman doesn't mean we can't. [She blows a strand of her black hair away from her eyes.] I feel we should continue as we are. I never did like plan number 1 in which we were supposed to discuss each problem serially. And I dislike plan number 2, with the screening committee of Jane and Dr. Ullman even more.

MISS JENSEN. I'd like to continue as is, also. I felt we were getting somewhere this past summer.

MISS WILLIS. I want to work as a large group. I feel I've grown, even though sometimes negative comments are aimed at me.

MISS REED. I feel we have made progress.

PSYCHIATRIST. Does anyone want to adopt plan number 2?

MISS GRAF. Last year was really better than I realized. We said the meetings were no good.

PSYCHIATRIST. This is exactly what we wanted to get at. Why didn't the issue of not liking the meetings come out in the open?

MISS THOMAS. You have to be able to think about them.

MISS FOSTER. I don't think we will get anywhere.

PSYCHIATRIST. Is there consensus in keeping an unstructured meeting?

MISS JENSEN. In the unstructured situation of last year I wasn't interested in the least. There was a lot of frustration due to irrelevance, yet I couldn't bring this up at the time.

MISS DREW. I told Jane I was sick of hearing about the student, Eleanor Gruen, and her problem. I wasn't interested.

PSYCHIATRIC NURSE. This problem was the reason for our proposal of discussing problems serially.

MISS THOMAS. I oppose having someone else decide what problems should be discussed. I want to do it myself.

PSYCHIATRIST. Okay. The purpose of plan number 2, in which Jane and I establish priorities, was based on faculty's problems. I don't know if we can move
in an unstructured situation.

MISS THOMAS. You and Jane scrupulously avoid voting for a plan. You are both
part of this group.

PSYCHIATRIC NURSE. Yes we are, Linda, but we have different roles.

PSYCHIATRIST. The following plan allows for compromise. We can meet as a large
group, in which each person presents a problem, but we screen it by not
getting into discussion until the group chooses the problem it wants to discuss.
Secondly, the large group may request a small group (younger or older) meeting at any time, or one member may meet with Jane and myself. Finally, the
group has the responsibility to decide what they want to talk about, and Jane
and I share this responsibility.

MISS NEWCOMER. I think there is an advantage to screening problems.

In this meeting group participation was more generalized than in the
previous meeting, though one member of the younger group completely
withdrew. Silences were minimal. The younger group members continued
with their note taking, mumbling, head nodding, and side comments, but
to a lesser extent. Basic issues and group differences were avoided. Some
members became entangled in side issues.

The psychiatric team's suggestion to divide the faculty group was responded to with agitation, anger, resentment, and superficial acceptance.
Faculty members seemed to fear that such a plan would create a split in the
faculty, which was a way of denying the existence of the current schism.

A central theme of this meeting was a three-way power play between the
younger and the older members, between the psychiatric nurse and the
psychiatrist, and between the faculty and the psychiatric team. Once again
problems pertaining to status needs became apparent. The faculty members
tended to deny the differences between the role of the psychiatric team
(especially that of the psychiatric nurse) and their own. They also tended
to frown upon individual differences in the name of group cohesiveness,
which became the guise under which pressure for individual conformity
operated. Several faculty members had expressed fear of conformity in the
previous meeting.

The fear of losing status in the eyes of students and each other was more
than likely tied to the fear of being stripped of all symbols of individuality.
The focus of this fear lay within the individual faculty member. Some
faculty members may have viewed individualism as being a corrosive of
professional ties and values and felt it to be irreconcilable with the group's
interests and welfare—an attitude that was similar to the one indicated in
their behavior toward the psychiatric nurse during the first year of the
project. The attempt to handle the fear of losing status might explain why
some faculty members retaliated against those in a position to withhold

recognition and appreciation from them. It is well recognized that the pattern of scapegoating is rooted in fear.

In such circumstances group cohesiveness became primarily a matter of fantasy and wishful thinking, having little to do with what was going on in the day-to-day relationships among the faculty members. Preservation of this fantasy grew out of the fear of change and resulted in frustrating the individual's need for acceptance, recognition, and personal growth. Anger, resentment, feelings of helplessness and impotence, resignation, and withdrawal were the inevitable sequel.

A few caustic remarks were directed toward the members of the psychiatric team. They were blamed for the current dilemma because of their recommendations for changes in the structure of the group meetings. Up until now, Miss Willis had supported the psychiatric nurse, but at one time during this meeting she withdrew this support. Because the members of the psychiatric team had failed in their efforts to be completely nonjudgmental in their analysis of the group interaction, the faculty members saw them as the cause of many of their interpersonal difficulties with each other.

The first sign of integration during the project appeared when the faculty members, insiders of the group, unified against the psychiatric team, the "outsiders." Gradually, some members began to expose their negative attitudes about the past meetings. Then, they began to reveal that, in retrospect, the meetings may have been more valuable than they had realized. As some of the members began to reappraise the situation, they came forth with more positive reactions. The meeting ended with the suggestion for a compromise.

Role of the Psychiatric Team. As the psychiatrist became more autocratic, the psychiatric nurse receded further into the background. Just when the faculty members were gaining strength through expressing their negative feelings, the psychiatric team introduced a recommendation that would split them again. It was with the hope of deflecting the faculty's hostility from herself, that the psychiatric nurse desired to separate the younger and the older groups. Nevertheless, the psychiatric team was forced to accept the faculty's decision not to split the group.

The psychiatric nurse's and the psychiatrist's overwhelming urge to help the faculty members work well together and their wish to function as mediators between the younger and the older groups became an obstacle to their recognition of the positive aspects of faculty interaction. It was just as hard for them to learn about their behavior and its impact on the group in the process of psychiatric integration as it was for the faculty members to learn about theirs. However, for genuine collaboration to occur the psychiatric team had to be in a position to discover its own maladaptive functioning. The necessity for this kind of awareness is what makes psychiatric integration and interdisciplinary collaboration so difficult.

THE STRUGGLE TO SOLVE A PROBLEM

October 13, 1959

PSYCHIATRIC NURSE. We decided last week that we would continue to work as one group, but that we would proceed by first identifying all the problems for discussion before going into any of them, and then as a group, we would decide which one to focus on.

MISS REED. I would like to discuss the problem of our inability to stick to decisions once we make them. When we make a policy for giving a D grade to a student, for example, we don't carry it out. [*Her piercing gray eyes appraise the group.*] And then there is the situation with the junior students. . . .

PSYCHIATRIST [*interrupts*]. I suggest that the the next speaker introduce another topic or say whether she wants to discuss this one.

MISS JENSEN. I feel that many times a decision has already been made by someone else and that we are just going through the motions of democratic process.

MISS REED. There have been occasions when I have carried out a decision in relation to a student only to learn it has been changed.

MISS THOMAS. I think this problem needs to be discussed.

MISS HUNT. I would like to discuss the topic.

MISS NEWCOMER. It seems to me that this problem can be broken down in many ways. It is only a symptom but we can only get into examples.

PSYCHIATRIST. This may or may not be so, but we do have to explore the problem to understand it.

PSYCHIATRIC NURSE. Another problem area we might discuss is the evaluation of student behavior.

MISS THOMAS. Do we first need to discuss a place where we can discuss students?

Miss Thomas' acidulous retort to the psychiatric nurse about first having to have a place to discuss students conveyed censure of the current structure, which had been imposed by the psychiatric team. (Perhaps she also was angry at the psychiatrist because the faculty members had had only desultory contact with him outside of these meetings.) She was inclined to view the discussion of student problems as the primary purpose of the faculty meetings associated with the integration project. This interpretation implied that she perceived the role of the psychiatric team as limited to working with the faculty on student problems. Unfortunately, because the members of the psychiatric team were preoccupied with the difficulties in intrafaculty relationships, at that time they did not follow this lead.

MISS JENSEN. Our relationship with the junior students is presenting problems. Then we . . . .

PSYCHIATRIST [*interrupts*]. Before we start discussing a problem we need to reach a decision about which one.

MISS DREW. I would like to discuss Maria Manning [*a student*], but this can be done elsewhere. It isn't urgent to discuss how the behavior of students fits into the evaluation.

Miss Thomas. Since Dr. Ullman and Jane made these stipulations that we have to choose a topic, then I choose number 1.

[*The group votes to discuss the problem of decision making.*]

Miss Reed. An example of the problem is whether we accept the decision about how many D's a student can get in clinical practice and still stay in the department.

Miss Jensen. This comes to a head when students are failed without having received a warning.

Miss Foster. Aren't we getting away from the real problem?

Psychiatrist. We need to get back to the topic. How do decisions get discarded?

[*The group is silent.*]

Psychiatric Nurse. Perhaps there is the feeling that many times a decision has already been made and that we are merely playing games by going through the motions of decision making.

Psychiatrist. The situation of wish-fulfillment that came up a couple of weeks ago in relation to Dot [*Jensen*] presenting a problem is an example of acting as though a decision had been made.

Miss Thomas. I still think Dot [*Jensen*] agreed to present a problem.

Miss Reed. We don't examine the far-flung implications of a decision. We are so impulsive.

Miss Jensen. We sure are, and it gets us into hot water with the students.

Psychiatric Nurse. Perhaps we are so dependent on approval from others and afraid of disapproval, we act as if we go along with a decision when we really disagree.

Miss Thomas. In the case of Gert Hall, no one could make up their minds about her.

Miss Foster. We have wasted hours in discussion of a decision that has already been made.

Miss Drew. We constantly act as if we have to have unanimous agreement with a decision, and then we proceed to act as if there is agreement, even though many times there isn't.

Miss Jensen. Some decisions shouldn't be given to us to make in the first place. Some decisions should be given as a dictum and not as a choice when there really is none.

Miss Vance. Suggestions such as the one that faculty members might invite the students to their homes for socializing and entertainment become decisions to which everyone is supposed to conform.

Psychiatric Nurse. But I wonder why we don't question these suggestions at the time they are given instead of acting helpless as though there is nothing we can do? We say nothing and then blame each other as the anger smolders.

Miss Foster. We quake at the thought of what we will hear in response.

Psychiatric Nurse. I am impressed by the relative ease with which we are frightened away from expressing our reactions and raising questions at the time decisions are under discussion.

Psychiatrist. Decisions seem to be made as though they are the solution to the problem.

PSYCHIATRIC NURSE. Didn't we see a demonstration of this right here when there was the assumption that Dot [*Jensen*] was supposed to present a problem? There was agreement on a nonverbal level, but it was not reached on the verbal. Once the so-called decision had time to incubate and there was the realization that we didn't like the proposed structure, the decision was thrown out.

PSYCHIATRIST. Jane is pointing to the difficulty in eliciting negative attitudes. This is especially true when the first person who reveals such attitudes does so in the face of previous attitudes that may have been unfavorable. Nevertheless, there are times when the negative attitudes may be more realistic and in keeping with what has occurred than positive attitudes.

Our focus is now on the broad problem of decision making. Our tendency is to focus on specifics with an effort to resolve them rather than use them as an example of the broad problem under discussion. Have we witnessed any of these factors right here in this group? How does this difficulty manifest itself in other areas? Do you want to continue with this discussion?

MISS NEWCOMER [*wrinkles her freckled brow*]. We have only scratched the surface.

This meeting was a portrait of the faculty's first endeavor to function within a given structure. The faculty members were noticeably inexperienced and undisciplined in functioning within an operational framework. Each member tended to wander into a maze of extraneous trivia, and the meeting time was frittered away as each competed with the other in demonstrating her knowledge of the topic.

Some member accepted guidance from the psychiatric team with a minimum of anxiety, whereas others were nettled by what they perceived as the team's interference with the democratic process, which they equated with absence of limits and structure. Regional outcroppings of blaming and of resistance against taking personal responsibility appeared.

At the same time the acting out of anger and resentment was decreased. Participation was less strained and flowed more freely. Some members continued to withdraw. Note taking and side comments were minimal. For the first time, fear of how others would react was referred to directly. Reference to wish fulfillment as a problem in decision making was responded to with irritation, annoyance, pensiveness, and reflection.

The suggestion by a member of the older group that decision making be the topic for discussion struck at a vital core of intrafaculty difficulty, because of this subject's close connection with personal responsibility, the concept of authority, and the democratic process. Several questions and principles were implicit in the discussion of this topic.

1. Are decisions ever made without asking the faculty about them when it should be consulted? Or conversely, is the faculty consulted when it should not be?

2. When should or can a decision be primarily administrative, and which decisions should be hammered out by the total faculty or a segment of it?

3. There is a difference between whether a decision should or should not be made by administration and whether the decision is a right or wrong one.

4. Administration might make more decisions than necessary, or fewer decisions in an effort to be democratic.

Although difficulty in making decisions is often due to interpersonal and emotional conflicts, these conflicts were not touched on during this meeting except for the reference to the fear of retaliation. Nevertheless, previous meetings had provided sufficient evidence that the faculty conflicts encompassed a broad range that included fear of making mistakes accompanied by fear of retaliation, desire to be ingratiating, resistance to change, unresolved attitudes toward authority, and the pursuit and maintenance of status.

Role of the Psychiatric Team. In the beginning of the meeting, the psychiatrist insisted on talking about what he wanted to discuss, but gradually, when the faculty members responded with silence, he gave ground and relinquished his power. At that point, the psychiatric nurse assumed the leadership and began to deal with the faculty members' concerns about a positive approach by focusing on the concrete; for example, she gave a specific illustration of how the faculty's decision making miscarried. This behavior on her part represented a new departure. Up until this time, the psychiatric nurse and the psychiatrist had assiduously avoided handling concrete issues because they had been engrossed in finding their place within the group.

The psychiatric nurse was more direct and to the point than she had been in the last few meetings. Her anxiety had been reduced considerably. She was more comfortable and sure of herself and her role, and in contrast to her previous oversensitivity, which had led her into all kinds of blunders, she did not take sarcastic comments personally and turn them in against herself. Her greatest fear was that the faculty meetings would terminate, and she handled it by bringing the problem into the open with the faculty. In the past the other faculty members had responded to the psychiatric nurse's anxiety and anger with disapproval and scapegoating, the very reactions she expected and feared. In this meeting, they responded to her increased effectiveness.

Following this meeting there was evidence that the faculty was beginning to stay with one issue and to discuss it in greater depth. Four consecutive meetings were devoted to the problem of decision making. As usual, however, the faculty did not come to any specific decisions, and the whole issue was left up in the air to be returned to time and again on those occasions when decisions misfired.

Disorganization within the Faculty Discussions

NEGATIVE ACTING OUT

Early in April, at the instigation of the psychiatric nurse, her group conferences with sophomore students were brought up for evaluation at the faculty meetings held in connection with the integration program. Generally this evaluation would not have taken place until some time in the summer when the evaluation of the integration program usually began. However, because the student conferences had reached an impasse, immediate intervention was required.

The impasse had come about because of the behavior of some of the participating instructors. From the beginning this participation had resulted in difficulties, and it finally reached a critical point. The meetings with students were tense and hostile.

Two faculty members struggled to define their role, responded to cues from the psychiatric nurse, and joined in the discussion whenever they felt it was appropriate. Three others sat passively on the sidelines and observed the psychiatric nurse without making any effort to participate. Three other faculty members, who had given other indications of attempts to undermine the integration project, acted out their negative attitudes toward the psychiatric nurse. They generally sat close to each other, exchanged sardonic grins, passed notes, and made audible side comments to each other. On several occasions they were successful in engaging some students in their ongoing interaction.

The faculty members' hostility toward the psychiatric team (probably because the team had assumed the role of sole authority and had taken over the decision making in the faculty discussions) was never brought into the open or clarified during the meetings. The basic issue regarding the faculty members' behavior in the student discussions with the psychiatric nurse was that these conferences provided one of the few opportunities for them to act out their negative reactions toward the psychiatric team. Because it was less threatening for them to attack the psychiatric nurse than the psychiatrist, they took a snipe at him through her.

For the purpose of trying to hold back and contain the crisis, the psychiatric nurse approached each instructor for an individual conference. As a result, some faculty members made a discernible effort to change their behavior. In the case of others, however, previous difficulties were further exaggerated. One instructor successfully evaded all the psychiatric nurse's attempts for an individual conference with her.

The students became more withdrawn in the unstructured discussions. They closed down on expressing their feelings and attitudes. The topics suggested for discussion were of a contrived nature rather than ones that had grown out of the students' interest and motivation to resolve problems.

As the weeks went on, the psychiatric nurse became more uncomfortable and felt uncertain about the direction in which to move. Accordingly, she asked for an early discussion and evaluation of the student group conferences. Six faculty meetings were devoted to this evaluation. Vignettes from three of these meetings are reproduced here.

REGIONAL ATTEMPTS TO DISRUPT STUDENT DISCUSSIONS

April 12, 1960
Two members of the older group are absent from this meeting, and one is completely silent throughout the meeting.

PSYCHIATRIST. The problem before us is should this type of conference continue in the integration program? What modifications do we need to make that will enable the experience to be beneficial to you personally?

MISS HUNT. I feel the student conferences should be more patient-centered. Up to now they have been student-centered, and therefore students won't open up.

MISS NEWCOMER. I think the emphasis on problem solving can be done in other ways. Students should be permitted to solve problems on their own without faculty. I don't feel the conferences with Jane should be continued. The same goals can be reached in other ways through clinical conferences.

PSYCHIATRIC NURSE. Monte and I aren't involved in clinical conferences with students except in our work with the individual instructors.

MISS NEWCOMER. Jane could serve as a resource person as necessary.

MISS THOMAS. There is no denying that we have had less time for patient care conferences. But I'm not wholly in favor of discontinuing Jane's unstructured conferences. We haven't had them long enough. It's too soon to know. I'm not able to state any modifications. We need to think about and clarify the goals first.

MISS DREW. I don't know how I feel. Sometimes I think the conferences should continue, and other times I feel like the rest of faculty. I think the choice of topics should be controlled. I don't feel students should discuss individuals—either faculty, nursing service personnel, or others. How were these hours used before Jane came here? Yesterday, the conference with her was helpful, but if the problem had not been brought up there, it would have been raised in my own clinical conference.

MISS HUNT. Students' attitudes and reactions about such things as the elimination of the capping ceremony won't get discussed in our clinical conferences.

[*The group is silent.*]

[*Miss Foster and Miss Newcomer exchange glances and make side comments to each other.*]

PSYCHIATRIST. Claire [*Foster*], do you want to express yourself on this?

MISS FOSTER. I agree with Ruth [*Newcomer*]. Students can solve their own problems.

PSYCHIATRIST. Do you think the conferences should be discontinued?

MISS FOSTER [*pauses*]. There's no reason for them.

Miss Graf. Can I come in here as an outsider who has not been in on the conferences? I asked one of the faculty how students took care of their problems before the integration program. She pointed out that students managed, but now that they have to fill in an hour every week, they find problems.

Psychiatrist [*tries to take a vote*]. Claire [*Foster*] and Ruth [*Newcomer*], how are you going to vote?

Miss Newcomer. This is a radical way to work with students.

Miss Graf. And the students don't seem to be getting much value from the conferences.

Psychiatrist. This is not the issue.

In this meeting two younger members joined forces and made a bold push to dispense with the student group conferences. This disruptive behavior was not merely a result of anxiety and being threatened, but it also stemmed from a desire to undermine the integration program. Miss Newcomer helped to widen the split in the faculty.

Some faculty members avoided facing their own attitudes and reactions to change and fear of loss of status. None of the participants was able to handle the situation. Individual defensive patterns included withholding, complete withdrawing from the discussion, using students as a rationalization for denying personal responsibility, and placing blame.

In spite of the melee, some members acknowledged their conflict and were willing to examine the problem and strive to resolve it. As these pockets of potential leadership began to open up, a splintering within the younger and older groups began to appear, which, paradoxically, opened the way for some group cohesiveness.

A Contest for Power and Prestige

April 19, 1960

Psychiatric Nurse. Since our meeting last week, I had my weekly seminar with the junior students who are having their psychiatric nursing experience. In the course of inquiring about faculty, they spontaneously asked about my unstructured group conferences with the sophomore students. In light of our recent discussions, I utilized this fortuitous event for their evaluation of the experience which these students had had the previous year. They were enthusiastic about the conferences and felt this experience was one of the most valuable in the curriculum. They were quick to add that they did not appreciate it fully until they were away from it for a time. They admitted that the experience was not easy or always pleasant, and that it takes time to catch on to the whole point of this kind of living experience in problem solving. They feel it has enabled them to relate better with all patients and authority figures, and has helped them to better understand psychiatric patients.

Psychiatrist. The student conferences with Jane alone were not abandoned last year in and of themselves, but rather because we were unclear about how they fit into the integration program and our goal of helping the faculty to learn and to apply psychiatric concepts. Jane's footwork and research into students' reactions indicate that this experience helps students in at least three ways. First, it softens and loosens up students in their relationship with the rest of faculty by giving them the opportunity to work through some of their problems with authority. It creates the greater possibility for faculty and students to be happier with each other. Second, it creates a receptivity to psychiatric nursing by imparting a spirit of meaning of behavior and how to handle it. Finally, it has greater value to succeeding classes as previous students communicate its value to them.

PSYCHIATRIC NURSE. For the past two meetings, faculty have expressed their reactions to the group conferences with students and have stated they would like the total emphasis to be on clinical material. Now I would like to clarify the way I see the situation and make a recommendation.

I feel it is important for students to have the opportunity to thrash out problems with someone who is not involved in evaluating them. Also, I feel it is just as important that I work closely with faculty. In consideration of these two factors, I suggest the following compromise for the fall.

1. Instead of working with students alone for the whole year, or having faculty with me, I would like to work with the students alone from September until January in unstructured group conferences.
2. After January, the focus would be changed to clinical conferences in which the faculty and I would participate as a team.

MISS NEWCOMER. Why should Jane be alone with the students?

MISS GRAF. Wasn't the purpose of faculty being brought in on the conferences because they did not feel as close to the students? Do we feel the students have improved? What will happen after Dr. Ullman and Jane leave the program? How does this experience with Jane alone help faculty?

MISS THOMAS. I was never concerned about what went on in Jane's conferences, but. . . .

MISS NEWCOMER [interrupts]. Why can't all the conferences be on a clinical level?

MISS HUNT. Faculty who evaluate students can't get into these kinds of problems.

MISS THOMAS. You know, Peggy [Graf], this is why we have the integration program in the first place. We thought we needed it.

MISS REED. I don't know how the other groups go, but I think my presence inhibits the students. There are just too many authority figures present. It wouldn't hurt for me to stay out. I feel the students think they will be evaluated on what they say and therefore it is difficult for them to bring in their problems. Jane can get at them because she doesn't evaluate. Also, in their evaluation of students, faculty members are bound to be influenced by what students say in the conferences, whether they want to be or not.

PSYCHIATRIST. The point has been raised as to why students can't bat out problems by themselves, and a certain aspect of this is true. In the student group conferences, we have a tool to help students deal with their neurotic interactions between themselves and patients. In caring for patients, students are up against neurotic interactions and therefore are receptive to deeper analysis of problems. From Jane's report, the conferences helped to wean the current group of students who are having psychiatric nursing away from attitudes of disdain and suspicion about psychiatric matters. Jane's and my only hope is that an aura will be established in which we have a faculty and group of students who are more receptive to psychiatry. We feel that students in all clinical areas need this kind of an experience with a psychiatric nurse and a psychiatrist. [*He asks for a vote from the group.*]

[*Miss Reed and Miss Thomas vote* for *the continuation of the unstructured conferences for one quarter. Miss Foster and Miss Newcomer vote* against *continuation of any unstructured conferences. Miss Hunt and Miss Drew abstain because they are not sure.*]

PSYCHIATRIST. Should we then explore the validity of the points that Ruth [*Newcomer*] and Claire [*Foster*] raise about these conferences holding the students back in their learning? Can whatever goes on in Jane's conferences take place in the nursing care conferences?

MISS NEWCOMER. These conferences are too radical. It's not as if there is no help available to students from faculty. Students can get it on an individual level and in groups when they feel it is necessary.

MISS WILLIS. Jane has taught me the meaning of trust when she had the meetings alone with the students. It's time for us to trust.

PSYCHIATRIST. Do we, as a psychiatric team, have anything to offer faculty other than to deal with psychopathologic behavior? Does the psychiatric nurse have anything above and beyond what the clinical instructor has to give in the area of dealing with patients' and students' emotional responses to illness?

To deal with patients who act out is a most difficult and complex problem and each instructor learns to handle this in her own way and pass it on to students. Deeper levels of handling, however, can be achieved only through resource people being brought in.

PSYCHIATRIC NURSE. I think the issue may be, what can the faculty and the psychiatric nurse learn from each other?

MISS NEWCOMER. The psychiatric nurse does not have a monopoly on behavior. There are other clinical areas that are concerned with behavior also, such as our own.

Once again a division of the faculty became apparent. The psychiatrist tried to force closure on the discussion by taking a vote; in so doing, he was repeating what the faculty had always done, namely, repressing the existing conflicts by making a premature decision.

In the vote pertaining to the continuation of the student group discussions with the psychiatric nurse, the group was divided three ways. Two older members voted affirmatively, two younger members voted negatively, and two other younger members abstained. It was a mirror of the deeper faculty schism.

Some older members were unsure about how to handle the younger members' negative behavior and further stimulated it by lecturing and moralizing. At the same time, differing points of view and sources of strength emerged in the younger group.

The Gentle Murmur of Change

The faculty members continued to attend the student conferences with the psychiatric nurse. With the exception of three members in the younger group, some obvious change occurred in their behavior. Participation in the meetings increased. The withholding of comments and withdrawal were reduced. Both the psychiatric nurse and the other faculty members were making some effort at collaboration. The students began to respond accordingly.

The changing attitudes were reflected when, prior to a meeting on this subject, two members of the older group came to the psychiatric team to tell them they would be unable to attend, but wanted to give them their vote for continuation of the student group conferences. Both of them voted for the compromise recommendation, according to which conferences with the psychiatric nurse alone would be held in the first quarter and would be followed in the remaining three quarters by clinical conferences in which other faculty members would participate.

April 26, 1960

Miss Hunt. Before we get started, I want to say to you, Jane, that for one who is supposed to be able to listen to others, you sure cut me off last week.
[*Silence*]

Psychiatrist. To return for a moment to the reasons for staying with the unstructured conferences with Jane alone, at first we couldn't justify these in terms of emphasis of psychiatric integration with the faculty. However, now we understand that faculty can be helped indirectly by helping students become freer in their communication with faculty. I know through my own experience with the students alone, in the team and tuberculosis nursing experiences, how positively they respond, reach out, and utilize such conferences.
[*Miss Foster nods her head and sneers.*]

Psychiatrist. I think it's time to take another vote.

Miss Foster [*lights a cigarette and inhales*]. I don't think the unstructured conferences with Jane will do any good. They defeat your own purpose. I can handle these problems with students. I think all the conferences with Jane alone should be eliminated.

Psychiatric Nurse. What is it you're so angry about, Claire? You were the person who last year pushed for the faculty to come into the conferences.
[*Miss Foster continues to write and does not answer.*]

Miss Drew. How would the clinical conferences that would take over in the second semester differ from those that the individual instructor has with Jane and Dr. Ullman?

Psychiatric Nurse. They would be quite similar.

Miss Willis. We've always been able to accept psychiatry here.

Miss Foster [*lights a fresh cigarette*]. I feel we should eliminate the unstructured conferences altogether. I don't feel that the presence of the clinical instructors with Jane is the problem. I have reasons to know this is so.

Psychiatrist. I would like to raise a point, Claire [*Foster*], about your negative contribution. The tenor of your contribution is so negative, so general, and so mysterious that it is unfair. If you have certain information about the conferences, it is not a private affair. It's as if we are trying to force something down your throat. You have been derogatory and hurtful to Jane and me as individuals.

Miss Foster [*withdraws into writing and her eyes fill with unshed tears*]. I'm not trying to cut out an experience, and I haven't meant to be derogatory.

Psychiatric Nurse. Claire, you have been derogatory to me.

Miss Newcomer. Students should have the choice of whom they want to go to with their problems.

Psychiatric Nurse. Because we have a psychiatric integration project it does not mean we assume that growth wasn't going on with students in their other classes, with their families, and so on. But the point is, does psychiatry and do Monte and I have something to contribute to both students and faculty?

Miss Drew. Can we hear about votes from Thelma [*Reed*] and Linda [*Thomas*]?

Psychiatrist. Both of them went along with the compromise and feel Jane should work alone with the students for the first quarter.

[*Silence.*]

Miss Drew. I feel the compromise is no good! [*Her brown eyes flash.*]

Miss Newcomer. What is the purpose of Jane's unstructured conferences? I don't like the method used, and it doesn't work with other clinical instructors.

Psychiatric Nurse. It might be helpful to summarize the recommendations thus far.

> 1. For the first two weeks in the fall, I would have the students alone in group conferences.
> 2. For the remainder of the sophomore year, I would participate with one instructor from each clinical area and her group of students.
> 3. By and large these conferences during the last three quarters would be clinically oriented, but also there would be the provision that students could discuss anything they want to bring up.
> 4. Those faculty who would not be working directly with me would be free to structure their conferences as they see fit.
> 5. Time would be arranged for the individual instructor and me to discuss what went on in the clinical conference.

Miss Vance. There are numerous times during this past year while in Jane's conferences that I felt I wanted to leave because I knew my evaluation of students was being influenced.

Miss Drew. I feel the same way as Esther [*Vance*]. I feel some topics should not be brought up in the group at all.

Psychiatric Nurse. The crucial issue here is whether students should have the opportunity and a person with whom they can discuss the problems that arise in their relationships with patients, faculty, nursing personnel, and other students.

Miss VANCE. I definitely think students should have this opportunity, but I don't think it should be with the clinical instructor who is too involved in evaluation.

Miss NEWCOMER. But the students are here to learn nursing.

The potential explosion erupted. Miss Hunt took the psychiatric nurse to task for having "cut her off" (which she had not done). Miss Foster openly attempted to destroy the psychiatric team's efforts in the integration program. She derogated the psychiatrist and the psychiatric nurse individually. When the psychiatrist interrupted her behavior, she responded with rage. A pregnant silence followed.

An older member expressed the belief that students should have these conferences, but expressed the opinion that leadership of such conferences was not the role of the instructor. A member in the younger group pointed to what she perceived as a contradiction between the goals of nursing education and the unstructured group conferences with the psychiatric nurse.

A RÉSUMÉ OF THE THREE MEETINGS

Until the meetings about the unstructured student conferences, the attitudes of some of the faculty members toward the psychiatric team and the integration program had been muffled in hypocrisy, ambiguity, and equivocation. The explosion during these meetings revealed more and more divergent points of view, and the existing schisms within the faculty and between the faculty and the psychiatric team became more evident.

Negative feelings toward and rejection of the psychiatric nurse came into the open. These attitudes were manifested primarily by three members of the younger group who had acquired leadership and power by default. It could not be taken for granted, however, that members of the older group were accepting the student experience or the psychiatric nurse on a deeper level. A combination of many complex factors may have been operating in their verbalized acceptance, including desire for approval by the psychiatric team, the fact that they felt less threatened than did the younger members with regard to problems of status, and the greater security they felt, because of the integration of their personal and professional roles as unmarried women and women with careers.

Although the general effect of the meetings was one of discord, a gentle note of harmony and change could be discerned amid the dissonance.

ROLE OF THE PSYCHIATRIC TEAM

These meetings became a test situation in which the faculty members seemed to be looking to see how the psychiatric team would handle destructive behavior in action. Were the psychiatric nurse and the psychiatrist genuinely committed to the integration program? Were they willing to "stick their necks out" for what they believed?

The burden of responsibility for deciding whether the student conferences were worth fighting for rested primarily on the psychiatric nurse. She had no doubt about the value of and necessity for such a student experience, but she was unclear about its relationship to the goal of helping the faculty members to teach and apply psychiatric concepts. For a time she was confused. She equated focus on faculty growth with elimination of whatever experiences might be unacceptable to the faculty, irrespective of the reasons for their rejection.

The students' enthusiastic and spontaneous responses to the group experience, plus one older faculty member's supportive and well-timed comment, "If you strongly believe in what you are doing, don't give it up at any cost," helped the psychiatric nurse to mobilize her inner resources and take a firm stand. When she shared her appraisal of the student experience with the psychiatrist, both were much more certain about how to proceed. Avenues of compromise that previously were unavailable to them began to open up.

In this series of meetings the psychiatric team began to intervene in the disruptive behavior of some faculty members. The psychiatrist dealt with elusive and disjunctive behavior when he interrupted Miss Foster's whispering and side comments by directly asking her for an opinion regarding continuation of the student discussions. Next, he suggested that the group explore whether or not the conferences were a deterrent to student learning. Finally, he pointed to the negative aspects of Miss Foster's contribution and left no doubt as to its personal impact on the psychiatric nurse and himself. The psychiatric nurse intervened in Miss Foster's disruptive behavior when she commented on Miss Foster's derogation and when she asked her why she was so angry.

When the psychiatric nurse and the psychiatrist made an issue about whether they had anything to contribute to the faculty and if so what, they were hunting for "bogeymen" because they were unable to understand why some faculty members were angry with them. The faculty members were not necessarly rejecting psychiatry and what it had to offer; it was much more likely that they were rejecting the psychiatric nurse and the psychiatrist because they had taken over the decision-making role.

During these meetings the psychiatrist retreated from his position of authority, and the psychiatric nurse assumed her legitimate role as leader. It was much easier for the faculty members to fight openly with the psychiatric nurse than with the psychiatrist because she had worked more closely with them in other situations and she was also more accessible to them.

FACULTY DERAILMENT

In the two months following the April 26 meeting, the faculty discussions centered on the evaluation of the clinical conferences in communicable disease and long-term illness nursing, team nursing, and public health nursing, in which the psychiatric nurse had been participating at the invitation of the instructors in these courses. The evaluation consisted of the instructor (in each case, one of the older group) and the psychiatric nurse telling the rest of the faculty about what they had been doing.

The next aspect of the integration program to be evaluated was the thirty-hour lecture-discussion course in psychodynamics that the psychiatric nurse taught to the sophomore students. As has been pointed out, this course was referred to by faculty members as "mental health classes." This course dealt with such subjects as anxiety, frustration-aggression, conflict, communication theory, and the illness process. Clinical situations from the students' own experiences were used to illustrate the various concepts. All the faculty members had been invited to attend any or all of the classes. Two instructors, one from the younger and one from the older group, attended regularly, and one from each group came sporadically.

The meeting at which this course was evaluated was the one in which the faculty finally reached the condition toward which it had long been heading —disorganization.

July 12, 1960

PSYCHIATRIC NURSE. Some of you have attended the mental health classes, and I would be interested in your reactions to them and how they might be improved. Also, I am interested in hearing from all of you how students are able to use the concepts.

MISS NEWCOMER. Students enjoyed the classes when a patient was discussed.

MISS JENSEN. The facts about the patient that students gave Jane in class were not true. They were distorted. [*She flips her blonde ponytail.*] Whatever suggestions she gave for handling the situation were based on distortions, and I had to tell the students they couldn't do such and such—whatever was suggested.

PSYCHIATRIC NURSE. You feel this put the clinical instructor in a bad light?

MISS JENSEN. I don't even know which patients are coming up for discussion in the class.

MISS THOMAS. Principles and techniques of interviewing need to come in sooner; by the time Jane gets to it, the students have already been doing it.

PSYCHIATRIC NURSE. If you recall, when the mental health classes started last year, everyone expressed realistic concern that students might become so involved with patient behavior that this would interfere with their learning basic nursing techniques. At that time all of you stressed the importance of not focusing on interviewing too soon, so that I have purposely played down interviewing until students had enough background in basic skills.

Miss Jensen. And it sure shows.

Miss Foster. By the first of the year, the students are interviewing in the outpatient clinic.

Miss Graf. I felt the mental health classes were dynamic and exciting, especially when the students discussed their reasons for going into nursing.

Miss Newcomer. I don't agree. I didn't learn anything, particularly about the students.

Miss Scott. Is there anything wrong with selecting a patient ahead of time? Also, would there be some value to discussing the students' distortions?

Psychiatric Nurse. The purpose of my presenting clinical situations in the mental health classes is to deal with students' anxiety and distortions rather than to come out with a clear-cut answer. Their distortions are an important part of the data.

Miss Thomas. Students feel that whatever you say is the way to handle a situation. They quote you, Jane.

Psychiatric Nurse. A student's own anxiety will lead her to clutch for pat answers and rigid rules.

Miss Jensen. The majority of students' class cuts have been in the mental health classes. Students don't find the classes valuable; they don't know how everything gets hooked together.

Miss Thomas. And it's not because they are going home. They use the time to work on care studies, and so on.

Miss Jensen. Students who are on the curriculum committee say they plan to cut the class because it is no help.

Miss Thomas. It may be due partly to the classes being held at the end of the day.

Miss Foster. It's not just the fact that it is at the end of the day.

Psychiatrist. If you checked the cuts in medical school, you would find that most of them are in psychiatry. There is a general aura around psychiatry, and our students are bound to become anxious, particularly since most of them are not going to become psychiatric nurses.

Miss Newcomer. Jane isn't teaching psychiatric nursing.

Miss Vance. Students tend to be awfully black or white about everything. Students have difficulty conceptualizing.

Miss Hunt. My students say they don't want to go to the classes.

Psychiatric Nurse. I can't get terribly upset about the students' reactions because they are not unusual. This happens even on the graduate nurse level. Since I don't rely solely on didactic teaching methods but emphasize the student's personal involvement in the classes, they are bound to become somewhat anxious. Boredom and indifference are not uncommon ways of dealing with anxiety.

[*Miss Foster and Miss Jensen exchange glances and nod their heads.*]

Miss Graf. The students participate more in this class than any other.

Miss Thomas. If Jane isn't concerned about it, should we be?

Miss Drew. I feel the students are cutting because they are not getting what they need.

Miss Jensen [*in a loud voice*]. Just how long do we have to wait for students to use mental health?

Miss Vance. The gap seems to be with faculty. We have to help students use what Jane is teaching; for example, to observe anxiety in the patient.

Psychiatric Nurse. Dot [*Jensen*], what do you mean by *use?*

Miss Jensen. One example is, all the students left a dying patient.

Miss Vance. Our students use the expression of feelings as an end in itself.

Psychiatrist. What does sift into the consciousness of students as a result of the mental health classes? Students explore their own concept of anxiety and how this interferes with clinical practice. What everyone is questioning here is what does the course do for the student and how can the outcome be evaluated objectively?

Miss Thomas. I would push up the content on interviewing. It might be a way of evaluating.

Miss Vance. The way you present the material in class, Jane, is terrific, but now I feel that you aren't concerned with its application.

Miss Scott. Shouldn't application come in care studies and patient-care conferences with the clinical instructors?

Miss Drew. In the clinical care conferences, the students completely withdraw.

Psychiatrist. In a personal psychoanalysis it takes years to change. Students' old patterns which are based on previous conditioning are much stronger than the pearls of wisdom that are new.

Psychiatric Nurse. Our goal is not to teach psychiatric concepts on a didactic level. There is a wide difference between having intellectual knowledge of the concepts and being able to apply them.

Miss Jensen. Shouldn't students be able to use these principles?

Psychiatrist. No. Knowing a principle does not enable the student to automatically use it. Application is another issue. It involves the nature of the problem, the setting, and various adaptations. I am getting the feeling that Jane's mental health classes are a fountain at which everyone bathes. The only place where Jane's classes come in here in our evaluation has to do with faculty's awareness of students' withdrawal and how to deal with it.

[*Miss Jensen makes side comments to Miss Foster.*]

Psychiatric Nurse. Dot [*Jensen*], I'm sure that what you have to say would be of value to the total group. It would be helpful if you would communicate so all of us could hear you.

Psychiatrist. The clinical situation is the place for the application of the principles.

Miss Thomas and Miss Scott. Other faculty have to help in making the applications.

Psychiatric Nurse. I explore reactions to painful, distressful situations. This then creates the *possibility* for change. It does not create change. The only thing that brings about change is necessity.

[*Miss Jensen mumbles audibly, makes side comments, sighs, and bobs her legs up and down. Miss Foster laughs out loud, chain smokes, and writes notes to Miss Newcomer. She leaves twenty minutes before the end of the meeting.*]

Psychiatric Nurse. Dot [*Jensen*], I am concerned with your attitude throughout this meeting.

MISS JENSEN. This year, students feel they want to leave classes for the first time. I don't think students felt this way two years ago.

PSYCHIATRIST. To expose students to a mental health program places a burden on faculty because such a program is more difficult and complicated than being autocratic. The problem is not whether students change, but whether they are more open and articulate? If so, this means faculty has to handle the situation differently.

MISS SCOTT. While I was on the ward with the students, they didn't want to care for patients.

MISS WILLIS. Formerly, nurses were able to change their patients when they didn't like them. Now, we keep students with patients to work through the problems.

PSYCHIATRIST. There is the factor of necessity. The nurse has to work with a patient.

MISS SCOTT. Sometimes the clinical instructor does exactly with a student what the student does with a patient. The instructor withdraws, so the insight doesn't work.

As the evaluation began, the younger faculty members focused predominantly on various limitations of the "mental health classes." They exploited the students' difficulties, confusion, and patterns of withdrawal from patients, possibly in order to alleviate their own anxiety and guilt feelings about not helping the students to utilize psychiatric concepts. Outbursts of laughter, raised voices, note passing, sneering, caustic side comments, and intimations that the students were not interested in mental health warped the evaluation process and turned it into an opportunity for attacking and blaming the psychiatric nurse.

Once again the problem of status moved to the foreground. Caught in the maelstrom of their fear of losing their unique position with students and being displaced by the psychiatric nurse, the faculty members were inclined to set up unrealistic expectations for students. They obviously were expecting the mental health classes to be a miraculous experience and the psychiatric nurse to be a magician rather than a teacher.

This situation was bound to have repercussions on the students, who could be expected to feel with faculty members in their uncertainty and negative attitudes about the mental health classes and to exploit these attitudes in the attempt to handle some of their own difficulties in dealing with the problems they were encountering with patients. Unless such exploitation and avoidance of nursing problems could be interrupted, a precarious situation was likely to develop in which the student and the instructor would utilize each other's insecurities to justify their own.

Accordingly, there were repeated attempts by the older members to short-circuit the disruptive interaction by emphasizing the faculty's role and responsibility in teaching the students to apply psychiatric concepts. Because some faculty members in the younger group perceived these attempts as indications that the older faculty members were against them, the current difficulties between the two groups were exacerbated. Any attempt to open up channels of communication was responded to with rejection, attack, derogation, and scapegoating. The psychiatric nurse was flailed with anger and contempt. The faculty schism was obvious, and it was also obvious that the members of the younger group had relegated the psychiatric team to the older group. The psychiatric team was completely alienated from the majority of the younger group.

The meeting closed with some younger members making derogatory comments to each other as they left, while other members (both younger and older) lingered on and talked to the psychiatric team. Disorganization of the faculty meetings was a reality.

Role of the Psychiatric Team. As the meeting unfolded, negative feelings about the psychiatric nurse were divulged. Whenever she pointed out negative behavior, this was ignored by the group. Conversely, when the psychiatrist did so, the group readily agreed with him. The psychiatrist did not set any limits on those participants who were attacking the psychiatric nurse. Nor did he understand, at the time, how his absence of limits had put the faculty and the psychiatric nurse into an untenable position. At this point the project seemed to be his alone, instead of his and the psychiatric nurse's.

The psychiatric nurse was therefore faced with three crucial questions for which she would have to find answers.

1. What problems were the faculty members having in seeking help from her, and what kind of barriers was she erecting between herself and the rest of the faculty.

2. How could she handle the situation so as to avoid participating in its irrational aspects and at the same time foster faculty cohesiveness?

3. How could the tide of the project be changed so that it would remain with the psychiatric nurse as well as with the psychiatrist?

Direct Confrontation and Intervention

For weeks faculty relationships had been at a breaking point. The faculty meeting room had become an arena in which a struggle for power was being waged. Three members of the younger group in particular were having a heyday as they engaged in an extensive diatribe against the psychiatric nurse. The older group seemed immobilized and unable to deal directly with the younger group's behavior. Both groups were looking to the psychiatric team for help in handling what had become an emergency.

The psychiatric nurse and the psychiatrist had made several attempts to intervene, none of which had brought about any lasting equilibrium. They realized it would take nothing less than an operation bootstrap to interrupt this self-paralyzing intransigence. To permit this situation to continue would be to subsidize the destructive behavioral pattern in which the faculty was imprisoned.

To galvanize the group into constructive action, the psychiatric nurse and the psychiatrist decided to work toward a clear confrontation in which each of them would present to the group his or her appraisal of what had been happening and its impact on himself or herself.

CONSENSUAL VALIDATION OF THE FACULTY SCHISM

July 19, 1960

PSYCHIATRIST. Obviously our timing must have been wrong in regard to the evaluation because we had a good deal to cover and there are some important features of the integration program that we have not touched on. I suggest in deference to expediency that we forget about that for the time being. I'm making this suggestion because in thinking about how the evaluation of the program has gone, I think perhaps we might profit most by looking at how we are evaluating it. In a sense we've made a real mistake because to really evaluate a program, everyone has to be involved in that program and concerned with evaluating it. I thought that this was something we could take for granted, but after watching the way the evaluation has gone, I'm not sure we were right in doing so.

I feel a little bit as though we went down to the oceanside and said, "Well, we're going to learn how to better handle the waves that are coming at us from the ocean," and so we begin evaluating the waves and how high and rapidly they're coming in. We delude ourselves into thinking that we've mastered the situation, but fail to realize that what we have left out of the account was the existence of an undertow. I, for one, have felt an undertow in terms of the feelings toward the program and what goes on in group meetings. To really do the situation justice, I think we have to consider what some of the negative feelings are about the program—those that have not been expressed directly, but come out indirectly through lack of participation or silence, or through occasional "pot-shots" that are not very constructive.

If you recall, when we began talking about things as a group two years ago, the very first problem to come to our attention was the fact that there was a split in the faculty. There were certain feelings about lack of communication, lack of democratic process, lack of due regard for deviant or diffident points of view, and so on. These problems had nothing to do with the psychiatric integration program because the program hadn't started yet. We felt that in a large measure these problems related to lack of adequate communication which involved all the things that people felt left out about and the inability to bring one's own point of view into the picture.

I refer to this because in some way I feel we're faced with a similar situation at this point, except now the integration program is involved. I feel that some sort of identification has been made along the same lines as two years ago, except that now Jane and I are identified with the older group. There is still an in-group and an out-group. It's a kind of un-unified state of affairs. If we're really going to go ahead with the integration program, I think we should forget the formal evaluation of the different aspects until we settle this problem. I think it is a serious matter.

[*Long silence.*]

PSYCHIATRIC NURSE. For several months now, I have felt separated and almost completely alienated from the so-called younger faculty members. Unfortunately, I do not sufficiently understand how this has happened or what it means, but I am deeply troubled about it. I am especially concerned about how I have contributed to the disruption of our group. I've arrived at the place where I am beginning to feel that I can't contribute anything without some form of value judgment and critical comment being passed. On numerous occasions I've sought out individual faculty members to try to explore the problem. In some instances the conference was most helpful, and in others, little understanding of each other was achieved. In one situation, all my efforts to get together failed.

I suspect that these negative attitudes must be sifting through to the students, especially in the unstructured group discussions where faculty are with me. I am concerned by what seems to be the reluctance to bring problems into the open and struggle together with them. I feel I have been pigeon-holed with the older faculty members. I have the impression that whenever they appear to support me this implies I am against the younger group. I sense that the younger members feel that I am no longer interested in their problems, that I can no longer look at them objectively, and that I am not interested in their welfare. For some time, I have felt completely cut off from you.

I have pondered long and hard on this problem. I feel as though the current situation closely resembles that which Monte and I entered three years ago. At that time the existing schism between the younger and older members was obvious. Now there also is a schism between the faculty and the psychiatric team. However, because of my professional identification with the faculty, my full-time investment in the project, and because I have become the main target for attack, I am sure I experience this estrangement from faculty more personally. Instead of the psychiatric integration program being the real issue under discussion, it seems to me, we are face-to-face with a crisis in which there are now at least two splits within the faculty. I feel it is crucial for me to become clear about how I have fed into the cleavage between the faculty and Monte and myself.

MISS DREW. I can't buy all you've just said. I think that there is a general problem that applies to the overall situation. However, my views on the integration program are quite well known, and I don't think they have changed in the past six weeks or six months as much as you indicate. As far as the student group conferences are concerned, they haven't gone along very smoothly, but I haven't felt any rift at all.

PSYCHIATRIC NURSE. Eileen [*Drew*], I agree that whenever we generalize, there are exceptions, but also I think that in our situation, the individual exceptions somehow manage to get lost or hidden within the all-pervasive group problem.

[*Long pause.*]

MISS SCOTT. Eileen, maybe you thought that there was a faculty chasm but that this does not necessarily involve you and Jane. Have you thought that there is a faculty chasm?

MISS DREW. I think it is quite obvious.

PSYCHIATRIST. I have been aware of this separation but I think before we can talk about it, we have to see if this is the general conception of the group.

MISS JENSEN. I think I would be very willing to go along with what Dr. Ullman and Jane have said. It is a very difficult thing to deny that a split has happened. The question is—why? For myself, I would say that I don't think that I've handled the situation well at all, and I'm not particularly proud of the way I've managed. At the same time I did the best I could under the circumstances. The most important thing for me is why has this happened?

PSYCHIATRIST. Well, I'd say that's the second most important, and I would say the first most important thing is, "Has a split happened?" We have not really gotten a statement to the effect that a split has happened. This is what has been holding us back. We have to acknowledge the fact that it has happened, that it exists, and that it's with us. Then we can explore why. Our difficulty has been that we have not explicitly acknowledged the existence of the chasm, how deep it is, and in what way it has involved the integration program. Until we do, we cannot get on with the question of why.

MISS WILLIS. I have the feeling throughout the spring there was a growing appreciation of many faculty members that they were moving along with Dr. Ullman and Jane. To me the rift was not as great as it was, but it is only since you've been in the meetings, Dot [*Jensen*], that I have noticed this feeling growing up again. Since the last two meetings, I felt we had gone backward instead of forward.

MISS THOMAS. It is like walking into a hurricane atmosphere. It seemed that during the last two meetings when Jane began to talk about what she had been doing, very grave differences of opinion became obvious. I was not aware of quite so wide a division until the week before last.

PSYCHIATRIST. I have a somewhat different feeling about it, and I guess that's due to not being misled by the surface appearance of things. Dot's [*Jensen*] return has brought the problem to a head, but our problem has nothing to do with Dot because she wasn't here. In other words, this is a problem that perhaps Dot might have been involved in had she been here. Perhaps she might have not. [*Some laughter from the group.*] Somehow she has become embroiled in the problem and, in a sense, has called our attention to it. I'm disagreeing with her role in it because I think if we're all grown up and if we're going to try and face the problem, we might as well try to face it as grown people, and really inquire into the attitudes—and I'm willing to be corrected if I'm wrong—of Claire [*Foster*] and Ruth [*Newcomer*]. I think Eileen [*Drew*] is right in that the only fair way to deal with this is not to generalize. We're trying to avoid personalities by generalizing.

I think Eileen has many reservations, doubts, qualms, and qualifications about the whole value of this program. I don't think that Eileen is free of those doubts at this point, but I don't think that it's our role that she be free of these doubts. It has been our hope that she would participate in the integration program towards deepening her grasp of what we were concerned with and to re-evaluate it after this experience. It's my feeling that she has been receptive to this experience, and has taken an objective attitude over and above her exclusive reactions. So that this is not the problem.

The problem is not whether anyone agrees with us or doesn't agree with us. The problem is if someone does not agree with us and does not express it and the disagreement is not known to us! This is the problem. We can learn from disagreements more than we can learn from agreements if they are expressed. We can't when they're not. And as I've said, this is where we've fallen off the track in trying to evaluate something because we're not sure to what extent everyone really wanted to evaluate.

MISS NEWCOMER. I will be interested in my feelings about mental health next year when the student group conferences are clinically oriented. This year I have had very little contact through students with mental health integrated in my own area. I feel we have a predominant role to play in behavior. Fifty per cent or more of the focus in our own clinical area is on mental health, so I think this has fantastic potential for mental health integration. However, the only contact I've had with Jane has been her sporadic attempts to establish rapport with me, and this happened very little, until recently. I don't feel our area has gotten integrated with mental health at all. My feeling has been that Jane hasn't admitted that our area also includes focus on behavior. I have felt that maybe she feels she has a cornerstone on behavior. Now I certainly agree that our area doesn't have a corner on behavior either, but that it is carried throughout nursing education and is a vital part of it. Maybe my view is not the psychiatric view but has more of a "relative behavior" orientation.

PSYCHIATRIST. Well, this is the way you feel, and it makes sense. But if this is the way you feel, you should have been shouting it from the rooftops.

MISS NEWCOMER. Well, perhaps, and maybe I'm wrong. But in my experiences as a young faculty member, maybe I haven't been able to shout what my feelings were.

PSYCHIATRIST. Well, perhaps some standoffishness, some difficulty in communication, some standing apart mentally may be involved. You didn't offer your feelings until you were really pulled in to do it. In other words, you didn't really approach the situation until it had something to offer, and then you were going to ask for it, but in a somewhat standoffish fashion. Just as in the case of what you say now. It would have been more helpful if it had been said six months ago, or four months ago, or at any point.

MISS NEWCOMER. It was said at the faculty group conferences.

PSYCHIATRIST. Well, let me ask this, was it ever satisfactorily resolved in your own mind?

MISS NEWCOMER. Not for this year, but for the next. I'm impatient to wait.

PSYCHIATRIST. Perhaps we're wrong, I don't know. I had the feeling that there was something bothering you that was never fully aired, but that it had its effect. I felt it was resolved partially when we did get down to the business of discussing and planning for Jane's student group conferences for next year.

MISS NEWCOMER. I thought this was constructive. I was delighted when students went to Jane for help with their care studies and also when three of the group conferences revolved around clinical situations. I feel integration is a two-way street and that Jane also has to indicate her interest in our area.

PSYCHIATRIC NURSE. It's been my impression that I have been pretty direct about my interest in your clinical area. I wonder if my lack of contact with your area has been confused with lack of interest. I asked Helen [*Scott*], for example, if I could work with her in her setting.

MISS SCOTT. It just so happens I asked for you.

MISS FOSTER. I never felt that Jane was not interested in my clinical area.

MISS WILLIS. Ruth [*Newcomer*], did you ever ask Jane for a conference to discuss this?

MISS NEWCOMER. No.

Miss Thomas pointed out the existing split between the faculty and the psychiatric team. In response to the psychiatrist's direct focus on her, Miss Newcomer, who had hitherto limited her participation to occasional comments and communication with her allies, became very much involved. She stated her attitude toward the integration program directly and simply. Both she and Miss Scott spoke about their feeling that the psychiatric nurse had stood outside of and apart from the group. In essence, Miss Newcomer seemed to be asking the psychiatric team, "Why don't you both forget you are experts and enter into a relationship with us on the level where we are and help us with our functioning as teachers. Why don't you play our game for a change, instead of insisting on your own?"

MISS VANCE. The problem that we are getting away from is how we became split as a group.

PSYCHIATRIST. The issue is not what clarification of the problem did or did not take place. Such clarification involves deep-seated attitudes toward cohesiveness or divisiveness. Perhaps the mechanics that are involved come out more sharply in Ruth's [*Newcomer*] clinical area. Nevertheless, there are three aspects to keep in mind.

1. We tend to handle problems in a way that leads more to divisiveness than cohesiveness.
2. This tendency existed before the psychiatric integration program began.
3. This tendency cuts deeper than the integration program.

MISS JENSEN. One of the problems is that we spend a great deal of time on where Jane can contribute, but little is said about the rest of faculty. There is the feeling that unless we have had the advantage of a mental health program, we have no business being here. There is continuous emphasis on going to Jane for the answers, especially when it comes to evaluation of students. Everything that relates to problems with students is taken out of my hands and I'm told to "go to Jane or Dr. Ullman." During the first year of the project was the last time I was told I did a good job.

Miss NEWCOMER. I don't agree. Jane has always shared student problems and during the first two quarters of the sophomore year, individual faculty were helped to handle the situations themselves.

PSYCHIATRIC NURSE. Ruth [*Newcomer*], I think you are pointing out the differences between collaboration and competition. Once we are straight on the difference, there no longer is a problem about whom the student goes to.

Miss THOMAS. Last year I felt shut out about students' problems, but I don't this year.

Miss VANCE. Is there an uncomfortable feeling that somehow Jane will lead us and the students down a path that we don't agree with?

Miss JENSEN. I've always gone along with what Jane and Dr. Ullman did.

Miss VANCE. The program was a threat to me at first. I didn't give either Jane or Dr. Ullman credit for being nonjudgmental. My awareness of their nonblaming attitude comes only in retrospect. Yet the anticipation of their being critical created problems for me in accepting them and the program.

Miss WILLIS [*to Miss Foster*]. Do you feel badly that you haven't worked with Dr. Ullman and Jane in the clinical conferences with students?

[*Miss Foster does not answer. She continues to write.*]

PSYCHIATRIC NURSE. This morning in the faculty meeting, for example, faculty was split right down the middle.

[*Miss Willis looks up in surprise at the psychiatric nurse and stops writing.*]

Miss JENSEN. I know, and I agree that it's immature behavior. But why does the undertow continue? [*She doodles.*]

Miss THOMAS. Well, for one thing, it would be more helpful to bring problems into the open rather than express them through this continuous note writing that goes on.

PSYCHIATRIST. You don't have to be paranoid to react negatively to the note writing and passing, regardless of the content of the note, when the purpose of the meeting is an open forum.

Miss THOMAS. Besides being destructive, it is impolite. In this group, we and not the students have the opportunity to discuss our problems.

Miss WILLIS. Are you objecting to this kind of meeting? Do you feel put upon? Dot [*Jensen*], are you saying you doodle because of lack of interest?

Miss FOSTER. Miss Willis, you have the tendency to take the blame for whatever happens.

Miss DREW. We are avoiding the real issue, which is the negative attitude toward the mental health program. I don't feel that these problems will get solved here in the group. I think they can only be dealt with on an individual conference level.

Miss HUNT. Right now, the faculty rift becomes apparent. I wouldn't dream of supervising older faculty, yet there are those older members who seem to supervise us younger members.

Miss JENSEN. An example of what creates the faculty split occurred when Catherine [*Willis*] said faculty worked well together as a group until I returned.

Miss WILLIS. You assumed that this related to you.

Miss JENSEN. Nevertheless, I feel that if I say what I really think, somewhere along the way I will have to pay for it. If you notice, Dr. Ullman was the only person who defended me.

PSYCHIATRIST. I hope you all agree that doodling is okay. It is communication between one's self and one's self, or in other words, it is an intrapsychic dialogue. [*The group snickers.*]

PSYCHIATRIST. This is quite different from note writing and comes through differently to others. Our problem is that we have an undertow. Eileen [*Drew*] is correct when she raises the difficulties involved in studying the undertow. In some instances, this can be done in the group or on an individual level. It is necessary to become aware of the undertow. Negative feelings entail personal responsibility toward whomever they are directed.

Perhaps one of the trends that Jane and I need to establish is to keep more in touch with the individual instructor, so we can be an outlet for the instructor's negative feelings. Then we have to consider seriously what Dot [*Jensen*] is saying about fear of having to pay a price for expressing negative attitudes. We have to shift from price paying, which only results in conformity. The answer must be an undeniable "no" to price paying. If it occurs, it must be proven so.

MISS SCOTT. It is not just what is said—it is the way in which comments are said.

PSYCHIATRIST. An individual should not be penalized even for destructive behavior.

MISS NEWCOMER. It is not fair to throw another person out. You did this to Claire [*Foster*], and she hasn't opened her mouth since.

PSYCHIATRIST. I reserve the right to say, "I don't like the tone of one's behavior," which makes the issue known and in the open.

Until this meeting, some older members had denied the existence of a faculty schism. In this meeting there was beginning to be some consensus within the group regarding the faculty cleavage, although the imputations directed toward Miss Jensen by Miss Willis for the current impasse served as a way of continuing to deny the former existence of the faculty split. Participation was more general, although one older member continued to remain silent throughout the meeting. The note writing and passing persisted and finally were commented on.

However, the hostility toward the psychiatric nurse was beginning to wane somewhat. Miss Foster stated that she felt the psychiatric nurse had always been interested in her clinical area, and Miss Newcomer and Miss Thomas both agreed that she had communicated with them about students' problems. Several members successfully redirected the group back to the initial issue.

A remarkable turn of events occurred at the end of this meeting. Miss Newcomer challenged the psychiatrist's behavior toward Miss Foster in the April 19 meeting. This was the first time that any faculty member, let alone a younger member, had directly confronted the psychiatrist with her perception of how he had been functioning. Voices of strength and leadership grew louder and clearer. The disorganization of the faculty meetings had uncovered the specific areas of divisiveness and cohesiveness.

Role of the Psychiatric Team. It also was the first time that the psychiatrist dealt directly with the faculty's negative reactions toward the integration program. In recapitulating what had led up to the impasse, he left himself outside of the group situation, however, by neglecting to focus on how he may have contributed to the difficulties. It was almost as if he, passively, had been put in the position of being scapegoated by the faculty.

The principal problem with the way the psychiatric nurse and the psychiatrist had functioned was that neither one had been sufficiently aware of the dynamics operating at the time. Because psychiatric integration and interdisciplinary collaboration were new learning experiences for the members of the team, just as they were for the faculty, an absence of awareness in certain areas might be presumed to be inevitable. The key issue in the psychiatric team's work with the faculty was not the fact that the disorganization of the faculty in these meetings had occurred, nor that the team members had made mistakes because of their unawareness of how their behavior had exacerbated the faculty schism, which fortified the disruptive aspects of the faculty interaction, but rather, the issue was the extent to which the psychiatric nurse and the psychiatrist were able to resolve the existing conflicts.

PICKING UP THE PIECES

Some weeks before the meeting just described, the members of the psychiatric team realized that they were faced with the problem of dealing with the hostility toward them. They had recognized that a different approach was crucial and had decided that one possibility for handling this kind of situation was for the psychiatrist to have individual conferences with faculty members, to provide them with an opportunity to air problems connected with the integration program that were too threatening for group discussion.

Also it was recognized that the faculty members may have resented the psychiatric nurse because they felt the psychiatrist belonged exclusively to her. Such a feeling, if it was present, would intensify the already existing difficulties. The psychiatrist had permitted the faculty members to act out against the psychiatric nurse for too long without setting limits. His individual conferences with faculty members would give them the chance to state directly whatever negative attitudes they had toward him and, in addition, would take some of the heat off the psychiatric nurse, who had been made the scapegoat.

The psychiatrist and the psychiatric nurse agreed that it was crucial to make it clear to the faculty that pertinent aspects of the conferences would be shared with the psychiatric nurse and the total faculty group. They also agreed to postpone making this recommendation to the faculty until the time when the faculty discussions were to be evaluated. Accordingly, the proposal was made in the following meeting.

July 26, 1960

This is the last faculty conference before the summer vacation. Two members from the older group are absent, one older member is taciturn throughout, and two others withdraw during a large part of the meeting.

The mood is pensive. The exchange of glances is minimal. Side comments and note passing cease. Communication begins to flow. Thoughtfulness and involvement permeate the discussion.

MISS WILLIS. Well, I'd like to say, Dr. Ullman, that I thought the meeting last week was a little trying for people who are trying to get through the end of the year. Would it be possible for us today to think about the approaches we might use in 1960–1961 in working with both you and Jane, and sort of get off the griddle that we were on last term? I think this would be helpful. I feel that we're trying to get through the year.

MISS THOMAS. I second the motion. I thought, too, that last week's meeting was very poor. I'm sure that Jane realizes how much stress people are under, but I think the meeting created a tremendous stress situation. I don't see that we resolved some of the big issues that were raised last week, and I think it would be wiser to start off on a fresh foot in the fall.

PSYCHIATRIC NURSE. You feel that my bringing up the attitudes and feelings I had about what was going on with faculty, when I did, was pretty poor timing?

MISS THOMAS. So it seemed to me. I've been aware of more stress within the faculty this week than at any previous time, but I'm sure the meeting didn't do anything to dissipate the stresses. I think it added considerably to them. Timing-wise, it wasn't right to add more stresses right now.

PSYCHIATRIC NURSE. I'd like to hear from some of the rest of you regarding your reactions to last week's meeting. Some of your feelings about the situation being made worse and this business of poor timing. I had not particularly thought of the timing. The problems had piled up for weeks and were beginning to come into the open. My own particular feeling was that to continue with the evaluations under these conditions would be a kind of farce, because as Monte mentioned in another meeting, we have been more preoccupied with placing blame than with evaluating the integration program. But I'd like to hear about how all of you see the situation of our timing.

MISS HUNT. I agree with Linda [*Thomas*], Jane. I know from my own experiences if anything unpleasant happened to occur on a Friday, it would hang over me the whole weekend.

PSYCHIATRIC NURSE. What was there about last week's meeting that was more upsetting than meetings just prior to this one?

MISS JENSEN. Well, I would agree that it was a very trying meeting, and that as a group, we were all tense to varying degrees. I would also agree that the timing was poor, but I don't feel that either Dr. Ullman or Jane had much choice as far as the timing was concerned. I think, as Jane said, it would have been a farce to continue with the evaluation, and I go along with this wholeheartedly. I'm not too sure in my own mind whether it's better to have things left unsaid and have tension, or whether it's better to have them said. I don't know which kind of tension is better. There's tension in either direction.

Miss Vance. My reaction was that although the timing wasn't good, the issue had to be dealt with, and fast. I have the feeling now that even though everyone has expressed how they feel and everybody has accepted the fact that there was a problem, we never got to the stage of being really intent on resolving it. I'm not sure that we necessarily have to lose what we gained by the discussion, which ended in acceptance of the problems. If we would be agreeable to the idea to try not to avoid the problems but keep them in mind, we might get somewhere. But I don't think we ever got to the point where anybody intended to really try to resolve them.

There was a complete shift in the quality of this meeting. The anxiety in the group had been considerably reduced. As a result of the disintegrative process, a radical change had taken place. For the first time in three years, the psychiatrist's power was effectively challenged by a member of the older group. Miss Willis took back her rightful authority. The conflict between the faculty and the psychiatric team was beginning to be faced and dealt with.

Psychiatrist. When the psychiatrist makes a mistake with a patient, the wisest policy, if he's really concerned with the welfare of the patient, is to recognize the mistake very quickly. I had some feelings about the last session, which I suppressed in the service of justifying what I did. Now your reactions and the point you raised make me examine these unquiet feelings, which is exactly what happens in a therapeutic situation. I would now evaluate these unquiet feelings as stemming from the fact that there were two things wrong with the situation.

One was that it was poor timing because it threatened to expose intergroup tensions when nothing could be done about them. When you can't help a patient, you do nothing to hurt him. Another element that added to my unquiet feelings has to do with the question of tactics. In thinking it over, and I think I was perhaps aware of it at the time, pinpointing the difficulties mainly in the direction of Ruth [Newcomer] and Claire [Foster] without ever having previously confronted either of them with my own personal feelings was unfair to them. Perhaps the problem might have been brought to the group only after some effort had been made to resolve it through some other tactics. And so I have found that I have to agree with Esther [Vance], who indicated the issues are there and they have to be met. But I don't think we've made it any easier for us all to meet them by bringing them up last time.

Now, actually, these problems have been developing over a period of time. From time to time Jane and I have thought of ways of coming to grips with these problems. In answer to Catherine's [Willis] question about approaching these problems in 1960 and 1961, there are two concrete suggestions that we want to make. Perhaps they may help to avoid this kind of difficulty and leave you with a clearer and more concrete idea of what our roles and aims are.

Next year I think I would like to meet individually with each member of the faculty and have an opportunity to follow the development of her own reactions to the integration program as they are in the process of developing rather than letting issues come to a sharp head. Now in order to do this, I think it would probably be necessary to make some inroads in our faculty routine. Jane and I suggest that we have a faculty meeting for an hour instead of an hour and a half, which would give me a half-hour to meet individually with a member of the faculty. In working with the instructors in this way, I would become acquainted with their uncertainties, their questions, their reservations, or their reactions to what is going on in the program.

The second point is that I think perhaps this is the time to pull the faculty together into a more focused approach on psychiatric concepts. We have a good deal of interesting material on tapes that hopefully will be transcribed. We hope to have some of the discussion with its general implications and key concepts abstracted, and then distributed for discussion.

Miss DREW. When you say "work with individual instructors," how do you define this?

PSYCHIATRIST. Well, I define it by first scheduling an appointment with an individual instructor and trying to find out what the instructor is getting out of the program; what the instructor is not getting out of it; what questions the instructor has about the various phases of it; and what the instructor feels she needs more of or less of, and simply getting to know more of the individual reaction.

Miss THOMAS. Were you thinking of these individual conferences as being with you and the instructor, or with Jane and you?

PSYCHIATRIST. No, I was thinking of the instructor and myself alone, because Jane has the opportunity to meet with the instructor.

PSYCHIATRIC NURSE. Yes, I think it's important that the faculty get to know Monte on their own terms without me being in there. After all, I had this opportunity and I think this is something that faculty should have also. What do you think?

Miss VANCE. I think it would be better, and it would also give the instructor the opportunity to deal with any personal issues that may come up.

PSYCHIATRIC NURSE. Because I am here on a full-time basis, of necessity Monte and I are bound at times to see the situation somewhat differently. Certainly I have my finger on the pulse of what goes on, but also it is more difficult for me to remain objective. Thus, I think it is important also for Monte to have the opportunity to meet with the rest of you so he can get various viewpoints.

Miss SCOTT. I think there's a little despondency here. I'm not sure, but by some of faculty's expressions I wonder if there's a feeling on the part of the instructors that there's a threat involved in these individual conferences.

Miss JENSEN. One question I'd like to ask is, does an instructor go of her own volition? Does she have a choice to go or not?

PSYCHIATRIST. Well, the last thing we want to do is to surround these conferences with any feeling of threat or compulsion. This seems to me to be simply an opportunity for either corroborating the fact that things are going along fine, that you're getting what you should out of this program, or that things aren't and why aren't they. If the faculty is agreed that they want to integrate the experiences in this program, the individual conferences would sort of follow in a voluntary way.

Miss VANCE. I think this is true, but I'm beginning to feel that people here are feeling that we're gradually being moved into a therapeutic session, and this is not what you proposed. It's not what anybody has said, yet. But I have a feeling of this kind of atmosphere coming on.

PSYCHIATRIST. I simply feel as individual instructors you've all been exposed to what we've done or not done and are reacting accordingly.

Miss REED. Dr. Ullman, a little while ago when you were asked, "Is there a threat involved here?" maybe other people heard the same thing I did, and that was, "Well, we'll tackle problem areas first." I think maybe unconsciously we are worried about this focus on problems. I think maybe this has been the trouble all along.

PSYCHIATRIST. Well, I think it would make more sense for those who perhaps are more deeply troubled about the program to seek conferences earlier. I think that would be up to them. I don't think when faculty see me should come from us. I think it is the consensus of the faculty that this is just another facet of an integration program designed to allow individual expression and reactions, just as we have had group expressions; and then leave it up to the faculty from that point on.

Miss VANCE. I think there are a couple of concepts here that may need some clarification. If I stretch it a little bit, in my mind I can perceive these conferences as a means of manipulation to sell people who have already made up their minds about the integration program and who do not want to change their minds on a particular point. For example, if I have the feeling I don't really believe in the integration program, the conference is a way to get me to change my mind. But I've already decided I don't want to change. I think there may be a tendency to build the conference into this kind of situation. I am perfectly aware this is not the intent, but this can happen.

Miss HUNT. I don't know why we spend so much time and attention on faculty. The integration program is for the benefit of students, and faculty is getting almost as much attention. I wonder what is the direct tie-up and how these meetings here help me to teach the students next fall. I don't see a direct tie-in or that I am any better for it.

PSYCHIATRIC NURSE. This, I think, is a legitimate subject for exploration. Maybe this could be investigated on an individual level, where you can follow your own train of thought and not follow somebody else's.

Miss THOMAS. About these meetings—because they are all on a voluntary basis you could end up this next year by missing many instructors.

PSYCHIATRIST. I think the conference is voluntary only in terms of arrangement in the order of working this out, but I think if faculty commits itself to it, then it is obligatory for everyone to participate.

Miss WILLIS. We're still in the integration program and it really is an experiment. I would see that the person might answer several questions in a conference with you and they might focus on four things: (1) How do I evaluate the integration program, (2) How can I work with students? (3) How can I work with colleagues? and (4) How can I work with patients? And then at the end of the year you might in this experiment find out where the needs are greatest. We don't know.

PSYCHIATRIST. Actually, this is the point. I hope to get more out of these conferences than possibly the instructor, because if I get something out of them, then I can bring it back to the faculty and understand their needs. My suggestion is not to set the conference up in any arbitrary way. If faculty as a group commit themselves to the program, then they commit themselves to seeing that each have this experience. That's all. When they do it depends on their own program and feelings about when they would like to do it. We might take any arbitrary order and have it flexible, and if something comes up, someone else can replace someone, or something like that.

MISS DREW. I think it's a worthwhile suggestion.

MISS THOMAS. I think the matter of mechanics, unless clarified, can become a way for faculty to get out of the conference.

PSYCHIATRIST. Different concepts and different interpretations have to be clarified because this is where we all could get in trouble with people interpreting a choice as being arbitary when it really isn't. The choice is within a framework, and if we commit ourselves to a program, then we do not have the right to say, "I choose not to do it." You do not have this right if you've committed yourself to this program. Actually this is as much a part of the program, say, as the obligation to participate in the faculty group, but I think because there are many factors around the time and scheduling that we have to leave the individual instructor with enough leeway to determine when she thinks it's most appropriate and best to have the conference take place. I think the needs here will vary greatly. Some will want it very early. Some will want more experience and then have it; some will want it when they are in the throes of a particular issue. I think that all we ought to do is announce that the time is available and we have to use it in this way.

During this meeting it was apparent that the faculty members had become integrated into a group. Several members identified the miscarriages that had occurred in previous meetings. Miss Reed, for example, referred to the team members' exclusive focus on the negative aspects of a situation. Once again, however, the psychiatrist completely by-passed her comment. Miss Hunt seriously questioned how the team's particular emphasis on the faculty would help her to become a better teacher. Miss Willis stressed the importance of helping faculty members to work better with students, colleagues, and patients. It seemed likely that the faculty members were telling the psychiatric team, "You should integrate with us; don't just make us integrate with you."

The faculty members were now able to explore all their feelings regarding individual conferences with the psychiatrist instead of just acquiescing in them. Some anxiety and suspicion colored the discussion of this. Fear of personal exposure was alluded to, and fear of being manipulated was stated directly. In believing that her mind could be changed in the individual conferences, Miss Vance endowed the psychiatrist with magic, right to the end.

The mechanics of scheduling the individual conferences was used as a means of avoiding them and thereby became a crucial issue. The psychiatrist demonstrated skillful leadership when he gave the faculty members no choice about seeing him individually. They made it quite clear that this was what they wanted. They forced him to say, "I want to see all of you."

MISS JENSEN. I wonder if it would be worthwhile, before we try meeting again as a group, if everybody saw Dr. Ullman alone, once, and then we started meeting again as a group. It's because we've reached a stalemate as a group that now we're going to meet individually.

PSYCHIATRIC NURSE. That sounds like an excellent idea.

PSYCHIATRIST. It's perfectly all right with me.

MISS DREW. I think it's a good idea, too.

MISS JENSEN. Then, too, I think after Dr. Ullman has seen everyone in an hour's conference and everyone's problems and satisfactions and dissatisfactions are more in focus, then he would be more aware of how much time he would want to spend with faculty again.

PSYCHIATRIST. That means suspending the rest of the evaluation which I think is the thing to do, really, because it will come out in terms of reactions of the individual instructors.

MISS THOMAS. I bet your voice will be so strong by then, Dr. Ullman, that everybody will finally be able to hear it.

[Burst of laughter.]

MISS WILLIS. I also think it would be helpful if some people could help the integration program along with Jane.

PSYCHIATRIC NURSE. I think this will gradually come as time progresses.

[There is a long silence.]

MISS THOMAS. I don't think we have had the time to talk to Jane.

MISS WILLIS. I think it would be very helpful if people would talk to Jane about the program—what's gone on in the past and what she hopes to do in the future. This way we may be able to help her, too. The other way we're seeking help for ourselves, and she needs support at this time and encouragement from all of us. I think it's a very difficult thing to be running a mental health project.

The suggestion that the group meetings be interrupted until the psychiatrist had seen each faculty member once, marked an auspicious occasion. There was unanimous and enthusiastic agreement. A little grace note of humor was introduced as some faculty members frolicked with the psychiatrist. This behavior suggested that each one had wanted him to herself.

At the close of the meeting an older faculty member beseeched the group to support the psychiatric nurse. The meeting ended with soft laughter and light chit-chat about vacation plans. The faculty members bid the psychiatrist goodby.

The disruptive pattern of interaction had been temporarily interrupted. The tide was stemmed. It is questionable whether this could have occurred without the intervention of the psychiatric team, poorly timed or otherwise.

Some potential sources of strength and leadership had been located. The next task of the psychiatric team was to focus on the positive aspects of the faculty members' functioning, to keep in tune with their needs, and to help them to further develop qualities of leadership.

Summary and Implications

During the stage of recoil there was exacerbation of the previous problems concerning status differences, attitudes toward authority, the democratic process and decision making, and matters related to approval and disapproval. As deeper feelings rose to the surface in regard both to the specific issues under discussion and to the integration process, individual defensive patterns emerged which, for a period of time, resulted in a heightening of existing tensions. Techniques of scapegoating, self-blame, withdrawal, denial, attack, and elusiveness were evidence of critical and resentful attitudes toward the psychiatric nurse and the psychiatrist. Many of these attitudes reflected aspects of the emotional byplay going on at the same time among the faculty members themselves. The bitter gulf between the psychiatric team and the rest of the faculty was widened and deepened. For a time, in the faculty group discussions at least, a state of disorganization prevailed.

In these disruptive situations the members of the psychiatric team had to be alert to the danger of assuming that attack on them from one quarter necessarily reflected the attitude of the total group. The intense and disjunctive nature of the irrational responses tended to obscure or obliterate the potential for a more constructive approach to dealing with the problem at hand. Although some of the faculty members did not always support the negative attitudes that were being expressed, they did not introduce a positive point of view either; possibly they felt that the venting of negative feelings should not be prematurely interrupted, and perhaps the fear of rejection by their colleagues and the psychiatric team contributed to their silence.

The psychiatric team might well have recognized that a stage of recoil was probably an inherent aspect of the integrative process in the situation with which they were confronted. According to two psychiatric nurses who have served as directors of psychiatric integration projects, their faculties went through several phases of the stage of recoil as described in this chapter, during the third year of their projects.°

Although the stage of recoil might well have been expected, one question that needs to be raised is: Could the disorganization during the faculty discussions have been avoided? A review of the ways in which the psychiatric nurse and the psychiatrist functioned in these meetings suggests such avoidance was possible. Among the factors that contributed to the disruption among the faculty members were:

1. Lack of real integration of the members of the psychiatric team with the faculty in regard to its professional responsibilities to students. During this period the psychiatric nurse's collaboration with the individual faculty members was limited to her work with two older instructors; therefore, the faculty as a group and the psychiatric nurse were unaware of what they had to give to each other. Except for the psychiatric team's participation with individual instructors in the clinical conferences, there was no integration of the psychiatrist with the faculty in any area of endeavor.

2. Insufficient focus on clinical situations during the faculty discussions. The psychiatric nurse's synthesis with the rest of the faculty started to evolve only when she began to concentrate to a greater degree on concrete issues that pertained to the faculty's professional responsibilities. When these responsibilities became the subject of discussion, both the psychiatric nurse and the psychiatrist felt more comfortable and performed with greater skill.

3. The psychiatric team members' lack of awareness and understanding of the extent to which they were taking the role of distant authorities without behaving as authorities by setting realistic limits on disruptive behavior. They should have taken a rational position toward the faculty members' negative acting out by consistently commenting on it but not interpreting it. Neither the psychiatric nurse nor the psychiatrist explored or clarified the extent to which the negative behavior was partly in response to the way they were functioning within the group.

Despite the lip service that psychiatric nurses and psychiatrists give to the necessity of functioning as participant observers in individual and group

° It might be useful to study if this pattern occurs with any consistency throughout the country, and if so, why? Several questions come to mind. Is it in the third year that the psychiatric nurse is most likely to resign from the school of nursing? If so, is there any way in which the problems that lead to her resignation could be anticipated? Do the problems differ in intensity when the psychiatric nurse works alone and when she works on a team? What kinds of help would be the most useful to her during this period? If she received the necessary help, could the rapid turnover of psychiatric nurses in integration projects be reversed?

situations, in this situation the members of the psychiatric team cast themselves primarily in the role of spectator-observer; hence, they were insufficiently aware of the impact of their behavior and how it had fostered the faculty's negative attitudes and the disjunctive forces that were operating within the group.

Realization of the fact that the reactive phase could have been circumvented in the process of psychiatric integration is not to suggest that the interpersonal conflicts should not have been uncovered. It is only through the recognition and exploration of conflict that the real issues which create schisms can be faced and understood. It does not follow, however, that in the facing of these issues, disruption of individual and group relationships must occur. In this situation the disruptive process, even though it essentially was limited to the faculty discussions, occurred because the existing conflicts among the faculty members and between the faculty and the psychiatric team were never recognized, openly faced, clarified, or understood within the group setting. Instead, the conflicts that related to the way the psychiatric nurse and the psychiatrist had been functioning were dissipated and displaced onto other areas, such as the problematic behavior of students. Although neither the psychiatric nurse nor the psychiatrist had made themselves sufficiently available to the faculty members on an individual level, the specific need for individual conferences with the faculty members arose because of the team's failure to deal with these conflicts in the group meetings.

Considering all the existing circumstances, was the psychiatric nurse's and the psychiatrist's intervention during the July 19th meeting poorly timed? Should they have waited to abort the disruption? Could they have handled the situation differently?

Once the schisms between the younger and the older members and between the faculty and the psychiatric team were evident, the team members were faced with the dissolution of the group discussions. The situation had to be handled. The psychiatric team's intervention entailed the calculated risk that the faculty members would completely withdraw. But all growth, after all, involves the acceptance of risk. The faculty's ability to mobilize itself sufficiently to become interested in making plans for moving in a new direction seemed to indicate that the psychiatric team had not aggravated the situation by arresting the disjunctive process. To the contrary, the team's intervention opened up new possibilities for change.

In spite of the existence of the interpersonal problems within the faculty prior to the advent of the integration program, the psychiatric nurse and the psychiatrist contributed to their isolation and rejection by the rest of the faculty. Many of their expectations were unrealistic, such as the expectation that the faculty would accept and grant approval to their suggestions with only minimal controversy. Like the faculty's unrealistic expectations of students—expecting the student to be now what she should eventually become—the members of the psychiatric team expected the faculty members to feel safe enough with them to expose and resolve their intrafaculty difficulties before the necessary groundwork of trust and confidence had been laid by the help which the team gave to individual members in their work as teachers.

How did the disorganizational process in the faculty meetings affect the relationships of the faculty members in other situations? What effect did this experience have on teacher-student relationships?

During the first three years of the project, the group discussions tended to remain an isolated experience. In the majority of situations (except for the unstructured student group conferences) in which the faculty members worked with each other, or worked alone with students, or worked with the psychiatric nurse, there was little if any carryover of the disintegrative process. From the faculty member's point of view, it was almost as if there were two psychiatric nurses working in integration. One was the psychiatric nurse whose participation in all faculty activities except for these group discussions was an effective one and who had thereby become an inside member of the group. The other was the psychiatric nurse who in these meetings pertaining to the integration project was inextricably linked with the psychiatrist and who was therefore viewed as an outside member of the group. Within this framework the psychiatric nurse was going through the complicated process of learning how to collaborate with the psychiatrist with whom she was competing. On the other hand, the psychiatrist, because he had had no opportunity to experience the faculty as a group or as individuals in other situations (except for the clinical conferences in which he and the psychiatric nurse worked with the individual instructors), appeared to be much more concerned with his relationship to the faculty than with his relationship to the psychiatric nurse. In this stage of integration it may be that in trying to create a place for himself within the faculty, he was competing with the entire group for authority.

Some faculty members already felt unappreciated and enmeshed in problems of status. One result of these dissatisfactions was that they tried to find an island of institutional safety and security by burying their individuality in the formation and membership in one of two corporate groups. As the group discussions revealed, many of the faculty members did not find the individual security or definiteness they were seeking in these groups. Instead, some members became further alienated from each other, from the psychiatric nurse and the psychiatrist, and from themselves. Frequently, individuality was the price that was paid for group conformity and safety, and the psychiatric nurse and the psychiatrist, because of their difficulties in establishing their respective roles, further reinforced these insecurities. They thereby became catalysts in bringing the faculty schism into the open.

In the stage of recoil was anything accomplished other than disorganization? Did any change occur? Was any growth achieved?

At the same time the tearing-down process of divisiveness was occurring and was exposed, several quiescent reservoirs of potential courage, strength, and leadership were tapped. The stage of recoil also was the period during which some faculty members burst forth from the cocoon in which they had so snugly embedded themselves. It was a time when they became better known to each other, to their students, and to themselves. It was an era in which the psychiatric nurse began to integrate with the faculty. However, the integration of the psychiatric nurse and the psychiatrist as an interdisciplinary team and the integration of the psychiatric team with the faculty remained a task for the future.

By upsetting the status quo, the faculty and the psychiatric team had prepared a soil in which individual creativeness, the roots of a unified group, could grow and yield a bountiful harvest.

Chapter Ten

INDIVIDUAL CONFERENCES WITH
THE FACULTY MEMBERS:
THE EARLY STAGE OF SYNTHESIS

... for we can only be said to be alive in those moments when our hearts are conscious of our treasures; for our hearts are not strong enough to love every moment.

THORNTON WILDER, *The Woman of Andros*

The stage of synthesis, or the resolution through change and growth, was the third and final stage of the integrative process among the faculty and the psychiatric team. It was the period during which the faculty achieved growth and reintegration at a level of greater maturity.

COMPOSITION OF THE FACULTY

More changes occurred in the composition of the faculty in the fourth year than at any other time during the project. An older member took a sabbatical leave during the first two quarters and returned in the spring quarter. A younger member resigned at the end of the first quarter and was replaced by Miss Newberry. A younger member resigned in the second quarter, and Miss Newell joined the faculty to replace her.

Throughout the stage of synthesis, plans were being made by the department of nursing to assume the total responsibility for teaching obstetric nursing, beginning in the fall of 1962 and psychiatric nursing and public health nursing in the fall of 1963. Meetings were held frequently and regularly to formulate the steps for implementing the new curriculum.

The Establishment of Equilibrium

At the end of the third year, because of the disorganizational effects of the faculty group discussions, the group meetings pertaining to the integration program were interrupted and interviews between the individual faculty members and the psychiatrist were introduced. During this hiatus in the meetings, the psychiatric nurse was involved in clarifying how her behavior had contributed to the disruption of the group meetings. She collected the available data concerning her unresolved needs, unrealistic expectations, distorted perceptions, and irrational modes of interaction. The psychiatrist assisted her with this task, but limited his efforts to her professional role. This period also was marked by conferences between individual faculty members and the psychiatric nurse.

Reducing Anxiety and Widening the Focus

The psychiatrist had individual conferences with each faculty member during the first quarter of the fourth year of the project. The purpose of the conferences was to siphon off some of the negative feelings among the group by providing an opportunity for the faculty members to air those problems and issues in relation to the integration program and the psychiatric team which in their opinion were too threatening for group discussion. At the beginning of each conference the psychiatrist made it clear that he would share certain pertinent aspects with the psychiatric nurse. He followed a specific line of questioning in order to elicit information about the difficulties in each faculty member's relationships with the rest of the faculty, with the psychiatric nurse and himself, and with students, and about problems pertaining to the curriculum. The quality of the responses demonstrated the psychiatrist's skill in effectively establishing individual relationships. This skill was due partly to his psychoanalytic training and experience.

The faculty members responded to the individual conferences in a variety of ways. Most of the instructors spoke freely and frenkly; in these instances, the psychiatrist experienced them more as individual persons than had been possible in the group. Two faculty members stated that the integration project had helped them to become more secure as people.

Some faculty members were extremely vague, and because they intellectualized about the faculty relationships instead of expressing their feelings about them, it was difficult to know how they really felt about the project and the psychiatric team. One member expressed contradictory attitudes. Another instructor was unclear about her relationship both with individual faculty members and with the group and about her role in the faculty discussions. Negative and rejecting attitudes permeated the conference with one instructor. Another instructor had little to say because, as she stated, she had remained uninvolved. Some faculty members referred to their desire for discussing psychiatric concepts, whereas others felt they did not need this kind of help.

The comments of the faculty members fell into three categories: those concerning the psychiatric team, those having to do with faculty relationships, and those pertaining to the students and the curriculum.

THE PSYCHIATRIC TEAM

The Psychiatrist. On the basis of one interview, it was difficult to get a clear picture of how each faculty member felt about the psychiatrist. One strength was mentioned frequently, namely, "It is a good idea to have individual conferences with the psychiatrist. It is the faculty member's first personal contact with him." The only limitation that was expressed was, "I resent his handling of a faculty member by calling attention to her behavior in front of the faculty group."

The Psychiatric Nurse. Feelings about the psychiatric nurse constituted a predominant feature of these conferences. However, comments about her strengths came primarily from members of the younger group. Included from these comments were:

She has helped me in teaching students how to care for critically ill patients.

She has helped me to learn how to help students to open up and how not to cut them off.

I learned a great deal from her in regard to evaluation, how to handle students and the value of giving recognition to students for their strengths.

She helped us to get through the barriers between the two faculty groups.

She is an excellent teacher. Her classes are stimulating. I have very positive feelings about her.

She helped me to learn how to accept criticism better and how to handle authority figures.

The psychiatric nurse's limitations as expressed by the younger group were as follows.

She stands between the two groups of faculty and she isn't sure where her loyalty lies. She has partiality but it fluctuates.

She uses too many superlatives and tends to dramatize and exaggerate.

A "mutual admiration society" goes on between her and some older faculty members.

Older faculty members give the idea that no one has anything to say about mental health except the psychiatric nurse.

According to the older group, her limitations were the following.

She seeks reassurance.

She doesn't give enough recognition to some faculty members' experience in psychiatric nursing.

Her enthusiasm for the emotional and psychological area of nursing sometimes overrides her interest in physical care, but she is trying to strike a balance.

The Psychiatric Nurse and the Psychiatrist as Partners. Opinions about the joint efforts of the psychiatric nurse and the psychiatrist tended to emphasize the limitations rather than the strengths of their efforts as a team. Two strengths were mentioned by the younger members, namely,

You both helped to get faculty members off their over-emphasis on time and helped to free the time schedule.

I have less fear that you want to change me.

The following comments about the team's limitations were made by the younger members.

You "railroaded" through the discussions and decisions in the faculty group.

You knuckled under the impact of the faculty schism and took sides with the older group against the younger group.

The older members present a united front and blindly follow you. They always agree with what you propose.

I feel as if the topics in group discussion are slanted and chosen ahead of time.

I came into the situation with the preconception that neither of you would listen to the younger members' comments.

You don't give sufficient credit to the younger group's comments.

Sometimes one or both of you "sat on" two younger members. It takes courage for a younger person to speak up.

THE FACULTY RELATIONSHIPS

Several good effects of the integration program on the relationships among faculty members were mentioned. The older faculty members' comments focused on group relationships. These were as follows.

In the overall picture, there is less of a gap between faculty members. We are more cohesive.

Relationships among the faculty members are closer.

The faculty members have come a long way in breaking down the barrier between them.

We are freer with each other.

The faculty members keep confidences better.

The comments of the younger members, for the most part, focused on the self. Among such comments were the following.

The group meetings are good, and I am able to say things now that I never could have said before.

There is less turnover in the faculty since the psychiatric team has been here.

The group discussions are good because they help you to look at yourself.

The following weaknesses in intrafaculty relations were mentioned by the members of the older group.

There is too much bickering about the group meetings.

Tension about the integration program arose in relation to new faculty members.

Among the comments of the younger members, the following were included.

No individual decisions are made and no individual recognition is given. There is individual anonymity.

The faculty members are not saying what they really believe in the group discussions.

The older group see the younger faculty members as being inexperienced and not understanding problems.

THE STUDENTS AND THE CURRICULUM

In connection with the integration program's effect on students, one benefit was mentioned by an older faculty member, namely,

Students talk more freely to faculty.

Mention was made of the following limitations of the integration program with respect to the students and the curriculum by the younger faculty members.

All the student group conferences with the psychiatric nurse should be clinically oriented instead of being unstructured.

The student group conferences with the psychiatric nurse were wasted.

Mental health is treated too differently from other areas.

Too many hours are spent on mental health.

The curriculum should be patient-centered and not student-centered.

Students are not able to apply what is taught in the mental health classes.

Students don't want to talk about what bothers them in a group.

I still object to the examination question about the patient who masturbates. There are other faculty members who feel the same way, but they do not say so.

The following comment was made by an older member.

Students have good relationships with patients but as a result, the quality of the patients' physical care suffers.

One of the most rewarding aspects of these conferences was the fact that the greatest number of strengths identified in connection with the integration project pertained to intrafaculty relationships. On this basis alone, the psychiatric integration project could be considered successful. Unfortunately, similar strengths with respect to the effect of the project on the students had not yet been recognized. The faculty members' responses revealed that they had displaced many of their negative feelings toward the psychiatric nurse in the group meetings onto the students and the curriculum. Regretfully, the conflicts regarding the roles of the psychiatric team and the rest of the faculty were never uncovered, nor were there any findings concerning how the faculty members felt about what the psychiatrist was or was not doing to facilitate or impede the group's functioning.

FACING ONE'S SELF

After the psychiatrist had completed his interviews with the individual faculty members, he and the psychiatric nurse conferred about her relationship with the faculty. Although the younger members were the ones who tended to emphasize the psychiatric nurse's strengths, some of them felt that her loyalty was divided between them and the older members, or that she had put up a wall between herself and them so that they could not come to her with their problems. Some older members felt that she tended to seek approval and permission from them before moving on her own.

The timing of this conference was perfect. It helped the psychiatric nurse to identify the impediments to her appropriate relationships with the other faculty members and marked a turning point in her approach to the solution of this problem. After the conference she was ready to break from the shell in which she had been hiding.

The faculty's comments about the psychiatric team's identification with the older group posed several disquieting questions. On numerous occasions the psychiatric nurse and the psychiatrist had been baffled by the older members' equanimity and acquiescnce. Had the team members sufficiently challenged the older group's agreement with them? Or had they avoided using this channel because the older members had sought them out? Had the team been guilty of accepting agreement without ascertaining if it was genuine agreement? Was the psychiatric nurse as objective about members in the older group as she was about those in the younger group? Were the younger members' feelings about the team's identification with the older group merely a projection of their own attitudes, or had the psychiatric nurse allowed herself to be drawn too closely into the administrative affairs of the older group, thus creating distance between the young group and herself?

As has been pointed out, insofar as the activities in connection with the integration project were concerned, the psychiatric nurse's position on the faculty differed from that of every other faculty member. These differences were threatening, especially to the younger members, but the threats had never been identified or dealt with. Instead, they had been aggravated by the psychiatric nurse's identification with the older faculty members.

The question arises as to why the psychiatric nurse had not dealt on an individual level with the younger faculty members' attitudes toward her. She had been afraid of their disapproval and rejection. Because all the members of the older group had worked closely with her during the second and third years of the project, they were more aware of what she was doing, how she functioned, and what she had to give. They had sufficient status in the situation, so that seeking help from her was not as threatening as it was for the younger members. In response to the younger members' competitive struggle with her, the psychiatric nurse had withdrawn. Her estrangement from the younger members had cramped their awareness of her as a person.

After this examination of her own failings, the psychiatric nurse took positive steps to bridge the gap between herself and the other faculty members, particularly those in the younger group.

The Demise of Anger, Fear, and Guilt

Because the psychiatric nurse, unlike the psychiatrist, was professionally identified with nursing in general, she had numerous opportunities to communicate and collaborate with the faculty members in areas that directly concerned them as nurse teachers and that were also less anxiety-laden than those directly associated with psychiatric integration.

Shortly after the individual faculty conferences with the psychiatrist were completed, an opportunity for the psychiatric nurse to confer with individual faculty members arose. A curriculum question which affected the entire faculty had been "settled" by a fiat issued by the older group. Once again the relationship between members of the older and younger groups was endangered.

Having learned that disenchantment with the democratic process foments the scapegoating pattern, the psychiatric nurse initiated an individual conference with each of the faculty members to seek their reactions and suggestions. This was the first time that she had conferred individually with some of them. A predominant theme of the conferences was the faculty members' sense of hopelessness about any possibility of a reversal of the curriculum decision. They were inclined to view the proposal as a *fait accompli* and felt helpless about doing anything except sit back passively and simmer inside.

For the most part the faculty members were quite candid in the interviews. Some of the older members were defensive about the position they had taken. Others in the older group, like the younger members, were dissatisfied with the decision itself, the way it was made, and the method of presenting it to the faculty as a whole. Such differences in point of view among some members of the older group were a further indication that the united front pertinaciously maintained by both groups had been pierced. As splinter groups were formed, divergent attitudes were revealed.

The faculty members felt safe enough to divulge numerous areas of controversy to the psychiatric nurse. Several members were mobilized to take constructive action. From this time on, the psychiatric nurse developed and maintained close contact with each individual faculty member.

From Competition to Cooperation and Compromise

During the time the psychiatrist was having an individual conference with each faculty member and in the period immediately following the resumption of the group discussions, two developments occurred which indicated that the psychiatric nurse and the psychiatrist had brought about something of a *détente* in faculty-psychiatric team relations. The first development concerned the faculty discussions. Near the end of the first quarter, when the psychiatrist was winding up his interviews with the faculty members, the instructors, one by one, began to drop into the psychiatric nurse's office to ask her if and when the faculty discussions would be resumed. The reasons for their expressed interest in and desire to continue the meetings may have included the following.

First, the members of the psychiatric team had demonstrated their respect for the group by their willingness to interrupt meetings. At the same time they had set definitive limits by making the individual conferences with the psychiatrist obligatory. Second, during the interruption of the faculty discussions, a faculty member's contact with the psychiatrist was limited to her one-hour individual conference with him. The group meetings were the only way for all the faculty members to maintain an ongoing relationship with him.

The second development occurred shortly after the group discussions were resumed, and it pertained to the faculty members' responses to the plan for their participation with the psychiatric nurse in the student group conferences. In the first quarter of the year, the psychiatric nurse had been meeting alone with the sophomore students. It had been agreed in the faculty discussions that in the second quarter the focus was to shift to clinical discussions in which the instructors would participate (see Chapter 6). When the time arrived for the shift to occur, not one faculty member showed up. After a prolonged waiting period, the psychiatric nurse sought out each instructor and reminded her about the new framework. Each one reacted with astonishment and spontaneously admitted she had forgotten about the change. In each instance the instructor and the psychiatric nurse laughed together about the "slip in memory." Words or explanations were unnecessary. In spite of some of the explosive discussions and vehement attitudes about the psychiatric nurse having the conferences alone, each instructor now seemingly was accepting the fact that the psychiatric nurse would work alone with students.

This turn of events was the consequence of several experiences. The most important of these, perhaps, was that during the stormy period when the instructors sat in on the student conferences, the shroud about them was penetrated. They also had had the opportunity to react negatively in the faculty discussions, where they were listened to and where a compromise had been effected. Finally, as the faculty members began to feel more secure in their role as teachers, they started to expand the boundaries of their own relationships with students and, as they were able to alter their professional relationship with students from an impersonal to a personal one, they achieved increased satisfaction. They probably no longer felt the need to move in on the psychiatric nurse's territory; they had created their own.

Looking to the Future

Beginning in the fourth year the psychiatric team endeavored to keep in close touch with the individual instructors. It had taken three years for the psychiatric team to learn the problems of faculty members and also to identify those that the members of the team had created. The psychiatric nurse and the psychiatrist had finished their individual explorations of problem areas and now knew what these problems were. They knew the levels on which the faculty members were functioning and were now aware of some definite needs of the students. On the basis of these understandings they established the following goals for the future.

1. Help the faculty members to focus on the strengths within the situation.

2. Give them a clearer idea of the level of interpersonal relations on which the group should operate regardless of their attitudes about each other.

3. Help them with problems that arise in regard to their role and functions as teachers through the application of psychiatric concepts.

4. Avoid trying to change their individual insecurities.

Chapter Eleven

THE WORK WITH THE FACULTY GROUP: THE EARLY STAGE OF SYNTHESIS (Continued)

All through the ages, from Moses down, the men who have never followed the opinions and ideas of the people around them are the men who have been building for the future. They have hewn steps out of the solid rock; they have worked in thorns and brambles and hard places that a stairway might be built for you and for me. They are like Moses, who, defying custom and habit and giving up ease and security, and having that faith which great mortals have, could see far off something better than the world had known.

CLARENCE DARROW, *The Attorney for the Damned*

In January, 1961, the group meetings reconvened. Three sessions of one and a half hours each were held a month; the fourth week was used for individual faculty interviews with the psychiatrist.

There was a shift from unprepared sessions characterized by diffuse discussions to ones of a more planned and selective character, and from an annual to an ongoing evaluation of the integration program. Each instructor presented to the rest of the faculty a summary and evaluation of her various experiences with the psychiatric nurse and the psychiatrist. Consequently, many of the faculty members became more personally involved in the project. Also, the existing problems were more apt to be identified as they arose. The focus of the discussions was on three subjects: (1) evaluation of student behavior; (2) psychiatric concepts; and (3) plans for the fifth and final year of the current grant. Upon the joint recommendations of the faculty and the psychiatric team, changes in the integration program were introduced as they seemed indicated from the faculty members' experiences with the psychiatric nurse and the psychiatrist.

A Redistribution of Power

The evaluation of students was chosen as the subject for the faculty discussions because the fourth and fifth years of the project were noteworthy for the prevalence of problematic behavior and adjustment problems among students. Major difficulties were being created by students who behaved in one or several of the following ways.

1. Remaining outside of the nursing situation by seldom becoming committed to caring for patients. These students often were described by their instructors as being detached, uninterested, negativistic, or placating.
2. Manipulating and controlling others, particularly authority figures, by challenging them or complying superficially and employing tactics of ingratiation.
3. Blocking out all anxiety regarding their professional and emotional problems.

The following is an illustration of the kind of problem that students presented.

> Roberta was in the second quarter of the first clinical year. Though she had a high intellectual capacity, she was close to failing in all her academic work. Her clinical performance was poor and she related with patients on a very superficial level. Whenever an instructor attempted to help her with her problems, she agreed quite readily that she had such problems; then at a later date, she used these problems as excuses for her poor achievement.
>
> There were no symptoms of presenting anxiety which created a block to the establishment of effective contact with Roberta either by a teacher or by someone undertaking therapeutic exploration. She had organized all of her problems along very shallow and ingratiating lines. Her need for approval was much greater than her desire for nursing. She was experiencing a sense of bankruptcy about her own ability to develop personally and so had to try to do something about manipulating the environment.

Problems such as these were being brought to the psychiatric team. In the case of this particular student, the psychiatric team suggested that first, it was imperative that the instructor avoid any reference to Roberta's problems, because she used them as a way of avoiding responsibility for changing her behavior. Second, it was crucial to make Roberta realize that she would undoubtedly fail if she did not show immediate improvement. Third, it was important to place the burden of responsibility on Roberta herself and to make it clear to her that whether she passed or failed was completely up to her.

The student problems were so prevalent that it was thought desirable to study them in the meetings of the total faculty as well as individual conferences. Accordingly, during seven consecutive weeks, the faculty discussions were devoted to the evaluation of student behavior. They centered on identification of the students' potential for growth, the degree of their motivation for nursing, the discrepancy between academic achievement and level of nursing practice, and the instructor's role in intervention.

SOWING THE SEEDS OF COLLABORATION

January 10, 1961

This is the first meeting since the summer vacation. Everyone exerts a special effort to be cooperative. Participation is fairly general. Those who remain silent appear involved and interested. There is some strain—or perhaps more an air of expectancy—about how the meeting will progress. Facial expressions are somber and musing.

PSYCHIATRIC NURSE. Well, I guess the first thing we ought to do today is to make some plans for the future. First we have to decide who will be working with Monte and me on a second go-round of clinical conferences with the students. Then also, we need to decide about who is going to participate with me in the weekly psychiatric nursing clinical conferences. Finally, we want to review the structure of our group meetings this year.

MISS DREW. I think I'd rather not have my second series of clinical conferences now, since I'll be working with Jane in the mental health content classes.

MISS REED. With my mixed-up schedule, I've been thinking about the possibility of working with Jane and Dr. Ullman for four weeks instead of the usual six.

MISS JENSEN. I feel that the six sessions are necessary. This experience is too important and valuable to be cast aside.

PSYCHIATRIST. Well, if Thelma's [Reed] schedule only permits working with us for four weeks, then perhaps Jane and I could work for two weeks with the students in small groups without an instructor.

Any decision about which faculty member will work with the psychiatric nurse and the psychiatrist was postponed. Some of the reluctance about volunteering for a second experience may have been a way of exerting pressure on the one younger member who had not yet worked with the psychiatric team.

PSYCHIATRIST. My conferences with the faculty members point to the fact that in some ways we have moved as a group and in some ways we haven't. Like President Kennedy, we didn't get a mandate. It was a close election, but we won. The faculty members did not feel the group meetings were useful.

PSYCHIATRIC NURSE. In the effort to improve the meetings we make the following recommendations.

> 1. The faculty members who are participating with Monte and me in the clinical conferences with the sophomore students and with the junior students in psychiatric nursing, and with me alone in all the other experiences, share their experiences with the rest of faculty. This will provide for an ongoing evaluation of the integration program.
> 2. Some meetings be devoted to discussion of psychiatric concepts.
> 3. One open meeting once a month be left for discussion of any pressing problems.
> 4. Every fourth week the faculty discussions be skipped so as to allow time for individual conferences with faculty members, with priority being given to those who are working with one or both of us in one of the experiences in the integration program.

Following this brief résumé of the psychiatrist's conferences, the psychiatric team asked Miss Jensen and Miss Scott to report to the total group on their experiences with the team. Miss Jensen agreed to report on her second series of clinical conferences with the psychiatric team (see Chapter 7), and Miss Scott agreed to evaluate her experiences in the psychiatric nursing seminars. A beginning basis for the ongoing evaluation of the integration program was thereby established. The group then moved on to the discussion of a problem involving a group of sophomore students.

MISS JENSEN. The particular group of students we are working with are extremely hostile. They show very little respect to either me or my colleague.
MISS VANCE. They are very difficult to work with in the clinical setting because they are self-centered and rude to the head nurses and staff.
MISS JENSEN. The juniors say they are very unfriendly.
MISS VANCE. They behave with a holier-than-thou attitude and act as though they are doing the nursing profession a favor. [*She pushes her long auburn hair behind her ears.*] There is a wide gap between the way they perceive themselves and the way they are functioning in reality.
MISS FOSTER. They continually talk and make side comments in the large core classes.
MISS VANCE. They try to corner the instructor into giving them the right answers.
PSYCHIATRIC NURSE. I am very much aware of this kind of behavior also, because it is happening in the mental health classes and small group conferences. What are your own reactions to all of this? What impact has their behavior had on your teaching relationships?
MISS JENSEN. I'm finding that I dig in harder on the students. I don't have as much patience and I don't look forward to teaching them.
PSYCHIATRIST. I am wondering whether I should meet with these students in small groups. During the first year of the project I had a very meaningful experience with the junior students when some problems arose. These students

are using the techniques of avoidance and they selectively inattended the important things that are being said. Then they deflect blame onto the instructor. In handling the students, the instructor needs to be aware of students' techniques in action rather than in review. The only way to deal with this behavior is through recognition of it and not accepting it. Yet at the same time the instructor has to be careful not to put herself in the position of not listening to students' real problems and discontents.

MISS JENSEN. There seem to be several ringleaders who pass on their negative attitudes to the rest of the class.

PSYCHIATRIC NURSE. Perhaps pointing out patterns of behavior to the troublesome students in your individual conferences with them would be helpful.

MISS DREW. Sue Eddy is a destructive leader.

MISS VANCE. Gerry Winston blames and criticizes everyone and everything.

MISS WILLIS. Patsy Fisher and Barbara Murdock transferred to the nursing department at the last moment.

PSYCHIATRIST. There is no point in getting into Sue Eddy's various problems, since she will only use these to further manipulate the faculty. She should be dealt with only in relation to the academic situation and each instructor should do the same on her own.

MISS DREW. Maybe we could use our clinical conference time this week to discuss this problem with the students. What do you think, Dot [Jensen]?

MISS JENSEN. Why, I don't see why not. Absolutely, that's what we'll do.

PSYCHIATRIC NURSE. Depending on how the conference goes, you might ask the students whether they want to meet with Monte, in which case they could decide whether to have the instructors present or not.

During this meeting the faculty members shared a common problem; all of them had had similar experiences with the students under discussion. Perhaps the timing of the student problem was fortunate inasmuch as it provided the faculty members with the opportunity to relate to each other on less personal and threatening levels. There was motion but no clutter, intensity but no shrillness. Side glances were exchanged to communicate agreement with what was being said. There was much smiling and nodding.

Instead of avoiding the problem of the students' behavior, Miss Drew and Miss Jensen took the initiative in uncovering the difficulty with students, and accepted the idea of collaborating with the psychiatrist with gusto. Their personal experience of living through the problem-solving process in faculty meetings and their individual work with the psychiatric team was beginning to be translated into the teaching process.

After meeting with the students, Miss Jensen called the psychiatrist to give him a report and to let him know the students wanted to talk with him the next day, with the result that the psychiatrist alone met with them to discuss the current problem. This was the first time that any faculty member had initiated contact with the psychiatrist without first having cleared with the psychiatric nurse.

Psychiatric Integration in Action

January 17, 1961

Psychiatric Nurse. Dot [*Jensen*] and Eileen [*Drew*], I'm sure the rest of the faculty would like to hear about what happened in your group meeting with the students last week.

Miss Jensen. In presenting the problem to students, we tried to emphasize our concern for the students rather than faculty's concern for themselves. Eileen [*Drew*] took the lead and started the conference. Initially all the students almost fell through the floor when we faced them with how we saw their behavior. They went on and on about how they "just love Eileen and me and the College." We pointed out that they have been rude, inattentive, and unable to work with staff and faculty. [*She plays with her lacquered fingernails.*] From the beginning, three out of the fourteen students agreed with our appraisal of the situation.

Miss Drew. I think this openness is new to the students because up to now the problem has been discussed only in the dormitory.

Miss Jensen. The ringleaders deny that anything is going on and continually fight what we are saying. A great deal of dislike toward them is beginning to crop up. We told the students that this is not just our opinion about their behavior, but that the total faculty feels similarly.

Psychiatric Nurse. It sounds like you had quite a meaningful experience. Did you get anything of value from the experience for yourselves?

Miss Jensen. I have more confidence in handling this kind of conference. When you see a problem, the best thing to do is to get it out on the table—get it into the open.

Miss Drew. We didn't terminate the conference at the end of fifteen minutes when the students were still denying the existence of a problem.

Psychiatric Nurse. How were you able to get them to open up? What did you do?

Miss Drew. We used concrete examples. The first time we reached the students was when we gave the incident of a student barging into an instructor's office and using her telephone without so much as a by-your-leave. [*The pupils of her brown eyes are dilated.*]

Miss Jensen. Dr. Ullman, how do you see the situation?

Psychiatrist. Well, it sounds as though one half of the class is in the dark and unaware of what is going on. One fourth of the class is taken by surprise, but can see the validity of the situation when it is pointed out, and the other one fourth are completely aware. The problem concerns some students who are unsure about nursing. They pick the mental health and growth and development classes and examinations to complain about because they are sufficiently ambiguous areas.

The spokesmen for the class are negatively and hostilely oriented individuals. Because those students who see the problem aren't strong enough to speak up, the others become leaders by default.

Psychiatric Nurse. I guess one of the primary issues for us to grapple with is how to handle these leaders by default.

MISS JENSEN. I have the uneasy feeling there is more going on and that the students wanted Eileen and me present when Dr. Ullman saw them, so whatever is happening wouldn't come into the open.

MISS VANCE. I think the hostility goes back to the students' gap in knowledge and how to use it. Jane periodically refers to the pain of learning.

PSYCHIATRIST. I get the feeling that the students who are making the most noise are feeling the most unsure. Learning in this situation involves using new skills and utilizing knowledge quickly. There is a whole series of different kinds of learning that can be utilized by students who are highly motivated. Low motivation for nursing frightens the instructor. When the student asks, "Why can't the experiences here be the same as they are on campus?" we need to ask why these students are unable to orient themselves to the nursing experience.

MISS JENSEN. I have the feeling that the faculty is the scapegoat for other problems.

PSYCHIATRIC NURSE. Can you get the other students who are inarticulate mobilized enough to say what is bothering them? As instructors, I think we need to help students to do this.

MISS WILLIS [*She adjusts her glasses*]. Some of the class officers said they are afraid of several students.

It would appear that in this meeting Miss Jensen was competing with Miss Drew for approval, especially from the psychiatrist. Miss Drew gradually began to fit herself into the presentation and discussion. Both instructors collaborated with the psychiatrist.

Some uneasiness permeated the meeting as the meaning of the students' problems remained curiously obscure. Fear of the students' acting-out behavior was reflected in the instructors' anger and helplessness in handling the situation. There was an upsurge of interest as problems became defined.

It was obvious that the faculty members had become more aware that to handle behavior in action both they and the students needed different skills from the ones necessary for teaching or learning didactically presented content.

HARVESTING THE FRUITS OF COLLABORATION

January 24, 1961

PSYCHIATRIST. In my second meeting with the students, closure took place. All awareness of problems was sealed off. I ransacked the building to find Dot [*Jensen*] or Eileen [*Drew*]. Finally I salvaged Jane, who put over the points of the problem very well. We all agreed, students included, to carry on for another session with Eileen, Dot, and Jane. Patsy Feinberg got carried away and stated that these conferences with us were a waste of time and were taking her away from nursing. I pointed out that this was a false dichotomy and part of nursing is to become aware of behavior.

PSYCHIATRIC NURSE. There is confusion about what the relationship with instructors should be. Students vacillate between wanting to be buddy-buddy with us and fearing evaluation. There was much effort expended in denying the existence of a problem.

PSYCHIATRIST. Sue Eddy was involved in intramural communication and side issues without any real participation. Patsy Feinberg kept trying to say, "I, as an individual, don't feel there is a problem," but she doesn't do this as an individual, but rather puts it that "the whole group feels this way." A bullying process is going on. None of the other students have a spokesman. I would like a vote of confidence to continue these sessions with the students, which means I will have to utilize Dot's and Eileen's time for their clinical conferences.

MISS DREW. At first I felt we were running this whole problem to the ground and that none of this was much use. Yesterday, however, Sue and Patsy were derogating the physician who was lecturing. I recommend that we continue with the discussions.

PSYCHIATRIC NURSE. This is the kind of specific that needs to be cited to students. Two students have set themselves up as intellectual avant-gardes, and as a way of bucking them, other students become stuffy and old-fashioned.

MISS JENSEN. Why do the other students buy this kind of behavior?

Miss Jensen's questions might appropriately be translated, "Why don't the older faculty members intervene when we act out?" Miss Jensen's and Miss Drew's positive response to the psychiatric team's intervention in the disintegrative process would seem to validate this point.

PSYCHIATRIC NURSE. I think that perhaps Sue and Patsy use the provocations, of which there have been several instances, of students' being cut off by the instructor. We get defensive, such as when I dismissed my mental health class when the badgering got just too much for me. Then these students focus on us personally rather than the initial provocation.

PSYCHIATRIST. Here we have a combination of "bad eggs" and problematic motivation. Perhaps we should wait until we see this through a little more before coming to conclusions.

PSYCHIATRIC NURSE. Yet faculty are faced with the realistic situation of having to evaluate students under these circumstances.

MISS JENSEN. I can't fail them on their behavior. They have certain basic skills. Telling them about their behavior won't help. They need insight.

PSYCHIATRIST. Perhaps it is too early to form a judgment, but I myself question whether these two students are capable of being professional people. There is an aptitude for professional behavior. The question is, is there a potential for professionalism?

MISS JENSEN. Patsy Feinberg doesn't want to care for patients beyond a certain time because when she is doing a care study she doesn't want to have to write any more about the patient.

PSYCHIATRIST. This is very important, and you have a definitive point.

MISS WILLIS. Does this problem happen in medicine, Dr. Ullman?

PSYCHIATRIST. The pressure of learning and staying in medical school during the first two years keeps the students in line. During the clinical years, there is some acting out.

The most effective treatment is to mobilize the silent students. We are interested in removing the blocks in their learning rather than trying to bait them and to be punitive. Other students are frightened to offer a contrary opinion because of the articulate aggression of these two students.

MISS VANCE. Should we work with the positive elements of the group by having a separate meeting with them?

In this meeting members of the older group were noticeably quiet as the younger members demonstrated that they had become surer of themselves. Side comments and periodic laughter punctuated the flow of discourse. There was even a note of hilarity. The psychiatrist participated in the byplay. The exchanges scintillated with friendliness and differed considerably from the derogation of previous years. Genuine concern about the student situation motivated the faculty members to stick with the problem at hand. As they explored the problem of students in greater depth, the complex issue of the role that behavior plays in the evaluation of students came to the foreground.

TRYING TO RELINQUISH THE BLUEPRINT

For the third time the psychiatrist met with Miss Drew's and Miss Jensen's group of students. In each instance, the instructor and the psychiatric nurse participated with him as planned. The students denied that they had been rude and attributed their behavior to exuberance and to impatience caused by intellectual curiosity.

The psychiatrist schematically demonstrated on the blackboard that curiosity is oriented toward appropriate behavior that involves two-way responsibility. He clarified the fact that impatience is related to excessive anxiety, which in turn leads to inappropriate behavior and thereby detours the search for knowledge. The meeting had obvious impact on Patsy Feinberg, in whom an observable transformation took place.

January 31, 1961

MISS JENSEN. After our conference with the students last week, Patsy Feinberg came to me and said, "Thank you for saving my soul. You and Dr. Ullman really helped." Patsy felt the real problem had been identified. She said that when Dr. Ullman drew the diagram on the blackboard and identified how students' impatience is related to excessive anxiety resulting in inappropriate behavior, that it hit straight home and was like having her own name flashed across the blackboard. Now she doesn't know what to do with her insight.

MISS DREW. Since our last group conference no one asks any questions during the medical lecture. There was one token gesture from Sue Eddy. I was very upset after last week's meeting with the students and I wondered if all of this is worth it.

MISS JENSEN. One of the juniors told me that when, as a team leader, she asked students who were doing nothing to help with medication cards, they refused.

PSYCHIATRIST. Eileen [*Drew*], what were you upset about? Your attitude about the problem seems to have changed.

MISS DREW. I feel that the emphasis on students' rudeness as being an expression of impatience merely serves as an excuse for the students. I am concerned that they will use this as a means to avoid real responsibility. There still are two students who did not say a word. Now I am aware that there is even a larger problem than I ever had realized.

PSYCHIATRIST. What do you think made you change your attitude since last week?

MISS DREW. Lois Reilly came to see me on Friday. She is so frightened now of doing something wrong that she doesn't do a thing without my okay. Then Barbara Murdock came to thank Dot [*Jensen*] and me for how much we helped. It's just as though the problem is all settled.

Some faculty members were now answering direct questions, as when Miss Drew responded to the psychiatrist. Some skepticism remained about the value of bringing problems into the open. Easy and immediate resolution of problems continued to be a hope and a fantasy, and at the same time Miss Drew seemed to fear a too-ready resolution. Areas of concern and points of disagreement were aired openly.

PSYCHIATRIST. Our goal is to try to re-establish some closeness between students and faculty with some minimal self-questioning being involved. We were trying to get students to the place of transferring their feelings of blame of faculty to looking at themselves. The point of the diagram was not to explain everything; it explained very little. Yet it may give the student something whereby she can begin to face herself.

There are several disturbed students in the group, so to have gone deeper into the problem would have meant a series of real group therapy sessions. Students' hostility is aimed at the total faculty. Their frustration is due to their denial of the problem and their fragmentation of the educational experience and their attitudes and behavior. Nevertheless, a remarkable transformation has occurred with Patsy Feinberg, who in the beginning felt nothing applied to her, but now feels we were talking directly to her. I came away with positive feelings that something had been done to heal the breach and get the students to look at themselves.

PSYCHIATRIC NURSE. A crucial question seems to be where do we go from here? Faculty's role involves making a decision regarding Sue's motivation for nursing. And this is no easy task.

MISS JENSEN. Take the situation of Rose Carey, for example. She annoys her classmates and it is easy to see why. She says she knew all along something was wrong in the class but she just couldn't speak out. On the clinical units, she functions in a maze of confusion, but at least she tries to use help.

There also are some problems regarding social regulations in the residence. [*Eyes meet and exchange significant messages.*]

The psychiatric nurse continued to refocus the discussion and encouraged the faculty to face the reality problem of having to make decisions about evaluating the students under discussion. When Miss Jensen mentioned the possibility of social problems in the residence, there was a complete shift in tone. One could also discern the contrapuntal strains of the worn theme of blame and scapegoating. It was too soon, however, to tell whether the underlying dissonance would break into full-blown cacophony. The atmosphere grew tense and some faculty members became defensive.

In the two weeks between this meeting and the one to follow, the discussion of the students' behavior continued.

Displacing Anxiety about Handling a Faculty Member

February 21, 1961

PSYCHIATRIC NURSE. The first item on the agenda that we have to take care of is to wind up the schedule for our work with the instructors in the clinical conferences. Esther Vance and Eileen Drew are already scheduled, so now Monte and I will be ready to work with you, Claire [*Foster*], in April.

MISS FOSTER. I don't know yet. I have to make out my total schedule for that quarter first before I can tell. [*She pokes a finger through her blonde braids.*]

PSYCHIATRIC NURSE. Perhaps you can work your schedule around the experience with Monte and me since you know now when that will be.

MISS FOSTER. I want to do the schedule first. [*She removes her rimless glasses and energetically wipes them.*] Then there are certain days I'll be away.

No decision was reached about Miss Foster working with the psychiatric team. Though an impasse continued to exist, Miss Foster's techniques of evasion were coming more and more into the open. The other faculty members were silent. The psychiatrist also withdrew. They were uneasy. Some closely watched the psychiatric nurse during the exchange, while others looked at each other, and still others lowered their eyes, and the psychiatrist doodled. There was audible sighing in the background.

PSYCHIATRIC NURSE. Eileen [*Drew*], you spoke to me earlier about some difficulty in evaluating Sue Eddy and assigning her a grade. Since evaluation time has come around again, this is probably a good time to discuss it.

MISS DREW. I don't know how to evaluate Sue. Her theory and academic work are okay. Her clinical performance is all right. Am I missing something? She's much more reserved the last three weeks since our conferences with Dr. Ullman. She is aware her behavior is under scrutiny. She is able to make a plan of care and to carry it out. She copes with most problems but not always in the best way. She is a little lax on technical skills and sometimes her physical care suffers. She writes good nurse's notes. She seems interested in the patient, although she is very disease-oriented, yet the patient doesn't get completely lost. She asks for help in implementing her plan of care. As a matter of fact, she uses me more now than she did during her clinical practice in fundamentals of nursing. She is no problem to staff as yet. One patient requested to have her again. She can be trusted to give safe care.

PSYCHIATRIC NURSE. Is there any aspect of her behavior that you would pick up as being problematic? There seems to be some discrepancy between what Sue verbally expresses about nursing and the way she behaves in the clinical setting.

Miss DREW. In the clinical conferences that Jane participates in, she has no interest in the discussion. Yet in the clinical area, she is interested in patients. Because of my need to give close supervision to two other students who are not safe, I have little time to spend with Sue. All I'm saying is that I have no basis to fail Sue Eddy and that she will be here for the next quarter unless she withdraws on her own.

Miss FOSTER. Yet we are constantly putting through students who have an up-and-down pattern of functioning. [*She exhales a cloud of smoke.*] Take Selma Kruthers, as an example.

Miss VANCE. I'm not concerned that we can't always be sure whether students can make it or not.

Miss REED. It's okay that Selma didn't leave until the junior year.

Miss THOMAS. I guess we just have to let Sue go along and if she hangs herself, then that's that.

PSYCHIATRIST. This is a complicated situation. We can't necessarily take Sue's professed attitudes as a fact. Perhaps she has some questions about nursing as a profession but still has some capacity to pass. Her derogation of nursing may not reflect her true feelings about nursing, but rather be derogation of faculty—her way of needling authority. This attitude is closely tied in with her own unresolved feelings about herself. She has a compulsive need to be derogatory. This may be a girl who is struggling with a real capacity for nursing. Her relationships with patients are real. Her attitudes toward nursing are more a reflection of her private problems; if she can keep these to herself, things might go more smoothly.

Perhaps Jane or I should have an individual conference with her to bring her compulsive derogation to her attention. Secondly, faculty's analysis of her problems should be made very clear to her. Eileen, what would you think about suggesting to Sue that she see me?

Miss DREW. I can do this very easily because I'm scheduled to have a conference with her anyway.

An analysis of the process of the meetings concerned with students' problems reveals two main features. One was the problem presented by Miss Foster's elusive response to the expectation that she would work with the psychiatric team. Miss Jensen, who had achieved a sense of accomplishment, growth, and satisfaction in her second experience with the psychiatric team, was vehement about the importance of the experience. However, her comment constituted the only attempt by a faculty member to intervene in the situation. The psychiatrist also abdicated his responsibility for dealing with this problem and he never handled it directly. Thereafter, the faculty members and the psychiatrist sat on the side-lines and passively watched the psychiatric nurse try to exact a commitment from Miss Foster.

The faculty members had dealt effectively with students like Sue Eddy before. The real problem, with which they most likely felt overwhelmed, was how to manage the anfractuous behavior of Miss Foster. Their preoccupation with Sue Eddy may have served as a displacement of feelings of helplessness in regard to Miss Foster's behavior. Previously, the definition of intrafaculty problems had been limited to the existing schism between the two groups. Now it began to be apparent that interpersonal difficulties also existed between members of the same group.

The second noticeable feature of these meetings was that the faculty members in the older group remained in the background. The situation represented a complete reversal of the one in the first year, when the younger members withdrew into passivity and submission and the older members dominated the situation.

Several questions might be asked about this reticence on the part of the older faculty members. Were they expressing their fear of the younger members' increased security and forcefulness? Was this a way of expressing disapproval of the younger members for bringing interpersonal difficulties into the open? In withdrawing, were they avoiding problems by pushing them underground? Was such withdrawal connected with the older members' conflict about democratic process as well as their fear of setting realistic limits on problematic behavior?

Or were the older members glad that at last the younger ones were expressing themselves because they wanted to hear what the younger group had to say? Would this account for the tense manner in which they held themselves, as if they were afraid they might break the spell?

Role of the Psychiatric Team

In this series of conferences the differences between the psychiatric nurse's and the psychiatrist's roles can be more sharply delineated. The psychiatrist identified the underlying dynamics that were operating in the situation. He clarified the student problem by pointing out that the aggressive students had become leaders by default only because those who disagreed were afraid and silent. Both the older and the younger faculty members at one time or another had found themselves in a similar situation in relationship to each other.

The psychiatric nurse, through her questions, tried to stimulate each faculty member to take responsibility for dealing with students' problems on an individual level. She encouraged Miss Drew and Miss Jensen to formulate what they did, how they did it, and what they learned from their experience.

The psychiatrist did not allow a competitive struggle to develop between Miss Drew and Miss Jensen and the psychiatric nurse. He supported and encouraged the instructors to handle the student conferences, but at the same time he included the psychiatric nurse. This was a most rewarding experience for all four—the psychiatrist, the psychiatric nurse, and the two instructors—particularly in light of the former alienation of the psychiatric team from members of the younger group. It served as a basis for more effective collaboration in the future.

The psychiatrist also helped to dispel any aura of mystery that might have surrounded his individual conferences with the faculty members, when he shared the results without giving specific details. Without becoming defensive, he stated that the faculty members had been unhappy with the group meetings; then he utilized their reactions to set up a future framework.

The psychiatric nurse emphasized eliciting a problem for discussion and collecting the data. She did this by seeking the reactions and opinions of the faculty members and supporting them in their efforts to communicate points of difference. Some faculty members had become comfortable enough with her to discuss openly and freely their problems in relating with her.

All these circumstances might have contributed to the faculty members' postponement of individual conferences with the psychiatrist, for they may have felt that these were unnecessary at this time. Both members of the psychiatric team referred to the fact that other issues seemed to take precedence over the interviews with the psychiatrist, but they did not press this point further.

During these meetings fear and uncertainty left the psychiatric nurse. She felt more comfortable and secure with the faculty and with the psychiatrist. She withstood Miss Foster's elusiveness. Though no decisions were made in the group (the psychiatric nurse worked this out with Miss Foster outside of the group) and the tension level was high, she kept returning to the dilemma. At least one thing was accomplished: the problem was in the open for all to see and experience.

The psychiatric nurse took back the integration project, which she so unceremoniously had handed over to the psychiatrist at the end of the first year; she was now able to share it with him. As in all relationships, collaboration had to evolve. There was no pattern for its creation. Like the other faculty members, the psychiatric nurse needed three years to work through the various steps in achieving collaboration.

Summary

During this phase large blocks of time were devoted to the discussion of student behavior, how to evaluate it and how to handle it. The faculty shifted from looking for ready-made solutions to students' problems to interest in learning more about the dynamics underlying the problematic behavior and included the desire to face issues rather than avoid them.

The faculty schism between members of the younger and older groups started to heal over. As relationships between the two groups improved, areas of disagreement between members of the same group became evident. Though there were occasional episodes of scapegoating and placing blame, the faculty members were assuming more responsibility for their own actions. They were less inclined to take comments personally and were more accepting of each other's personal idiosyncrasies.

Chapter Twelve

THE WORK WITH THE FACULTY GROUP: THE LATER STAGE OF SYNTHESIS

===============

Is the knowing all? To know, and even happily that we meet unblessed; not in some garden of wax fruit and painted trees that lie in Eden, but after, after the Fall, after many, many deaths. Is the knowing all? And the wish to kill is never killed, but with some gift of courage one may look into its face when it appears, and with a stroke of love—as to an idiot in the house —forgive it; again and again . . . forever?

ARTHUR MILLER, *After the Fall.*

The final phase of the faculty discussions was marked by a study of two psychiatric concepts, based on an exploration of the ways in which the faculty members were themselves experiencing these concepts. Strictly speaking, this study was begun in the closing months of the fourth year. However, because it extended well into the fifth year, it is appropriate to describe it against the background of the other events that were taking place during the fifth year.

Context of the Meetings

FACULTY CHANGES

As in other years the integration process was somewhat affected by changes in the faculty group. In the fifth year of the project, one instructor took a sabbatical leave during the first two quarters and returned in the spring. Another instructor resigned and was replaced by Miss Newberry. Two members of the younger group were promoted from the rank of instructor to assistant professor. One of these members also received tenure, but she was not appointed to the Executive Committee.

WORK ON THE BOOK

The fifth year's activities were to a considerable extent shaped by the fact that the psychiatric nurse and the psychiatrist were on partial leave for the purpose of organizing the data from the integration program for use in writing this book.* It was obvious that a curtailment of their other activities would be necessary, yet both of them were convinced that they could not absent themselves entirely from the situation for one year without seriously jeopardizing their relationship with the faculty and the progress they had achieved thus far. They agreed that the psychiatrist should be in the situation for two hours a week and the psychiatric nurse for a minimum of four hours a week.

The psychiatric nurse had mixed reactions to this allocation of time. The opportunity to write up the psychiatric integration project represented the fruition of a long-cherished dream, but she was concerned about how the project would be affected by her partial absence from it. She was confident that the other faculty members had the ability to carry on the program, but she had some misgivings about whether they were sufficiently motivated to do so. She was also troubled about having fewer contacts with the other faculty members. She was concerned, on the one hand, that they might feel abandoned by her and, on the other, that they might begin to feel no need for her in the future. These reactions constituted a clear case of the separation anxiety which is bound to occur in any positive relationship.

In a project of this kind, the psychiatric nurse's willingness to become involved sufficiently to care about the other faculty members is a vital part of the integration process. Some psychiatric nurses may underestimate or even discourage or completely bypass this basic aspect because they may think of involvement as being incompatible with objectivity. They may fail to connect, or avoid or resist connecting, involvement in a situation with caring about the people in it. If the psychiatric nurse perceives herself as a savior of nursing education by way of psychiatric integration, she may become too preoccupied with self-aggrandizement. It follows that she will view caring as a one-way and close-ended process that emanates from the rest of faculty, but from which she herself is immune.

Contrary to the pessimistic expectations of the Skidmore project director, the work on this book proved to be a cohesive, rather than a divisive, influence on her relationships with the other faculty members. The time for

---

* At this period of the project, the psychiatric nurse and the psychiatrist had planned to collaborate on the writing of this book. Owing to the pressure of more immediate commitments, the psychiatrist was forced to withdraw from co-authorship before the book was begun.

writing the book and for the necessary solitude had not yet come. It was first necessary to collect further data—a task which required the cooperation of the other faculty members as well as the students.

In the process of working for four years on an empirical level with the faculty and the students, the psychiatric nurse thought she had identified various trends that were operating in the faculty and student groups. However, during the fifth year as she worked on this book, she found it necessary to formulate and validate what, up to now, had been a mixture of hunches, hypotheses, rumor, and some facts. In the effort, therefore, to create a partial basis for a better understanding of faculty and student interaction, she thought it might be helpful to learn something about the cultural, social, and professional values and past experiences that the faculty members and the students were bringing with them to the department of nursing. In particular, she believed that some information about their hopes and aspirations, areas of self-mastery, various prejudices and biases, and vested interests might shed considerable light on the problem of unrealistic expectations and motivations and goals for nursing and teaching.

Accordingly, in September and October of the fifth year, the psychiatric nurse interviewed individually all the faculty members and fourteen students selected from the senior, junior, and sophomore classes, as well as four members of the class that had graduated in 1961. The selection of the students and graduates was based on two criteria: religious preference and status of relationships with men. The Protestant, Jewish, and Roman Catholic faiths as well as students who were married, engaged, "going steady," and "unattached" were equally represented. The following areas were broadly touched on in the interviews: geographical origin of students and faculty members (see Chapter 4 and Appendix B); educational and work experiences; racial and religious attitudes; short and long-term goals (marriage vis-à-vis a career); perception of psychotherapy; view of the curriculum; and evaluation of faculty-student relationships.

The time was ripe for the interviews. The relaxed, give-and-take quality indicated that the psychiatric nurse had secured the trust and confidence of the faculty members and that the differences in roles were less of a barrier. Some faculty members utilized the interview as an opportunity to express personal as well as professional problems and to seek help in handling them. Work on this book, therefore, was used as a way for faculty members to talk about problems that did not come into the open in the faculty group. There is no question that but for the writing of the book these interviews never would have occurred. Thus, the preparation of this book became an instrument of change.

Through these interviews the psychiatric nurse experienced each faculty member in a highly personal way. The immediate change that followed seemed to indicate that this had been a mutual experience. The interviews created a denouement not in the writing of the book, but in the integration process itself.

The faculty members also became involved in the preliminary work on the book through the psychiatric team's periodic reports to them. The team proposed these reports as a means of providing the faculty members with an opportunity to make suggestions. The faculty members responded to this proposal with spontaneous enthusiasm and interested anticipation. Some surprise at the psychiatric team's willingness to share the planning of the book was conveyed in an older member's comment, "Well, all I can say is that you both have a lot of courage to take on such a project with this group." It seemed rather clear that this faculty member was expressing some appreciation of the anxiety and interpersonal difficulties that such discussions might engender.

OTHER INTEGRATION PROJECT ACTIVITIES

The psychiatric nurse's anxiety about the discontinuance of some of the integration activities proved to be unfounded. Several faculty meetings were devoted to the discussion of plans for implementing the psychiatric integration program during the partial absence of the team. At these meetings, the faculty members had an excellent opportunity to discard any or all of the aspects of the integration program. Instead, they took it for granted that the various experiences would be continued, and directed the discussion to the way in which the responsibility for these experiences could best be divided between the psychiatric team and the other members of the faculty. It was decided that the psychiatric team would continue to meet with the faculty once a week and would be available for individual conferences. The work that they had been carrying on with students would be divided between them and other faculty members.

In particular, both members of the psychiatric team would be available for conferences with individual students who were referred to them by the instructors. These students were to be seen first by the psychiatric nurse, who would decide if further referral to the psychiatrist was necessary. This was a pattern that began to evolve in the fourth year.

As for the other activities with students, it was decided that the leadership of the unstructured group discussions and the teaching of the course in interpersonal relations could be turned over to another faculty member. The faculty group selected the instructor who had collaborated with the psychiatric nurse in the psychiatric nursing and the public health nursing clinical conferences. This decision was based on the time this instructor had available and the other faculty members' recognition of her special knowledge of psychiatric concepts and skill in handling group interaction.

Emphasis was also placed on the fact that she was free from any responsibility for the evaluation of student performance during this period. This emphasis indicated substantial growth on the part of those faculty members who earlier had resisted this principle, partly because it made the psychiatric nurse's role different from their own. The ability of the faculty members to accept the difference in role without viewing it as a reduction of their own status probably was related to the feelings of increased status that had resulted from their growth in self-acceptance and self-worth, accompanied by beginning attempts to give individual recognition to their colleagues.

OTHER FACULTY PREOCCUPATIONS

The fifth year was also characterized by intensive work on the plan for the new curriculum. This planning took so much of the faculty members' time that during a period of four months it was necessary to suspend the integration project discussions. Also, the competition among the various nursing specialty groups for curriculum time, a natural concomitant of a major curriculum revision, made itself felt in intrafaculty relationships. The work on curriculum, along with the integration project activities, might therefore be viewed as part of the background for the faculty discussions on psychiatric concepts.

The Concept of Anxiety

When the integration program was launched, neither the psychiatric nurse nor the psychiatrist made any specific plans to study in a structured way what psychiatric concepts were being taught in the nursing courses of the Skidmore program. However, during the psychiatric nurse's orientation period, when she was functioning as an instructor in medical nursing, she repeatedly attempted in curriculum meetings to work with the faculty on psychiatric concepts. During this period the faculty members in the younger group resisted any material connected with psychiatric concepts and the learner's role. Such comments as "I've been teaching this for years in all my classes," "We've had all of this stuff before," and "I don't need any help" temporarily thwarted such explorations. The younger faculty members obviously equated theoretical knowledge of these concepts with the ability to apply them in nurse-patient situations and to teach them in an experiential framework to students.

During the psychiatric nurse's participation in curriculum development and in the team's work with individual instructors, however, a general but rather clear picture of what psychiatric concepts were and were not being taught gradually emerged. Certain aspects of the following content were taught by the majority of the instructors in their courses: human needs of well and sick persons; communication as it pertains to interviewing techniques; stress as it relates to emergency and disaster situations; and role—the nurse versus the student. It was also possible for the team to ascertain the depth to which this content was taught and the teaching methods that were utilized. The concepts of anxiety, frustration-aggression, conflict, and such defense operations as withdrawal, resignation, hopelessness, projection, and scapegoating were not dealt with in any detail prior to the clinical course in psychiatric nursing.

These findings caused the members of the psychiatric team to consider again the request of some of the other faculty members, particularly those in the older group, that the faculty meetings in connection with the integration program be utilized for a study of psychiatric concepts. The net result of this reconsideration was a decision to undertake such a study. In line with the psychiatric team's belief about how psychiatric concepts are learned, the method selected for the faculty's study was the experiential one, in which "the person in the role of teacher uses the experiences of faculty and students to help them to recognize, describe, analyze, validate, and synthesize the meaning of their experiences" (1).

The exploration of psychiatric concepts was first begun in June of the fourth year of the project. The concepts of anxiety and aggression were studied during the remainder of the five-year period. These particular concepts were chosen because they seemed most closely related to current intra-faculty tensions, interpersonal and communication difficulties, and defense patterns. The psychiatric nurse and the psychiatrist deliberated about each of these concepts and added dimensions to each other's thinking before presenting it for group discussion. Because an understanding of anxiety is basic to learning about all other psychiatric concepts, the psychiatric team agreed to present it as the first concept for group study. Three meetings were devoted to the exploration of this concept.

EXPERIENCING THE CONCEPT

June 27, 1961

Curiosity, expectancy, and eagerness radiate through the group. Two older members, Miss Vance and Miss Scott, are absent. A few members sit on the side lines, burying themselves in note taking. One older member is flushed and hides her face with her hand. She stays in the background for most of the meeting.

PSYCHIATRIC NURSE. Well, today is the day! You probably won't believe it because I hardly can myself, but we finally are going to start discussing psychiatric concepts.
[*There are giggles, smiles, head-nodding, side comments of "At last," and "Good!" The members of the group take out pencils and paper.*]
PSYCHIATRIC NURSE. In deciding where to start, Monte and I concluded that since anxiety is part of all living, and all of us have experienced a great deal of it

together, this would be a good place to begin. Maybe we'd better start out by defining it. How would you define anxiety?

MISS HUNT. A student is anxious when she is afraid of being dropped.

PSYCHIATRIC NURSE. This is because fear is connected with a direct precipitating cause and therefore it differs from anxiety.

MISS NEWELL. It's a feeling—an emotion.

MISS JENSEN. It has an intangible quality; a sense of uneasiness and vagueness. It is negative when it overcomes you, but sometimes it helps you to get things done.

MISS REED. Anxiety is diffuse. I'm not sure that people know what makes them anxious.

MISS JENSEN. The cause is unconscious; it's repressed. What people complain about is not what causes the anxiety.

MISS REED. Have we said it is an uncomfortable feeling?

MISS JENSEN and MISS THOMAS. It's not acceptable to be anxious.

MISS THOMAS. Anxiety involves one's status, such as students' concern about nursing.

MISS REED. It is a gnawing, nagging feeling.

MISS JENSEN. It leads to illogical thinking.

PSYCHIATRIC NURSE. What is the quality of the situation in which anxiety occurs?

MISS DREW. There is a threat to one's self.

PSYCHIATRIST. We see then that first, anxiety is a feeling, which therefore links it to other feelings such as guilt, love, rage. It is different from any other feelings in that it arouses a sense of helplessness. Other feelings occur in relation to the environment. With anxiety, we don't know how to relate to the environment. This is what makes it so painful. There is less pain when other feelings come in, such as anger, avoidance, and so on, because at least something is coming in from the environment, be it positive or negative.

Earlier, Jane referred to some differences between anxiety and fear. Fear is not associated with helplessness. The individual can flee, fight—in other words, can do something. The object of fear is identifiable.

[*A great deal of note taking is going on in the group. Several members appear to bury themselves in writing.*]

PSYCHIATRIST. There are positive and negative aspects to anxiety which relate to its expediency or inexpediency. The negative aspects relate to the pain and the ways it interferes with constructive action. Mild or anticipatory anxiety serves a constructive end because it orients the individual to danger. There is tension and alertness. Whatever contributes to the threat usually is not known. Reactions to situations are not always clearly understood because they are threatening.

PSYCHIATRIC NURSE. To get clear about the meaning of being threatened, what are some situations in which you feel anxious?

MISS NEWELL. I'm overly cautious about driving. I have been in an automobile accident.

PSYCHIATRIC NURSE. The anxiety is communicated in not wanting to take a chance.

MISS JENSEN. What can she do to overcome it?

PSYCHIATRIST. It can be handled in any idiosyncratic fashion. She can refuse to drive, which is withdrawal, or use gradual solutions such as driving in and out of the driveway.

MISS JENSEN. Take skiing, for example. I always get anxious.

PSYCHIATRIC NURSE. I know what you mean, Dot [Jensen]. But there is a real danger of breaking your neck. [Spontaneous laughter.]

MISS THOMAS. I'm not interested in hearing about driving. [She tugs at an earring in her pierced ear.] I want to focus on anxiety around the students' behavior.

PSYCHIATRIST. There are objective and subjective components in both situations of driving and skiing, though in Marie's [Newell] example of driving, there is more subjectivity or less realistic basis for fear, which means there is more of an element of anxiety.

PSYCHIATRIC NURSE. Sometimes we find it difficult to understand why a person gets anxious when the objective facts do not warrant it.

PSYCHIATRIST. This involves one's values. You cannot stop anxiety through using words, but only through changing one's self.

PSYCHIATRIC NURSE. Perhaps we can see how anxiety comes up in handling students, parents, and so on. How about some examples of our relationships with students and each other in which differing values create anxiety?

MISS HUNT. Students get caught between the patient and the instructor and having to meet the expectations of both.

PSYCHIATRIC NURSE. Conflict of values always arouses anxiety and a feeling of helplessness. What values are operating in Audrey's [Hunt] example?

MISS THOMAS. The student feels the instructor doesn't understand, which may be irrational. Then she orients her own values toward what she thinks the instructor wants, and she can't fulfill the needs of both.

MISS NEWELL. When a student who has failed says, "Goodbye," I feel completely paralyzed, trapped, and helpless. I want to escape.

PSYCHIATRIC NURSE. Maybe we feel that somehow we should have been able to prevent the student's failure and feel guilty about not doing so.

MISS DREW. I share Marie's [Newell] feelings. I shudder every time I have to disqualify a student on my service. [She twists a blonde curl around her finger.]

MISS JENSEN. Is it a case of questioning our own judgment? Do we wonder, "What right do I have to say a student hasn't got what it takes to be a nurse?"

MISS DREW. I worry about how others—student's peers, parents, authority, and so on—will see my failing a student.

PSYCHIATRIC NURSE. I guess we would all agree that evaluation time is a mass demonstration of anxiety.

MISS JENSEN. How do the poor students who haven't failed feel?

MISS THOMAS. Evaluation is especially difficult when you don't like a student. There is anxiety about your own subjectivity.

MISS FOSTER. There is confusion between liking, not liking, and her quality of work.

MISS DREW. I am concerned that even though we say a decision about a student is a faculty decision, the burden still rests with the instructor. I continually ask myself if I'm being fair, especially when the student's whole life is involved.

PSYCHIATRIC NURSE. We seem to be talking about the anxiety that comes from taking individual responsibility for making a decision, as well as anxiety connected with the possible consequences of our action.

MISS JENSEN. We have to be clear about our own responsibility.

PSYCHIATRIST. Two sources of irrational anxiety emerge. In evaluation, you are called upon to take an individual action. One of the unfortunate trends in our culture is the stress to conform. Taking an action such as disqualifying students does separate the instructor from the rest of faculty and from the students. It is true one has to be without bias. The instructor may not like a student and have to disqualify her, but this does not mean that bias necessarily is operating. Bias can operate, or we can bend backwards to avoid it and perhaps ignore a student's bad points.

The second source of anxiety is the instructor's irrational need to be liked. This results in conformity, which is always threatened by individual action. The irrational need for approval is augmented.

MISS WILLIS. Don't we need to be sure we did everything to help the student to help herself, such as the various methods of teaching?

PSYCHIATRIST. This is an objective component and a rational expectation, but it is not necessarily a source of anxiety. If one expects one's decision to be one hundred per cent sure, this is an impossibility.

MISS THOMAS [*to Miss Newell*]. I think in your own situation you feel sorrow when students leave.

PSYCHIATRIC NURSE. Frequently anxiety will occur when feelings of sorrow and compassion are aroused, because we are not supposed to have these feelings—especially in the American culture.

MISS JENSEN. I don't feel we can experience the same depth of pain when a student is disqualified as the student herself does. After all, we won't be fired. We don't have to face parents.

PSYCHIATRIST. It is just as painful when one takes an individual action because one is a separate self, away from the group.

Interest was demonstrated from the beginning of the meeting. The majority of the members participated in defining anxiety. Healthy competition was motivating and operating. However, it took a while for the members to get warmed up and to feel sufficiently secure to give examples of anxiety from their own experience. Security operations against their own anxiety included giving such superficial examples as skiing and driving a car. Miss Thomas bristled with annoyance and refocused the meeting on faculty concerns. Miss Newell brought up the touchy and recurring predicament of students who fail.

No better situation could have 1 een chosen for exploring the nurse teacher's anxiety, because it is one in which she is faced with an inevitable and often unresolvable role conflict. First and foremost she is a nurse and, as such, is responsible for the safety of patients who are nursed by the graduates from the program in which she is teaching. Therefore, when there is any question whatsoever about a student's ability to give safe nursing care, she cannot let the student have the benefit of the doubt and give her a passing grade. On the other hand, as a teacher, she has a great emotional stake in the welfare and happiness of her students and is therefore tempted, in the case of a student whose performance is border-line, to resort to the criteria that are sometimes utilized for promoting or graduating students in other types of educational programs—"She is trying," "She has shown some progress," "She may improve after graduation and should therefore be given a chance."

In the past, the faculty had consumed hours in trying to come to grips with this anxiety-laden problem of how to evaluate students. The discussions had generally been slanted toward and limited to an identification of the faculty members' own goals and expectations. Although the faculty members had reacted to each other's evaluations in various ways, the personal impact on one member when she had to fail a student never came into the open (see Chapter 8).

In this meeting, instead of dealing with the concept of anxiety from a purely theoretical viewpoint, the faculty members struggled to discuss it within the framework of intrafaculty relations. There was evidence of an underlying desire to understand their own behavior. Several younger members revealed their guilt feelings about failing students. They helped the group to approach evaluation from an entirely different level, that of personal anxiety. Feelings of compassion for each other surged forth.

The psychiatric nurse and the psychiatrist were clear about their roles and were complementary to each other. They clarified the fact that the anxiety experienced by the instructor when she fails a student stems from having to take individual action that is incompatible with group conformity. This principle illuminated a trouble spot in intrafaculty relations that periodically had been touched on, namely, depreciation of individual differences accompanied by group pressure to conform.

The meeting ended with reaffirmation of the pain involved in failing a student.

A WASTELAND RE-EXPLORED

July 11, 1961
An area too raw and painful to touch on has hovered over some faculty members for three years to obsess them in every student-evaluation conference. In this meeting, fear about expressing feelings becomes secondary to the desire to understand what happened and how the situation miscarried, and to begin to resolve the problem.

Participation is spontaneous and lively, although one younger and two older faculty members continue to withdraw and withhold their reactions. Some faces are animated. Some are perplexed. Others appear like masks and hide what is going on inside. With the exception of two older faculty members, no one takes notes. Occasional doodling becomes an outlet for anxiety.

PSYCHIATRIC NURSE. It's been two weeks since we had our beginning discussion of anxiety. Since Esther [*Vance*] and Helen [*Scott*] couldn't be here, it might help to summarize briefly what we covered.

1. We decided that anxiety is a feeling that emerges when the self feels threatened. It differs from other feelings such as anger, love, and guilt because it involves a sense of helplessness, which is the aspect that makes anxiety so painful.

2. We differentiated anxiety from fear and saw how fear is not associated with helplessness because the object of fear is identifiable and therefore we can do something about it, such as fighting against it or running away from it.

3. We also mentioned that anxiety can be useful when it is mild and alerts us to a problem. We talked about the objective and subjective components in situations that arouse anxiety and related these to rational and irrational expectations.

4. Finally, we discussed numerous examples in which we experience anxiety. This brought us to the evaluation of students and particularly to the faculty's anxiety associated with failure of students. We ended up by pointing out that to fail a student requires the faculty member to take an individual action and that because of lack of conformity she is separated from the group. Such separation will always arouse anxiety.

Today we are going to talk about what we do in our situation when we are anxious, and the various techniques we develop along the way for handling our anxiety.

MISS JENSEN [*in a side comment to the psychiatric nurse*]. Very good summary, Jane.

MISS THOMAS. Well, one thing we do is we come to evaluation conferences and attach another grade to a student whose whole history of performance is a failure. [*She pushes aside a strand of her black bangs.*]

MISS NEWELL. We escape the problem.

MISS VANCE. It's avoidance in making a decision.

MISS DREW [*her brown eyes snap*]. I wasn't escaping when I raised the problem in the first place.

MISS SCOTT. Do we ever give an F grade to get back at a student because we are glad to get rid of her?

PSYCHIATRIST. It is easy to understand realistic anxiety in which realistic circumstances make us helpless regardless of what we do, such as in war or someone attacking us in the park. We get into trouble not because there is a realistic threat to our physical selves, but rather a threat on a social level. Anxiety need not occur if a change occurs within the individual.

We need to ask ourselves what conscious value systems are involved? What unconscious value systems are adhered to that we are not aware of? What values, conscious and unconscious, is this situation of grading a student tampering with?

Grading a student has to do with taking responsibility and standing out alone and subjecting one's self to the possibility of criticism from faculty and parents. In handling the situation the uncertainty is not necessarily in regard to the basis and reality of the F grade. The anxiety is in terms of the possible repercussions.

Miss Jensen. Does the situation change when you get acceptance from the group?

Psychiatrist. To the extent that you are not clear about the student, the group helps if your own conviction deepens. If you are anxious and the group makes the decision, your anxiety is only postponed. Anxiety should not be confused with doubt. When one is certain and there still is anxiety, one needs to ask, "What is behind what appears as doubt?"

Miss Jensen. Fear of the consequences. [*She tugs at her blonde ponytail.*]

Psychiatric Nurse. Fear of disapproval from other faculty members, particularly those who are in authority. Also, there is the desire to be liked by the students.

Miss Vance. Feeling guilty is often at the bottom of the doubt or anxiety.

Psychiatric Nurse. When one tries to clarify the basis for anxiety, often the issue itself becomes secondary and allaying one's anxiety becomes primary.

Psychiatrist. In taking a particular action, there also is the value of approval and support from parents, faculty, and so on. One is in a difficult spot. In defining areas of legitimate support, you have to be clear on whether your decision or course of action demands total agreement. When you don't get support from the group, you have to ask yourself, "Am I clear? Who is right?"

[*Much interaction goes on as Miss Jensen makes side comments to the psychiatric nurse and asks her if she should bring up the old problem of the student, Kay Fried. The psychiatric nurse strongly encourages her to do so.*]

Miss Jensen. Well, here I go with the "Kay Fried Incident." [*She pauses briefly; her blue eyes scan the group.*] You can even see by faculty's reactions right now the feelings that are involved. At the time I failed the student, I felt complete rejection from the group. I felt that faculty saw me as incompetent. I didn't trust my own feelings, even though at first I was sure.

Miss Vance. The original problem got lost and sparks flew. I doubt that this would ever happen again.

Miss Thomas. This is an example of where the group felt differently about Dot [*Jensen*] than she supposed they did.

Miss Vance. There was tremendous concern that the student would evoke retaliation, that she might feel there was insufficient evidence.

Miss Newell. This causes me anxiety all the time. Students' values seem so different from faculty's, and the latter are the ones who make the value judgments from their own frame of reference. I don't go along always with what faculty does. But I can't say anything and this makes me nervous.

Miss Scott. Why can't you say something?

Miss Jensen. I'm not anxious about flunking the student. I'm anxious about the response of the group.

Psychiatric Nurse. How does this past anxiety-laden situation operate in the present in terms of our inability to deal with new or different group responses? Do we act now as if the old situation is continuing in the present? How much does the anxiety that is attached to the past experience of Kay Fried obscure and distort what is going on in the present?

Miss Jensen. I still feel the sting of that experience.

PSYCHIATRIST. This is a complicated situation, and therefore we must be aware that such a decision will have repercussions. It is possible for an individual instructor to become preoccupied with other than real issues. Such preoccupations also can go on with the group. The result is a clash. The individual instructor feels cast out. The group's responsibility is to help the instructor in terms of the rational aspects instead of supporting her irrational preoccupations. Dot [*Jensen*] had the feeling, "If I take a stand, the roof will fall in." And it did —at least enough to make Dot feel alienated.

MISS THOMAS. I felt we should have had more concrete evidence to back up the student's failure.

PSYCHIATRIC NURSE. I told Dot [*Jensen*] at the time that I felt negatively about how she handled the situation because I felt if she was sure and certain about the student failing, she should have brought this to the student's and the faculty's attention sooner.

[*Miss Jensen nods in agreement with the psychiatric nurse.*]

MISS SCOTT. Everyone, not only Dot, was ostracized. [*She smooths her chestnut upsweep.*] All of us ostracized each other.

PSYCHIATRIC NURSE. Faculty was divided into two camps on the issue. If you supported one, you lost the support of the other. At that point, I didn't know what to feel, because either way, it seemed to me I would end up alienating someone. [*Laughter.*]

MISS DREW. This is one of the reasons why I was uneasy about presenting a student for discussion six weeks ago. Dot [*Jensen*] warned me that if she went along with what I said, the situation would be serious.

MISS JENSEN. I thought I'd be fired.

MISS WILLIS [*her brown eyes open wide*]. I am disturbed that after all this time you couldn't discuss this with us.

GROUP [*several members in chorus*]. But that's the whole point! She couldn't! This is the way anxiety operates. She felt helpless.

PSYCHIATRIST. Dot's inability to communicate had to do with her anxiety and irrational feelings. Dot felt she was thought of as the chief bungler. I am sure that there were some feelings among the group that Dot had been banished.

MISS VANCE. I saw it as a bungling of the whole problem. [*She strokes her long auburn pageboy.*] There was no system, plan, or policy for handling the problem.

MISS SCOTT. The rest of faculty also felt anxious and guilty. I know I did. [*Her gray eyes look sad.*]

PSYCHIATRIC NURSE. Dot's own anxiety blocked her in experiencing what the rest of the faculty was feeling. In turn, our own anxiety cramped our awareness of what Dot was feeling. If we can't resolve anxiety, we use the group not for clarification, but instead as a means of buck-passing, evasion, avoidance, denial, and withdrawal.

MISS THOMAS [*exhales her cigarette with a deep sigh*]. We haven't mentioned this problem for three years.

PSYCHIATRIST. How might this situation have been handled? How should Dot have presented the student situation to the group so not to trigger off feelings in the group?

Dot presented the problem in terms of—a situation has come up with me about the failure of a student. The grade is not the issue, but because there are no policies worked out to handle this kind of situation, I am in an untenable position by surprising the student. Then the issue becomes a collective problem, not the failure of the student, but the absence of channels to handle it. If the problem is handled at this level, Dot's lack of foresight is no more or less than that of the total group. Since faculty operated on the grade level, any suggestions for different methods of handling was seen by the individual as questioning her judgment.

This faculty experience was an epochal one. It was the first time since the Kay Fried incident had occurred three years before that several faculty members together openly faced and dealt with their own anxiety and feelings of helplessness regarding student evaluation. Inordinate fear of group disapproval and rejection had kept the lid fastened on the caldron. Once the lid popped off, those instructors (one younger and one older) who were most directly involved in the incident discovered that some of their colleagues also had deep and mixed feelings about it.

In spite of the anxiety, the discussion was kept going by support from the psychiatric team and by the support that the faculty members were beginning to give to each other. At the same time, the freshly cemented relationship between the younger and older groups began to give way. Once again difficulties between them broke out. Nor was all serene among the older members. Miss Vance began to chip at some other older members as she pointed to the absence of a policy or a specific plan regarding failing students.

FEAR OF RETALIATION

In the interim between the foregoing meeting and the next one, several curriculum meetings were held to make plans for implementing the new curriculum. The new curriculum design made it necessary to reduce the time spent in several clinical areas. Controversy reigned. Although each faculty member had committed herself orally to the new design, when it came to her own clinical area, she was reluctant to let go of hours. An older faculty member who was being pressed to give up additional time from her area announced to the group that she would resign rather than do so. It was on this note that the following faculty discussion opened.

July 18, 1961
The atmosphere is strained. Silence hangs heavy. Some faculty members squirm uneasily. Others stealthily eye the tape recorder.

PSYCHIATRIC NURSE. Last week we discussed the defenses against anxiety and did so within the framework of student-evaluation. We saw that anxiety is an outcome of tampering with one's own or another's conscious and unconscious value systems. We pointed out that in the case of student-evaluation, anxiety is not necessarily about the validity of the grade, but rather is related to the possible repercussions from others.

This brought us to the re-opening of the famous, or more properly, the infamous "Case of Kay Fried." Feelings that have been smoldering underground for years came to the surface. As we aired our feelings we learned with some surprise that Dot [*Jensen*] was not the only person who has felt guilty about the whole incident. I was impressed that many of our feelings were more similar than different. The defenses against anxiety that we used in that situation included evasion, avoidance, buck-passing, scapegoating, and withdrawal.

[*There is silence and a long pause. All eyes are turned down; there is much doodling and sighing.*]

Miss Scott. Last week we said we wanted to continue the discussion of anxiety.

Miss Thomas. There's not much more to discuss. [*She taps her long tapered fingernails on the arm of her chair.*] Maybe we should move on.

Miss Vance. Yet out of this kind of situation we can set up policies.

Miss Hunt. Does the College always counsel parents of students who fail? Why do we do this?

Miss Scott. In this department, personal attitudes and motivation play an important part in evaluation. This is hard for parents to understand and swallow.

Miss Vance [*twirls her glasses*]. I feel there's a fundamental difference between the way Dot [*Jensen*] and I saw the bungling and the way administration perceived it. As instructors we felt the bungling was on the part of administration. Administration felt the bungling was on the part of the instructors.

[*Miss Willis leaves the meeting, not to return.*]

Miss Thomas. In the end, there was no disagreement about the student's failure. Difficulty arose when the student was not told the reality of her precarious position while she was in the clinical experience. She had not been told of her status in a face-to-face contact. Dot [*Jensen*] didn't have any specific data written down to use as a basis for backing up the failure.

Miss Jensen. I didn't become aware of Kay Fried's deficiencies until the last two weeks of her experience. I had had conferences with her and told her that her work was unsatisfactory. I conferred with Esther [*Vance*] and told her that the student would fail.

Miss Thomas. In terms of anxiety, it is too bad, Dot, that you couldn't find out how the rest of the faculty felt about the whole thing.

Miss Vance. I feel that this discussion is going as it is because Dot keeps being mentioned. Also, I personally, as head of the course, had no part in making administrative policies.

Miss Thomas. I too, had nothing to do with parents, and so on.

Miss Scott. What is happening here today? There is much more tension. [*She adjusts the chestnut knot on top of her head.*] I am very uncomfortable. Last week I felt much more comfortable during the discussion. I thought we had really resolved something. Today, the meeting is tense and blamey.

[*Psychiatric nurse, psychiatrist, and Miss Jensen nod in agreement.*]

Psychiatrist. Esther [*Vance*] seems to have some unresolved feelings, whereas Dot [*Jensen*] was comfortable.

MISS JENSEN. I felt there was still more to discuss, yet after Jane's summary, I
wasn't sure what there was left to discuss. I have some unresolved feelings.

PSYCHIATRIC NURSE. I'm not sure why we had the need to come back to the discussion. But it has taken on the tone of scapegoating which seems to be a recurrent theme among us.

MISS NEWELL. I got the feeling that Esther [Vance] feels some guilt and just
couldn't get it out.

MISS VANCE [stops wiping her glasses as she nods in the affirmative]. Yes, I felt
terribly guilty about the whole situation.

MISS JENSEN. Esther tried to communicate, but no one would listen. Esther was
the only person who supported me either verbally or nonverbally.

PSYCHIATRIST. What bothers you now, Dot?
[Miss Drew tries to say something. Miss Foster leaves the meeting, not to return.]

MISS JENSEN. I don't know.

PSYCHIATRIC NURSE. Yes, Eileen [Drew]?

MISS DREW. I don't see how hashing over three years ago helps.

PSYCHIATRIC NURSE. Are we displacing all our anxiety on the "Kay Fried Incident"? What is going on between us right now?

MISS DREW. I, too, feel something is going on right now, but I don't feel free to
discuss it.

PSYCHIATRIST. You seem to be talking about something splitting the group.

MISS THOMAS. There are problems now, but they aren't creating a split.

PSYCHIATRIST. We need to settle what confusions about the "Kay Fried Incident"
are left unresolved. Dot [Jensen], I thought you wanted to continue the discussion of anxiety, but you wanted to continue the discussion of Kay Fried's evaluation. Why?

MISS JENSEN. I got an intellectual understanding of the situation, and I did get
clearer about Helen's [Scott] and Jane's feelings. But I still feel the group blames
and scapegoats me, though I don't feel blameless.

MISS THOMAS. Don't you feel this could have happened to any of us?

MISS JENSEN. I was louder about the problem. I could have been quiet and by-
passed it.

MISS NEWELL. Do you feel solely responsible for Kay Fried leaving?

MISS JENSEN. Yes.

MISS DREW. This is an individual responsibility and not totally a group responsibility. There is a much broader problem—the whole area of failing students.

PSYCHIATRIST. What could you [Dot Jensen] have picked up from last week? You
were an instrument in the absence of a policy.

MISS JENSEN. Now I can answer your question, Dr. Ullman. I don't think policy
had a thing to do with this problem.

MISS THOMAS. Yet with a policy, there are certain steps to take to prevent this
kind of problem from occurring.

MISS JENSEN. Even with a policy, a student who is not doing well can get missed
by not coming to your attention.

PSYCHIATRIST. Certainly it is possible to miss a student even when there is a policy.

What then is bothering you? If another instructor had been caught in the same problem, would she have had an easier time?

MISS JENSEN. Another person would have some rough times too.

PSYCHIATRIST. Well, then, what is bothering you? Why do you have personal feelings about this? Why is there a state of irresolution?

MISS THOMAS. Dr. Ullman's questions seem legitimate.

MISS NEWELL. Dot, are some of your own feelings of scapegoating self-imposed?

PSYCHIATRIST. This is important. Marie [*Newell*] is in a position to pick up various nuances because she is new on the faculty and has not gone through this experience with us. I also get some feeling of your scapegoating yourself. Last week we were able to discuss this problem without pointing a finger. This raises the point of your own expectations of scapegoating.

MISS NEWELL. Somehow, Dot, I feel you expect this. Faculty do trust you.

MISS SCOTT. Dot, you had a feeling that you may have goofed. Does this feeling exist in some current situations?

MISS VANCE. No one has worried about my residual anxiety.

PSYCHIATRIC NURSE. Esther [*Vance*], that's because you got out rather clearly how you feel. With Dot [*Jensen*], she hasn't. We have to take pot luck guesses about how she feels.

MISS JENSEN. I don't mean to do that.

MISS VANCE. I just got tired of sending warnings on students who were doing poorly and of all the discussion without really discussing the problems at all.

PSYCHIATRIST. Last week we did not get embroiled in whether the problem was a clinical or administrative one, but rather, we saw it as a matter of policy.

[*Miss Jensen is called out of the meeting five minutes before its termination.*]

MISS VANCE. I left the meeting last week, feeling the theme was "Be kind to Dot," so I decided more discussion was needed.

MISS THOMAS. Perhaps we picked up Dot's feelings of scapegoating.

PSYCHIATRIST. We must see problems in perspective. When issues are relived there still will be some old feelings stirred up. If there is the feeling that this discussion takes a slant on the original issue through scapegoating, that is one thing. However, I felt that last week the distress was looked at plainly and in light of what happened. If you feel that the same scapegoating went on in this group today that occurred around the original issue, then certainly we should look at it. But if not, then why the discussion?

There were several interruptions during this meeting. Miss Willis left over an hour before the meeting ended; Miss Foster left shortly thereafter. No explanations were given. Neither one returned.

Instead of continuing to discuss anxiety, Miss Vance returned to the evaluation incident, and Miss Thomas attempted to go off onto another topic. As the meeting gathered momentum, scapegoating and blaming took over. The scene that had occurred during the student evaluation was re-enacted. Miss Vance and Miss Jensen distorted the original problem of absence of a policy on evaluation into a struggle between administration and clinical instruction. A decisive stage was reached when for the first time a faculty member intervened. Miss Scott pierced the circular pattern of scapegoating by reacting openly and directly to what was happening and questioning what it meant.

The group as a whole became mobilized and moved in a more positive direction. The focus was on Miss Jensen, who continued to take the "Kay Fried Incident" personally. Three younger members continued to retreat and passively observed what was going on.

In these three meetings, the responsibility for failing students became the framework for the exploration of anxiety. Anxiety was directly connected with concern about disapproval and rejection from other faculty members, parents, and even the students. The student incident was also used as a vehicle for focusing on the split between the two faculty groups. Fear triggered off the defensive pattern of scapegoating. Anxiety was no longer just a theoretical concept. It had been taken down from the bookshelves and given its rightful place in the living experience of the faculty members.

Some faculty members began to take responsibility and initiative in the meetings. For the first time one faculty member pointed out another's difficulties. A few faculty members began to identify some of their own defensive maneuvers such as escaping the problem and avoiding making decisions.

The discussion of anxiety also set different defense patterns into motion, such as when the chorus of younger members enunciated some of the dynamics of anxiety to deal with Miss Willis, who responded by withdrawing from the discussion. A pattern of faculty interaction began to emerge. When any member of either faculty group was direct about what concerned her, some older members tended to retreat. This response was bound to engender feelings of guilt and fear of being punished for speaking one's mind. It became apparent that the faculty schism between the younger and the older groups had its roots in the realization that when the chips were down, it was the older group that had the power and authority.

Role of the Psychiatric Team. The goal of the psychiatric team was for the faculty members to learn the concept of anxiety through the process of identifying it in the ongoing interaction. The team members' sharing of their own attitudes and reactions was well timed. It was only through such sharing that faculty members could personally experience each member of the team.

Throughout these discussions the psychiatric nurse gave most of her attention to the group interaction process by involving the members in the discussion. When she discerned an undercurrent that seemed to interfere with resolution, she asked the group if some extraneous anxiety-arousing phenomenon was being introjected into the current discussion.

Perhaps at no time in the entire integration program were the special contributions of the psychiatrist so dramatically demonstrated as in his exchanges with Miss Jensen. Relentlessly, she distorted and exploited the student situation so as to lash out at the older faculty members. Unremittingly, the psychiatrist pulled her back from her excursions and detours, and he did so within the context of the educational problem and the group inter-action.

The Concept of Aggression

During the first months of the fifth year, the plan for further discussion of psychiatric concepts was dropped because of the faculty's preoccupation with problems related to student behavior. During this period neither the psychiatric nurse nor the psychiatrist exerted sufficient pressure to continue the discusisons on concepts, but tended, rather, to allow the rest of the faculty to chart the direction and establish the focus of the meetings. In accordance with the faculty's apparent wishes, the meetings were spent in the discussion of social and academic regulations, student government, the honor system, the establishment of policies for the psychiatric referral of students, and an occasional progress report on the plans for the book. A large block of time was devoted to the discussion of how to handle students exhibiting problematic behavior.

After these meetings had continued for some time, several of the younger faculty members started commenting to the psychiatric nurse (outside of the meetings) about their discontent with what they described as "the constant rehash of students' problems." They felt that some instructors were uneasy about making their own decisions regarding students and were becoming overly dependent on the psychiatric team. They expressed impatience to move on to further study of psychiatric concepts because they had found the previous discussions on anxiety "so fascinating." This desire to increase their knowledge of psychiatric concepts was significant in view of the fact that it was these faculty members who had so long resisted studying these concepts.

The general state of intrafaculty relations constituted another reason for resuming the study of psychiatric concepts. All through the first sixteen weeks of the academic year 1961–1962, while the new curriculum was being planned, the faculty members grumbled to each other privately about what they did not like in it. Instead of a single split—namely, that between the younger and the older group—the rift was much more diffuse. Individual members spoke about each other with indignation. The mounting aggression and hostility rolled in like a fog.

At the beginning of the second quarter, the psychiatric team decided that the time was propitious for making an effort to recapture the earlier enthusi-asm and harmony. Such an effort required that the faculty members begin to face their aggression toward each other, how it was being expressed, and its impact on the educational program.

An opportunity to bring up the subject of aggression occurred during the meeting of February 20, 1962.

Effort toward Redirection and Withdrawal from Authority

February 20, 1962

Psychiatric Nurse. Since we're getting into the spring of the year, Monte and I thought it might be a good idea to review our original plan and structure for the group meetings. We had agreed to spend one or two meetings a month on discussion of psychiatric concepts, one meeting every six or eight weeks on a progress report of the book; one week was to be left free for individual faculty conferences with Monte and the other week to be left open for whatever we wanted to discuss. Since we haven't gone along with the plan, we thought it is important to find out about your reactions to the meetings this year.

Miss Thomas. We seem to make schedules only to break them.

Psychiatric Nurse. Dot [*Jensen*], you have expressed some feeling about the meetings. What did you have in mind?

Miss Jensen. I'm referring to our constant rehashing of students. By now, I think we're capable of handling a lot of these problems ourselves without taking up all this precious time in the meetings.

Miss Scott. When we do discuss students, we go on and on and on. We keep giving examples of the same point that has already been elaborated on.

Miss Thomas. In the case of trying to decide whether we should drop Rita Salzman or not, we didn't even resolve the problem after all the discussion we had here, and so we had to call an Executive Committee meeting to come to a decision.

Miss Willis. We know the authors [*the psychiatric nurse and the psychiatrist*] have been busy collecting data for the book. This is the fifth year of the project, and I think as a faculty we want more guidance in terms of psychiatric concepts and reading.

Psychiatric Nurse. I have felt uneasy about not focusing on psychiatric concepts as well as dropping the individual conferences with Monte. Do you think the evaluation of students has become a kind of ritual?

Miss Foster. We evaluate students in the regular faculty business meeting before our group discussions with you [*the psychiatric nurse*] and Dr. Ullman. We get nowhere and when faculty are already under pressure, this waste of time in this meeting is no good.

Miss Jensen. Maybe student evaluation has become a ritual and we tend to lean on Dr. Ullman and Jane for support. Maybe we use students as a way of avoiding more painful problems.

Miss Willis [*peers over her blue-framed glasses*]. We just aren't organized enough.

Psychiatrist. Perhaps Jane and I gave up the planned structure too easily because we've been wrapped up in plans for the book. Originally we saw the psychiatric concepts as coming out of the transcribed tapes, but this proved not to be very workable. We can present some theoretical material, however, and relate it to our problems. We gave up the plan of individual conferences with me too soon. These conferences are one way to provide opportunity for faculty members to discuss problems of the total faculty group but which may not be appropriate for total group discussion.

The faculty members were dissatisfied with the progress of the group meetings. Instead of sitting on their feelings, once the psychiatric nurse had introduced the problem, they expressed their attitudes openly and without blame. They were clearer about what they wanted from the meetings and from the psychiatric team and were more direct in seeking it.

Miss Willis. An associate of the college asked me what we are doing in the department of nursing and wondered if we were "psychoanalyzing all our students." We have to interpret what psychiatric integration is all about.
Psychiatric Nurse. It sounds, Catherine, like you're asking for help here.
Miss Willis. He said this in a loud voice, in a public place, for everyone to hear. I was so embarrassed. And he kept at it.
Psychiatric Nurse. How would you label this behavior?
Miss Jensen. If he had been genuinely concerned, I doubt he would have used such poor judgment and have done what he did in public.
Miss Hunt. If I were in his place, I would be concerned with the problems of the department, but he didn't seem to be.
Miss Scott. Was this his way of avoiding any discussion of plans for future expansion and fund-raising by taking the offensive?
Miss Reed. I still feel he was concerned about the department, but that he is being pushed to do this.
Miss Hunt. Maybe the college is concerned whether they are better off with or without a mental health project.
Psychiatric Nurse. I'd like to hear how some of the rest of you see this.
[*Pause.*]
Miss Thomas. And what about you, Jane? You're a member of this faculty.
Psychiatrist. Reports on the psychiatric integration program are useful in creating good will, but in this situation they wouldn't have helped. This was irrational behavior with no attempt to correct his own misinterpretation. The behavior had a quality of aggression. It carried a threat. It was an act of personal aggression, namely, "I'll put her on the spot first." The problem is money and the budget and the real communication was "aggression." Whenever one relies on a stereotyped and burlesqued way of responding, it is usually a mask for aggression. Masked aggression entails a substitution of the real problem with stereotyped generalizations whether this is about Negroes, Jews, or whatever.
Miss Scott. How might Catherine [*Willis*] have handled the situation?
Miss Thomas. I'd have asked him, "Why do you ask me this question here?"
Psychiatrist. If you had concerned yourself only with the objective facts, namely, the real problem and his masked aggression rather than also your subjective feelings, effective handling would have evolved.

Miss Willis' encounter with an associate of the college and his aggressive remarks about the psychiatric integration project provided a practical framework for a beginning exploration of aggression. The psychiatric nurse picked up the fact that Miss Willis was asking for help. In the beginning the problem was dealt with on a concrete and stereotyped level. Miss Scott, however, clearly identified the dynamics of the encounter and perceived that the reactions to the integration project were merely a symptom of the real problem.

The participation during this discussion was one-sided. Members of the older group were the most active. Five members, one from the older group and four from the younger group, remained silent; only two younger members contributed at all. Some faculty members appeared interested and involved as they savored the new experience of studying psychiatric concepts as they operate in action. Some sat stiffly at attention. Others appeared detached, preoccupied, and indifferent. Unresolved attitudes toward authority figures were acted out according to the entrenched pattern of withdrawal.

Despite prodding by the members of the psychiatric team, the silent members remained silent. Possibly, some members of the younger group tended to disengage themselves from any problems with administrative overtones because they failed to see that these problems had any particular relevance to their own functioning. Their behavior may also have been a way of expressing their ambivalent reactions toward some of the older faculty members.

As on previous occasions, Miss Thomas responded with anger when the psychiatric nurse tried to elicit responses from the silent members. She never exhibited this reaction, however, when the psychiatrist made similar attempts. Role differences between the psychiatric nurse and the other faculty members were still not sufficiently clarified or accepted. Nevertheless, at this stage, the psychiatric nurse did not fall into whatever role the other faculty members were trying to create for her.

AGGRESSION AT A DISTANCE

February 27, 1962
As the meeting begins, a thoughtful mood pervades the group. Some of the members engage in avid note taking. Faces are wrinkled in concentration.

PSYCHIATRIC NURSE. It's been some time since we've taken up psychiatric concepts for discussion because so many other issues kept coming up. Several months ago we discussed anxiety in some detail. Last week, Catherine [*Willis*] presented a situation that provided us with the opportunity to see aggression in action. Today we're going to continue the discussion of aggression. First, we have to define it.

MISS THOMAS. Aggression is when someone says, "I don't like you."

PSYCHIATRIST. Oh, you don't, eh? You're not going to get out of this so easily. [*Members of the group laugh.*] Then aggression is a direct or indirect expression of hostility.

MISS DREW. It's a negative response to a situation.

MISS HUNT. Aggression exists when there are ill feelings between two people. When the person has disturbed feelings, he is the aggressor.

PSYCHIATRIC NURSE. How would you define the nature of the disturbance?

Miss Jensen. When an individual or a group tries to dominate and inflict their will on another person or group.

Miss Newberry. It is a negative expression of hostility.

Miss Foster. It is a physical, verbal, or nonverbal attack on someone due to negative feelings.

Miss Reed. It is dominating another person or group. Aggression contains some anger.

Miss Scott. There is a compelling feeling of tightness, a sense of compulsiveness resulting from frustration and anger. It can be directed inward or outward. It results from some threat to one's own integrity.

Miss Willis. It is a forceful, negative reaction by a forceful person to any positive suggestion.

Psychiatrist. Does the term *aggression* primarily refer to a feeling or to an activity between two or more people?

Miss Thomas. It's a form of activity.

Psychiatrist. Yes. It is a technique of relatedness that has roots in certain feelings. Is hostility synonymous with aggression?

Miss Thomas. Aggression isn't necessarily negative.

Psychiatrist. Are the concepts of domination, control, and manipulation a clue to the nature of aggression?

Miss Thomas. When students are being forceful with patients, they are aggressive, and this is positive.

Psychiatrist. Is aggression identical with forcefulness? Is aggression ever positive? Is all domination negative?

Miss Thomas [*laughs*]. You're splitting hairs! [*She is called out of the meeting and returns in about ten minutes.*]

Psychiatric Nurse. What is the difference between aggression and forceful self-assertion?

Miss Willis. Aggression is attack on an individual, whereas leadership is good for me.

Miss Scott. Aggression is destructive; leadership is constructive.

Psychiatrist. This brings us to the matter of motivation. In aggression, the individual is acting in terms of self-interest. In leadership, he acts in terms of others, in someone else's interest, even if that person is unaware of his own strength. Aggression implies derogation of people.

Psychiatric Nurse. In such derogation, people are dehumanized and treated as "things." But are there any situations in which aggression (a negative response) is rational and appropriate? Are there situations in which there are no other alternatives?

Miss Hunt. In war, destruction, derogation, alienation, and so on are necessary for survival.

Miss Willis. And look at all the psychiatric casualties we had after World War II. [*The group is silent and pensive.*]

Miss Newberry. But I thought the desire to hurt someone is conscious and that this would be aggression.

Psychiatrist. Aggression always involves derogation. Anger is not necessarily derogatory; aggression always is. The action itself betrays the intent.

Perhaps we ought to get to some of the roots of aggression. Whenever the need for an aggressive act arises, it grows out of the soil of anxiety, insecurity, and helplessness. Aggression is used in problems that cannot be handled productively. Some individuals capitalize on aggressive techniques. Our culture and business world reward aggressiveness.

PSYCHIATRIC NURSE. The helplessness that arises from anxiety makes an individual feel powerless and out of control, so that aggression becomes a way of gaining power over others through dominating them. The tragedy of aggression is that it further alienates people from each other.

MISS WILLIS. Russo-American relations is a good example.

PSYCHIATRIST. Aggression is a substitution for love and intimacy. Karen Horney spells out very clearly how we relate to people. She states three directions [2]:

1. Moving toward people in terms of submission.
2. Moving away from people in terms of withdrawal.
3. Moving against people in terms of domination.

MISS JENSEN. Is part of maturity learning to deal with one's angry feelings in a positive way?

PSYCHIATRIC NURSE. When the child is not allowed to express behavior, he develops aggressive techniques.

MISS THOMAS. Are you suggesting that the child should be allowed to express his anger? Would you give an example?

PSYCHIATRIC NURSE. Well, the youngster who hasn't been permitted to get his anger out balloons himself to the extent that no one else exists. Or a youngster will develop some aggressive techniques toward other kids when he is not allowed to express anger with children.

MISS NEWTON. Is tactlessness the same as aggression?

[Miss Foster leaves the meeting, not to return.]

PSYCHIATRIST. Not always. If the tactlessness is continuous, then this is aggressive behavior.

Now we come to self-aggression, which is the effort to make one's self disappear. Such aggression is expressed in irrational self-depreciation and derogation. This is quite different from the fleeting, transitory feelings of pressure that all of us experience. Self-aggression is being intolerant of one's own feelings of hopelessness, accompanied by the attitude that one should always be right, happy, and useful. Such intolerance leads to feelings that things will never be any better. In other words, self-aggression is being intolerant of one's own need to be human.

MISS HUNT. You see this in alcoholism.

MISS JENSEN. We see self-aggression in relation to failure of students.

MISS HUNT. And how about in accident proneness?

PSYCHIATRIC NURSE. Unfortunately, we have to stop now. We will continue the discussion of aggression next week. I think it would be useful to get into some concrete incidents in which we personally have experienced aggression from another person. Second, we will focus on describing the behavior, our responses and feelings, and, lastly, how we handled the aggression.

At the beginning of this meeting, Miss Thomas and the psychiatrist quipped and frolicked and engaged in byplay about the differences between forcefulness and aggression. The other faculty members chortled.

The emphasis of the meeting was on the clarification of aggression as a negative mode of interaction. The use of such terms as *domination, attack,* and *destructive* underscored the negative quality of aggression. Participation was general and flowed freely.

The group did not examine the ways in which aggression was being expressed in intrafaculty relationships, although Miss Jensen referred to the failure of students as an instance of the way in which faculty members were turning aggression in against themselves. She may have been thinking about her own experience during the discussion of a student's failure when another member of the younger group pointed out to her that she was submerged in self-imposed scapegoating.

On the whole, the process of this meeting showed that the faculty members were growing in their ability to conceptualize and formulate ideas and experiences.

Aggression *in Vivo*

The final faculty conference in the fifth year of the project took place in April. During the interval since the meeting of February 10, there had been a spring vacation and two meetings in which the progress report of the plans for this book had been discussed.

During this period also, the faculty was working on the new curriculum plan and had been setting up various subcommittees to implement it. As the curriculum planning took shape, the tension between two faculty members—Miss Foster and Miss Scott—mounted. The entire faculty had been aware of this tension for some time, and several faculty members had consulted with the psychiatric team about the problem. Miss Scott felt completely excluded from any participation with Miss Foster, whose clinical area was closely connected with her own. Miss Foster felt that Miss Scott was unduly critical of her. Neither one was able to talk out the problem directly with the other or to reach any resolution.

The psychiatric team had planned to continue the discussion of aggression by identifying how it was operating among faculty members themselves. The team was prepared for some resistance through evasion and avoidance, but it had not anticipated eruption of the problem between Miss Scott and Miss Foster.

April 6, 1962

The meeting opens with further discussion about the formation of subcommittees. Because of the pressure of various deadlines, the psychiatric team is told that the faculty meetings associated with the integration project will have

*to be temporarily suspended. The psychiatric nurse is asked to participate in
the work of several of the subcommittees. The first portion of this meeting is
spent in organizing a schedule that will enable her to work with the other
faculty members, see students who are referred to her, and use the meeting
time to work with the psychiatrist on plans for the book.*

Miss Scott. Clair [*Foster*], I would like to plan with you. [*She looks through
Miss Foster.*] When are you going to start planning?

Miss Foster. Sally [*Newberry*] and I haven't even had a chance to decide or
discuss what we are going to teach or to draw up any kind of a schedule. We
have to do that before we can bring anyone else in. [*She stubs a half-smoked
cigarette, lights another, and mumbles to Miss Newberry.*]

[*There is general silence as well as doodling, exchange of glances, sighing, and
pencil-tapping. Miss Scott withdraws into silence. The group continues discussing curriculum matters and subcommittees.*]

Psychiatric Nurse [*interrupts*]. I think we ought to get back to what you were
saying a few minutes ago, Helen [*Scott*]. I don't think the subject was finished.
Do you have something more you'd like to say about your planning with
Claire [*Foster*]?

Miss Scott [*pauses*]. I want to know, Claire, if I will be in on the planning of
your course. I am angry because I am never part of it.

Miss Jensen. It is awfully difficult to deal with students unless you know what
goes on in the curriculum.

Psychiatric Nurse. I've been thinking a great deal about this business of sharing with each other. In taking over my unstructured group conferences this
past year, Helen [*Scott*] has become more involved in the curriculum and with
students. This has implications for the integration program next year. Upon my
return on a full-time basis, I don't know yet whether or not I see myself as
functioning alone with the students even in the unstructured group conferences.

Miss Foster. I'm teaching until 5:00 every day. [*She mumbles to Miss Newberry,
then blows on and cleans her glasses.*] My area is not the only one that is
divorced from the rest of the curriculum. I don't know what is going on either
in some other areas.

Miss Willis. Sharing is part of curriculum planning, so Claire, will you please
make arrangements to include Helen [*Scott*] in your planning? [*She twists a
gray curl around her finger.*] What possibilities do you have for time?

Miss Foster [*Her blue eyes are fastened on her doodling. There is a long pause.*]
I can have the meetings on Mondays.

[*A long silence.*]

Psychiatrist. In terms of the concept of aggression, this is what we are very
much involved in. We ought to try to see how aggression operates in this context
and identify the various defenses used in responding to it. We observed that
one faculty member felt aggressed against and then the other responded with
aggression. To feel aggressed against and then be called the aggressor involves
anxiety.

In pointing out the defenses against anxiety, I don't wish to cast a poor light
on either Claire [*Foster*] or Helen [*Scott*]. Claire responded to the anxiety by

getting lost in the activity of doodling. Helen withdrew and waited for someone else to pick up the ball. Jane picked it up, and then Helen stated she was angry. She still waited for the group to take over the problem for her, which it did.

Claire became defensive and construed the situation as one in which she is being aggressed against. This defense is not practical or feasible. If you proceed along the line that faculty "are infringing on us," you get caught up in focusing on concrete factors, such as time, pressures, and so on, which are rationalizations and not the issue. The real issue is whether faculty believe in sharing and this issue has to be decided on its own merit.

The interplay that went on evokes defenses which are not always rational. When this problem was exposed to the group, the group was pulled in two ways. The exposure helped to bring about a statement of the issue and a clarification of the issue. Clarification broke down, however, when Claire [*Foster*] resigned her position because of the overwhelming numbers in the group and pressure from them.

Miss Scott. But what is the point of going to the planning meeting when you feel you aren't wanted? And I still feel I'm not wanted.

Miss Jensen. I'd like to hear some of our own reactions to this.

Miss Vance. I feel Dot [*Jensen*] turned to me and took sides. [*She uncrosses her short legs.*] I disagreed with this concept of sharing everything during the introduction to nursing course.

Miss Jensen. There could easily have been a struggle between Eileen [*Drew*] and myself because we work so closely together.

Miss Willis. I came in and stated to Claire that I thought Helen should be asked to join in the planning.

Miss Jensen. Helen has a stake in the planning because of her own teaching area. [*Flips one long fingernail against another.*] I have a different stake in the joint planning and I rose to Helen's defense.

Miss Vance. I think we began to take sides.

Miss Jensen. I feel the issue just got tabled.

Psychiatric Nurse. Actually, the group dropped the problem between Helen and Claire. Instead, we got caught up in the mechanics of setting up meetings. [*Miss Reed nods in the affirmative.*]

Psychiatric Nurse. Not everyone has expressed herself. We need to hear from the others.

[*Silence.*]

Psychiatric Nurse. How about you, Linda [*Thomas*]?

Miss Thomas. I support Dot [*Jensen*]. I agree that there is a need for sharing.

Miss Hunt. I thought Miss Willis suggested to Claire that Helen join her and that the interplay was between Catherine [*Willis*] and Claire [*Foster*]. [*Members of the group point out interaction was between Miss Scott and Miss Foster. Silence.*]

Psychiatric Nurse. What are your reactions, Thelma [*Reed*]?

Miss Reed. I don't want to talk to the point. [*She hugs her tiny waist.*] It makes me too anxious. There was a struggle. The group was taking sides.

PSYCHIATRIST. Claire [*Foster*], to what extent do you feel the issue is resolved?
MISS FOSTER. I'll have the subcommittee meetings on Monday.
PSYCHIATRIST. That's not what I asked you. How do you feel about it?
MISS FOSTER [*Holds her blonde head*]. I don't know.
PSYCHIATRIST. Eileen [*Drew*], how do you feel about the situation?
MISS DREW. This has been a serious problem of long standing. We still tried to
    dump it. It came to a head today. [*Her brown eyes look soulful.*] I felt very
    uncomfortable and still do.
PSYCHIATRIST. Why?
MISS DREW. I don't think I can go into it here. [*She crosses and uncrosses her
    short legs.*] I don't want to.
MISS SCOTT. Intellectual acceptance doesn't change the feelings. I still feel bad,
    but I'm not sorry we explored the problem.
MISS THOMAS. I am concerned about feelings being made worse, now.
PSYCHIATRIC NURSE. There is always the reality of various splits and group dis-
    affection coming to the surface.
PSYCHIATRIST. Even surface acceptance of the principle of bringing the problem
    into the open can be helpful. If it can't get resolved, then we can look to why
    it isn't being resolved.

At this meeting the hitherto submerged rumbling fulminated into an open
altercation. The misunderstanding between Miss Foster and Miss Scott was
so great that their relationship broke down in the presence of the group. The
atmosphere seethed with anger, hostility, and rage. The faculty members
tried to escape the hot issue by fleeing to the hinterlands of curriculum
matters.

The psychiatric nurse took the responsibility of not allowing the crisis to
take place underground. This was no easy task. Because she was cognizant
of the various details and intense feelings that surrounded the situation, she
anticipated an explosion. She looked pleadingly toward the psychiatrist,
hoping that he would execute the ticklish job for her. He avoided her glance
and nonverbal adjuration. It was up to her to decide whether she would
escape with the rest of faculty or would assume her rightful role and responsibility.

She and Miss Jensen pointed to the principle of faculty sharing, an action
which could have been interpreted as taking sides with Miss Scott in her
controversy with Miss Foster. Miss Foster became defensive and resorted
to such rationalizations as the pressure of time and the fact that other faculty
members were not sharing either. Miss Willis prematurely ended the problem-solving process when she importuned Miss Foster to set a time for
meeting with Miss Scott. Miss Foster relented.

A power struggle was being waged between members of the older and
younger groups. The domination by some members of the older group, which
was responded to by submission on the part of the younger members—a persistent behavioral pattern—was now in bold relief.

The tension mounted. Rage was expressed through livid coloring, mottled necks, quivering voices, suppressed tears, and obsessive doodling. At the peak of feeling, the psychiatrist moved in quietly and calmly by injecting the sobering comment that the faculty members were demonstrating aggression.

The faculty members responded quite openly and freely about the way they had facilitated or impeded the handling of the situation. Without becoming defensive, they agreed that they had taken sides. Several members withdrew. The psychiatric nurse tried to elicit responses from the silent members including Miss Thomas, Miss Reed, and Miss Drew. They remained guarded. Miss Thomas expressed fear that the problem would be aggravated by having been brought into the open; however, for the first time she did not become angry with the psychiatric nurse for attempting to get her to express her opinion.

Immediately following this meeting and for several weeks thereafter, several younger and older faculty members discussed their reactions to it with the psychiatric nurse. There was general agreement among them that Miss Foster's inclination to compete with the other faculty members for the students' approval rather than to collaborate with them, and her tendency to withhold her reactions and opinions and pertinent information about students and the courses she was teaching, were long-standing problems which were barriers to effective faculty planning. The rest of the faculty also felt that Miss Scott had a legitimate basis for taking issue with Miss Foster. However, several faculty members disapproved of Miss Scott's approach. They thought the problem should not have been presented in the group until Miss Scott had faced Miss Foster alone with her personal feelings. They felt that if such an encounter had resulted in a fruitless endeavor, then with Miss Foster's full knowledge, and only then, was Miss Scott justified in bringing the issue before the total group. This attitude was in marked contrast to the faculty members' earlier appraisal of interpersonal problems. Its manifestation indicated the degree of growth and synthesis that had occurred.

INTERRUPTION OF THE FACULTY DISCUSSIONS

Because of the ongoing curriculum revision, at the request of some older members the faculty discussions associated with the integration project were suspended for the remainder of the fifth year—a period of four months. The meetings were resumed in the sixth year, which, however, goes beyond the purview of this book. Some younger members privately told the psychiatric nurse they were disappointed about the interruption of the group meetings. The issue however, was not questioned within the group.

The lapse was an unfortunate one inasmuch as it occurred during a period when more than ever the faculty needed an opportunity to discuss the impact of all the ongoing problems and pressures related to the implementation of the new curriculum. Once again, the younger members were unable to rally their forces and stand up to the older group for something they themselves supposedly believed in and wanted. Instead of facing their difficulty in taking responsibility, the younger members blamed the older group.

The psychiatric team's chief avenue of communication with the faculty as a group was now closed off. They were in touch with faculty problems only to the degree that the psychiatric nurse put together bits and pieces of information volunteered by individual faculty members. The psychiatric nurse and the psychiatrist continued to have periodic individual conferences with instructors about students who had been referred to them. In these individual contacts, when problems of the group were confided to her, the psychiatric nurse urged the faculty members to request resumption of the meetings.

Summary

How can one commend the faculty members adequately for having engaged in a search that cut to the bone? Through teaching and learning psychiatric concepts, they were incited to contemplate the past and confront the present. Resolutely, they filtered their spate of ideas and feelings concerning each other's behavior as well as their own. One of the most gratifying aspects of their change and growth was their desire and struggle to relate the psychiatric concepts to their own experience rather than to study them from a purely intellectual point of view. It is probable that the faculty took so readily to discussing concepts on an experiential level because the focus in the faculty group meetings had been on the identification of professional problems and the establishment of free communication.

At the conclusion of the faculty meetings associated with the integration project, the faculty and the psychiatric team had come a long way together. Many faculty members had discovered something essentially new in the concepts they had "known" before.* They had set a firm foundation on which to build further understanding of psychiatric concepts.

Much of the force of power and status differences was crippled, the resistance to change hobbled. The beginning of a higher order of explicit communication aroused and sustained hope for a creative future. When, for instance, the grant for the psychiatric integration project was renewed for another six years, such faculty comments to the team as, "Congratulations, you both deserve it"; "Now we can be sure you will be with us"; and "This

---

* Gardner Murphy describes the process of making new connections as "canalization" (3). He has stated, "Canalization entails a world of discovery, not a gliding through endless well-worn grooves. The making of the grooves is the canalization process, and new grooves can always be made."

is a basic aspect of the nursing curriculum," were further indication that the integration project belonged to the total faculty.

Through all the pain and joy of ordering the chaos, new depths of strength, fecundity, and imagination were stirred among the faculty members, the psychiatric nurse, and the psychiatrist. They were ready to begin to freeze the change.

REFERENCES

1. Dewey, John. *Experience and Education.* New York: The Macmillan Company, 1947, pp. 39, 96, 108.

2. Horney, Karen. *Our Inner Conflicts.* New York: W. W. Norton, 1945, pp. 48–95.

3. Murphy, Gardner. *Human Potentialities.* New York: Basic Books, Inc., 1958, p. 67.

Chapter Thirteen

INTERDISCIPLINARY TEAMWORK

. . . when the future that we can now foresee deviates so markedly from all that we hope and all that we value, we can by our example, and by the mode and the style with which we conduct our affairs, let it be apparent that we have not abandoned those hopes nor forsaken those values; we need to do this even while concrete steps, to which we resort to avert more immediate disaster, seem to negate them.

J. ROBERT OPPENHEIMER, *The Open Mind*

In a large majority of the psychiatric integration projects that have been or are being conducted in baccalaureate degree programs in nursing, the psychiatric nurse works alone or with periodic consultation. Judging from the reports of such projects in the literature and at conferences, psychiatric nurse-psychiatrist teams are a rarity. Moreover, examples of nurse participation in interdisciplinary collaboration are by no means as profuse as one might gather from the literature. The oft referred-to "doctor-nurse team," for example, has frequently lacked the elements of true collaboration; traditionally, it has consisted of a totem-pole structure in which the physician has the power for major decision making and the nurse's task is primarily to follow his orders. Again, much of what has been labeled "interdisciplinary collaboration" in studies of nursing education and nursing practice has consisted of the utilization of members of other disciplines primarily as consultants or trouble-shooters whose principal function is to study nursing problems and to offer recommendations. Unfortunately, many of the team situations in which social scientists and nurses have come together to study a nursing problem have deteriorated into a competitive struggle for status.

The psychiatric nurse–psychiatrist team that was responsible for guiding the Skidmore project, on the other hand, represented a truly collaborative enterprise. For this reason, a fairly detailed description of how the two members developed this collaborative relationship may be useful in the development not only of similarly composed teams in other psychiatric integration projects but of interdisciplinary teams in other nursing projects.

Considerations in the Establishment of a Team

This is not to suggest that an interdisciplinary team is essential, or even desirable, for every psychiatric integration project. The goals of the project, the problems that must be handled within the particular setting, and the kinds of methods that are necessary to handle them determine whether the project should be guided by a psychiatric nurse alone or whether consideration should be given to putting it in the hands of an interdisciplinary team and, if so, what disciplines should be represented on the team. If these criteria indicate the desirability of utilizing a team approach, other factors should be taken into consideration before a final decision is reached—the professional and personal maturity of the psychiatric nurse and the availability of qualified members of other disciplines who are willing to collaborate on a nursing problem.

The experience in the Skidmore project, however, indicated that in deciding upon the personnel to conduct a psychiatric integration project, two reasons for including a psychiatrist might well be given considerable weight. The first of these reasons would apply to all psychiatric integration programs.

The goal of psychiatric integration is to develop the ability of nursing students to give comprehensive nursing care by helping them to handle patients' emotional responses effectively and to intervene on problematic behavior. Nursing care is based on a nursing plan, which in turn is based on the patient's health needs and the medical plan when one exists. Moreover, one of the criteria for evaluating nursing care is the degree of homogeneity in the patient's health needs, the nursing care plan, and the medical plan. For this reason, as well as the fact that all emotional problems, if pursued in any depth, cut across disciplinary lines, a psychiatric integration project in nursing could profitably utilize an interdisciplinary approach that involves both a psychiatric nurse and a psychiatrist.

Again an interdisciplinary approach might well be used when there are indications that one segment of a problem (such as curriculum change) requires study within a broader context than the original definition of the problem might suggest. Because the integration of psychiatric concepts into the baccalaureate nursing curriculum has implications for change which reach far beyond the mere juggling of a curriculum, it is questionable whether psychiatric integration is a problem that can be dealt with in depth without examining the larger context. In the Skidmore project the exploration of other segments of curriculum development—such as the degree of the faculty's knowledge of psychiatric concepts and the ability to apply them, the responses to change, the distribution of power and its effect on the communication process—was not visualized at the beginning of the project; on the contrary, it was the existence of the psychiatric team that influenced the level on which the psychiatric nurse and the psychiatrist worked and the methods they used. What was originally conceived of as a project focused on curriculum development and teaching faculty members and students evolved into a participant-observational study of how faculty members and students function within a particular organizational structure. The psychiatric team, therefore, was required to deal with the problems of communication, decision making, and status relations among the faculty members, and with the impact of these on the faculty members, the students, and on themselves. In such a situation, because of the differences in orientation, training, and role definition, the psychiatric nurse and the psychiatrist are bound to make different kinds of observations. One purpose of the psychiatric nurse–psychiatrist team is to identify the interrelation between these different observations (10).

Prerequisites for a Team Relationship

If a team approach is decided on, it is important that all those who are involved in setting up the integration project recognize that a team is more than a collection of people working on a common problem. The recent fanfare about group work in educational, professional, and business communities often creates the illusion that "groupiness" is a virtue in and by itself and that visible solidarity and surface consensus are creative. In reality, as Joseph W. Eaton has pointed out, "It can be the cradle of mediocrity" (5). What distinguishes a team from other groups are the collaborative relationships that are developed among the members.

As has been stated, such a relationship characterized the psychiatric nurse–psychiatrist team associated with the Skidmore project. However, the coordination of the psychiatric nurse and the psychiatrist into a collaborative team did not occur automatically or spontaneously; as in every other interpersonal relationship, the process was a developmental one. An examination of how it evolved indicates that certain basic elements for such a development were present from the start.

ROLE DIFFERENTIATION

In the report of a research project on interdisciplinary team research, Margaret Barron Luszki has defined an interdisciplinary team as follows (9).

An interdisciplinary team is a group of persons who are trained in the use of different tools and concepts, among whom there is an organized division of labor around a common problem, with each member using its own tools, with continuous intercommunication and re-examination of postulates in terms of the limitations provided by the work of the other members, and often with group responsibility for the final product.

The phrase *different tools and concepts* in this definition indicates the first requisite to the development of an interdisciplinary team—a recognition by all the members that each of the disciplines brings to the group knowledge and skills that are essential for the work at hand and that cannot be provided by any of the other disciplines represented. Such recognition enables the members to determine which team member is best fitted to assume leadership in making each of the decisions and in implementing each decision. Without such an understanding, attempts at collaboration are likely to result in one of two outcomes: either to be stillborn because "one profession [carries] out assigned tasks which may or may not lead to professional understanding of the essential differences which are inherent in two professions" (1) or to suffer an early death in a struggle for power.

As has been pointed out, the first of these outcomes is by no means unusual in a physician–nurse relationship. In the particular situation of a psychiatric integration project in which a psychiatrist is included on the team, it might well occur if the psychiatrist does not recognize psychiatric nursing as a specialty, but instead sees the role of the nurse in the psychiatric setting as primarily that of the provider of physical nursing care. The psychiatrist with such a viewpoint would tend to equate the abilities of the psychiatric nurse with those of the other nurse faculty members, in which case he would be unable to see how she could make a special contribution to the psychiatric integration project.

Such a problem did not arise in the Skidmore project. True, the psychiatrist's most recent experience in working with nurses had been as a resident in psychiatry some twenty years before, at which time the role of the nurse in the psychiatric setting was to a considerable degree limited to the custodial aspects of nursing care, such as the giving of medications and the administration of such "quieting" measures as hydrotherapy, restraint, and seclusion. However, he was aware that something new and different was going on in psychiatric nursing, and he had some vague ideas about the expanding role of the psychiatric nurse. Because of his readiness to accept psychiatric nursing as a specialty, plus the psychiatric nurse's ability to demonstrate her specialized skills, there was no question as far as the two members of the psychiatric team were concerned about the uniqueness and essentiality of the psychiatric nurse's contribution.

The second outcome of insufficient role differentiation—that of a struggle for power—is most likely to occur if the nurse member of the team is one who believes that the psychiatric nurse's role includes practicing individual and group psychotherapy in the same way and with the same goals as the psychiatrist. Among such nurses, verbal communication is perceived as the nurse's most important tool, and physical nursing care, as well as the nurse's participation in all the other activities involved in day-to-day living, is spurned as a crutch of unenlightened psychiatric nurses. It might be surmised that the nurse who subscribes to this viewpoint does not, to her way of thinking at least, need a psychiatrist on her team, and if she were to find herself on a team with one would be likely to compete in what she regards as a commonly held domain.

This viewpoint was not—and is not—held by the psychiatric nurse in the Skidmore project. Her concept of the psychiatric nurse's role with individual patients and groups of patients evolved from three frameworks (11): first, the traditional role and functions of the nurse in giving bedside and physical nursing care; second, the role of the public health nurse in giving bedside care, providing health teaching, and giving health supervision to patients and their families within the home setting; and third, the role of the "therapeutic assistant" or "helper" with psychiatric patients in the community, as described by Silvano Arieti (2) and Paul Federn (6).

The premise of her perception of the role and functions of the psychiatric nurse is that no one treatment modality in and of itself is superior to another in terms of therapeutic relevance; instead, all aspects of the total treatment program must interact in a way that will add up to more positives than any single aspect. When this happens, a therapeutic milieu is created, and it is this kind of setting rather than any one aspect of the treatment program that helps the patient to move toward recovery. Were this not so, the patient could receive individual and group psychotherapy on an outpatient basis and would not have to be admitted to the hospital in the first place.

Second, the nurse has a unique role in the creation of this therapeutic milieu because in relating to patients she has at her disposal the daily activities of the patient's living—bathing, dressing, eating, playing, sleeping, toileting—which, because they are primitive and close to the fundamental processes of living, may, as Weber has stated, "be more meaningful and therapeutic than the verbalizations of the psychotherapist. In our development, movement, touch, sight, and smell have meaning and convey reassurance long before words do" (13).

This recognition of the unique aspects of psychiatric nursing enabled the psychiatric nurse in the Skidmore project to see that she could bring something to the psychiatric integration project that could not be supplied by the members of any other discipline—a knowledge of how psychiatric concepts can be utilized in everyday nursing care activities. Secure in this recognition of her own specialized contribution, she had no need to deny the psychiatrist's unique contribution: an extensive knowledge of different aspects of human functioning—physiological and psychological—and a specialized knowledge of group and individual psychodynamics, and the influence of unconscious motivational factors. She recognized that because of his intimate and long-term contact with many patients and his diagnostic ability, he was in a better position than she was to understand and link behavioral patterns to psychodynamic formulations (13). In other words, just as the instructor in medical nursing relies on the physician for the diagnosis of an organic disease, so the psychiatric nurse relied on the psychiatrist for the diagnosis of an emotional disorder and the interpretation of the accompanying behavior.

This perception of the boundaries between the roles of the psychiatric nurse and the psychiatrist did not, of course, result in an immediate identification of the ways in which the psychiatric team's organized division of labor should be accomplished. Rather, it served as a framework for the differentiation of their functions, which was an important phase of the process through which they eventually achieved a collaborative relationship.

COMPATIBILITY IN ORIENTATION

The Skidmore psychiatric team also possessed the second important prerequisite to the development of a collaborative relationship—compatibility in philosophical and theoretical orientation. Neither the psychiatric nurse nor the psychiatrist had a strong vested interest in a highly developed theoretical structure and conceptual system, and both had a solid orientation toward the interpersonal concepts of psychiatry and some acquaintance with the interactional concepts of sociology. Consequently, throughout the project they were generally in agreement regarding an overall theory of behavior and the definition of such concepts as anxiety, frustration-aggression, conflict, role, communication, and illness. In the approach to psychiatry, neither one was exclusively concerned with psychopathology, and they both tended to emphasize self-concept, cultural variables, environmental factors, participant-observation, interpersonal processes, and communication. Moreover, their interest in and motivations for working in the area of applying psychiatric concepts to the care of medical, surgical, and pediatric patients in the hospital and home were similar.

A second factor that influenced their behavior as a team was their common philosophy of education and learning. They both believed that the goal of education is the liberation of rational faculties and that the basis for rational behavior is understanding. They did not assume that knowledge is the same as understanding; rather, they viewed knowledge as did Aldous Huxley when he said, "Some of it is correct knowledge, some of it is incorrect knowledge, and some of it only looks like knowledge, and is neither correct nor incorrect; it is merely meaningless" (7).

Lastly, the psychiatric nurse and the psychiatrist agreed for the most part in their overall approach to people and in their attitudes toward living and the world at large. Because of these agreements in fundamental matters, neither team member ever felt that he was compromising himself and was therefore never in the position of wanting to subtly sabotage the integration program.

Congeniality of Temperament

As Clyde Kluckhohn has pointed out, interdisciplinary research is above all an interpersonal situation, and the smoothness and strains must be analyzed in terms of the individual personalities as well as the structure of the situation (8). It is therefore important, if not essential, for the members of a team to be personally congenial.

That such congeniality does not depend on similarity of temperament was demonstrated by the personally pleasant working relationship that developed between the psychiatric nurse and the psychiatrist in the Skidmore integration project. The psychiatric nurse was inclined to plunge into a problem in an attempt to get things accomplished, thus delaying her evaluation until her action was completed. The psychiatrist tended to proceed with much more caution and to size up the situation before taking action. The psychiatric nurse acted as a catalyst to get the psychiatrist moving when he seemed to be holding back unduly, whereas the psychiatrist functioned as a positive restraining force in slowing down the psychiatric nurse. Thus, the fact that their approaches were complementary was beneficial to the project.

Selection of the Team

As has been previously stated, because of the difficulty of securing a psychiatric nurse who was qualified to direct the Skidmore project, the Skidmore faculty had employed the psychiatrist before the psychiatric nurse. Understandable as this action was, in the circumstances, the psychiatric nurse and the psychiatrist did not have the opportunity to learn about each other's background before employment or to judge whether they could work as a team. That the psychiatric nurse and the psychiatrist had a similar orientation and the personality factors necessary for effective collaboration was purely happenstance. Disharmony might easily have been the result. There is no such thing as "shotgun collaboration" (3).

It must be admitted, however, that judging from her initial reaction to the idea of working with a psychiatrist, the psychiatric nurse might not have sought help from one or, if she had done so, she might have asked for it on a consultative basis. As has been pointed out, no great need for the continuing services of a psychiatrist was immediately apparent to her; yet it was because a psychiatrist was on the team that the project assumed the shape that it did, thereby making his services indispensable. And let it here be said that despite her original ambivalence, the psychiatric nurse found that the psychiatrist's presence on the team immeasurably enriched not only the project but her own experience in it. Were she to direct another such project, she would recommend an interdisciplinary approach.

The fact remains that in future projects of this kind some procedure for employing personnel should be worked out whereby the risk of an incompatible group would be reduced. One solution might be for the faculty of the educational program in question to decide, on the basis of its evaluation of the situation, whether it wishes a unidisciplinary or an interdisciplinary approach. Both the decision and the reasons for it would be made known to the person being considered for the position of project director; in the event of his disagreement, he would state his reasons and rebut those of the faculty. The faculty would then re-evaluate the situation and come to a final decision—as would the prospective project director. If the decision were for an interdisciplinary team, the person employed as project director would have a voice in the selection of the other members of the team.

This method has particular relevance for psychiatric integration projects. Its application would not only be reasonably likely to result in a real team, but would have the virtue of allaying the psychiatric nurse's concern about whether another specialist was being brought in to "bring her up to mark." She would know that the faculty wanted a team, regardless of what psychiatric nurse was to head it, and her participation in the selection of the members would be a symbol of the faculty's trust in her judgment.

The Process of Collaboration

Although the psychiatric nurse and the psychiatrist came to the Skidmore integration project with the prerequisites for collaboration, they had to work out and worry through many problems before they became organized into a team. They had to establish effective communications. They had to evaluate their respective abilities and, in the light of this evaluation, to further refine their roles in each of the project activities. Finally, they had to learn to orchestrate their efforts sometimes at the cost of foregoing a solo display of virtuosity, so that in every situation they would be working in concert. Moreover, they had to solve these team-centered problems while they were working with other people whose reactions to each of them could not help but affect their relationships with each other.

This impact from other than team members was particularly pronounced in the activities in which the faculty as a group was engaged. The fact that for a considerable period of time the other faculty members were reluctant to acknowledge any difference between their status and that of the psychiatric nurse, whereas they accorded the psychiatrist leadership status, made it difficult for the psychiatric nurse and the psychiatrist to establish a balanced relationship between themselves—one in which the leadership of the team would not be static but would shift from one to the other in accordance with their relative qualifications for dealing with the problem at hand. That this attitude on the part of faculty members was able to make such an impact on the relationship between the psychiatric nurse and the psychiatrist was because of the psychiatric nurse's own uncertainty about her appropriate role when working with the faculty as a whole.

The boundary lines between psychiatry and psychiatric nursing (at least according to her concept of psychiatric nursing) furnished sufficient guidance for the psychiatric nurse to distinguish her role from that of the psychiatrist in those activities involving the students and the individual instructors. In the conferences with individual students the psychiatrist had the physician's role of evaluation and diagnosis, and she had the psychiatric nurse's role of supporting the students, identifying their problems, and referring them, if necessary, to the psychiatrist or to other faculty members. In the work with groups of students and with individual faculty members, the psychiatrist was the scientist—the parent source of psychiatric content. It was the responsibility of the psychiatric nurse to reformulate the psychiatric concepts within the context of nursing and to help the students and the instructors to apply them in their nursing and teaching practice.

When it came to working with the faculty as a group, however, the psychiatric nurse was less certain about her role and that of the psychiatrist and the way in which their roles differed. It was within the framework of the team's activities with the faculty group, therefore, that the process of collaboration largely took place. For this reason this context has been selected for tracing the various steps of the process. Because this subjective account is being written by the psychiatric nurse, the process will be described in terms of her movement in the direction of a collaborative relationship.

Like the progress of the faculty members toward synthesis, the journey of the psychiatric nurse toward a collaborative relationship with the psychiatrist was marked by three stages. These might be described as the stage of independency, the stage of dependency, and the stage of interdependency. It took three years for the psychiatric nurse to reach the destination of interdependency.

STAGE OF INDEPENDENCY: PERIOD OF COMPETITION

At the beginning of the project, because of the psychiatric nurse's disappointment about being expected to collaborate with the psychiatrist, plus her professional insecurity in the unexplored territory of psychiatric integration and her uncertainty about her role in the project, she set out to prove to herself that she was perfectly capable of functioning on her own, without the psychiatrist. In her desire for autonomy she attempted to avoid working with the psychiatrist. He was not involved with the faculty in its regular activities and was therefore not aware of the problems associated with these activities except as she reported them to him. In her need to feel powerful in a situation in which she felt rejected and not in control, the psychiatric nurse withheld from him such information as the faculty's dismissal of her suggestions for improving certain aspects of the curriculum.

However, her show of independence and her withdrawal also served as a mask for her desire to lean on the psychiatrist. In her belief that he could redeem her from the rest of the faculty, she began to bring to him her problems in relation to the total faculty. In other words, the psychiatric nurse's attitude was a double-edged one—"I'll do this all by myself even if it kills me, but it won't kill me because the psychiatrist is going to save me." Like the other faculty members, the psychiatric nurse tended to overevaluate the power of the psychiatrist and to underestimate her own.

During the first year the psychiatric nurse frequently felt that the psychiatrist was uninterested, unmotivated, and generally not very helpful to her. There were times when, although he had been alerted by her to some of her problems, he acted as if they did not exist. Often he did not become actively involved in an issue until it had reached proportions that were serious enough to jeopardize the life of the project. On these occasions he often reacted as if he had not heard about the problem before. The first year, therefore, took on the quality of a perpetual emergency, in which the psychiatric nurse kept alerting the psychiatrist to the existence of a fire and even pointing out the smoke to him and he tended to respond only when he heard the screech of the fire engine sirens.

It is possible that to a certain extent at least, the psychiatrist's unwillingness to risk the smoke of the conflagration was a refusal to respond to the psychiatric nurse's feelings of helplessness and her bid to hide behind him. A large part of his resistance to becoming involved in intrafaculty problems, however, might well be attributed to his expectations; when he first joined the project, he perceived his task as principally one of orienting students to the emotional aspects of illness and envisioned his role as almost entirely that of teacher.

His background may also have played a part in his hestitancy to deal with the problems of the faculty as a group. Because of his psychoanalytic orientation, he was accustomed to dealing with problems on an individual rather than a group basis. Because he had never taught in a nursing program or in any undergraduate program, he was less aware than was the psychiatric nurse of the strength of the nurse teacher's influence on the young nursing student and of the close correlation between the teacher's feeling of security among her colleagues and an effective student program. Moreover, as a member of a profession which seldom has to accept a subordinate place in any organization, he was less aware than was the psychiatric nurse of the obstacles to individual security that can be imposed by a hierarchal structure. Finally, his involvement with the Skidmore faculty had been by no means as extensive or intensive as that of the psychiatric nurse, who had been participating in the regular faculty activities, so he was not as cognizant as she was of the manifold obstructions to intrafaculty communication.

The full import of these differences in the team members' background had not been recognized at the beginning of the project, nor could they have been until the psychiatric nurse had had an opportunity to become oriented to the situation and realized that the program called for more than a teaching approach. During the first year, however, it became apparent that the differences had implications for a further role differentiation— because of them the psychiatric nurse was better qualified than was the psychiatrist to assume leadership in certain areas of problem identification. On the other hand, the psychiatric nurse recognized her need for the psychiatrist's help in approaching the problem of intrafaculty relationships— thus her feeling of dependency.

It should be pointed out, however, that had a collaborative relationship existed between the psychiatric nurse and the psychiatrist at this time, the two could have worked out the approach to the intrafaculty problems and their separate roles in working with the faculty, and it would have been seen that each team member needed the other in this work. In other words, had the two been operating as a team, the psychiatric nurse's need for the psychiatrist's help would have been linked to an interdependent, rather than a dependent, relationship.

STAGE OF DEPENDENCY

The first real step in the collaborative process was taken at the end of the first year when, at the suggestion of the psychiatrist, the psychiatric nurse and the psychiatrist worked together in drawing up and presenting to the total faculty a blueprint for the integration project. During the preparation of this blueprint, the psychiatric nurse assumed her appropriate role as leader in the task of problem identification, thereby demonstrating progress in the refinement of roles. Also, because the plan called for an expansion of the scope of the project to include a participant observational study in which the psychiatrist's contribution would be essential, the psychiatric nurse, in proposing the study, was in essence declaring her willingness to relinquish autonomy in favor of a collaborative relationship.

Unfortunately, the collaboration had not reached the point where the two members could plan their appropriate roles in the presentation of the blueprint to the faculty. Had they done so, the psychiatric nurse might have conceded that in the best interests of the project the psychiatrist should make this presentation. Instead, the presentation was made by both of them, with results that might have been predicted—each time a suggestion was offered by the psychiatric nurse it was rejected, only to be accepted when recommended by the psychiatrist. The faculty members had invested the psychiatrist with superior status and authority, and the status factor was effective in "selling" them the program.

Not only should the psychiatric nurse have been prepared for this behavior, but she should have been willing to face the reality that she and the psychiatrist did not enjoy equal prestige. As Caudill and Roberts have pointed out, the psychiatrist is generally cast in a superior position by society and has a higher wage scale and standard of living than do the members of other disciplines (4). Certainly this distinction holds in any comparison of psychiatrists and psychiatric nurses.

The psychiatric nurse might further have realized that her situation was by no means an uncommon one; it is rare for a group of people to enter a team with equal status, particularly when they represent different disciplines. However, such status differences in the eyes of society or even the other people with whom a team may be working (in this case, the faculty members) need not pertain in the team members' relationships with each other. If at the outset of an interdisciplinary project the members of the lower-status disciplines can face their situation as one of the inevitable facts of life, instead of perceiving it as an injustice of which they are the victims, more possibilities for effective collaboration are opened up.

Although the psychiatric nurse might have been invested with this wisdom at the beginning of the project (as it is hoped the psychiatric nurses who read of her experiences will be), she had not acquired it at this point in the integration project. Nor had she integrated her individual goals into the goals of the team to the extent that she was happy that someone on the team—and therefore the team—had been successful in getting the blueprint adopted. All that she could see was that an activity that had been conceived by her and that was to be carried on in a program of which she was titularly the director had been accepted primarily because of the psychiatrist's efforts. To make the pill more bitter, this apparent rejection of her leadership was caused by a status prejudice on the part of members of her own profession.

The psychiatric nurse was likely to react to this situation in one of two ways. As lower-status personnel sometimes do, she might have attempted to decrease the distance between the two disciplines of psychiatric nursing and psychiatry by encroaching on the traditional role and functions of the psychiatrist, thus slipping into the role of psychotherapist. Instead of circumventing her confusion and anxiety in this way, however, she chose another path—that of withdrawal. She handed over what she considered the most important part of the integration project—the faculty discussions—to the psychiatrist. Her response to his bid to be included in the project, which at first had been a positive one, was in effect changed to, "Here, you can have the project. It belongs to you anyway."

However, the blueprint incident resulted in one permanent step in the direction of psychiatric nurse, psychiatrist teamship. While the psychiatric nurse and the psychiatrist were working on the blueprint, their interpersonal relations improved and progressed to a high level, which was maintained throughout the project. The basis of this positive relationship was mutual respect, strong motivatioin, a feeling of comfort about the differences between their contributions, and an eagerness to learn from each other. Beginning in the second year, they maintained regular personal contact, and these increased as the project progressed.

Nevertheless, the psychiatric nurse was unable to carry over this feeling of being on equal terms with the psychiatrist from the intrateam situation to the faculty meetings. During the second and third years, she hid behind the psychiatrist. She also was dependent on the support of faculty members and saw them as hindering all effective action. In her dependency and sense of helplessness about initiating action and creating a climate for change, two major currents had reached their confluence—her need for approval and fear of disapproval, and her awareness that because the faculty members perceived her and reacted to her autistically as a symbol of change, she was a potential scapegoat on whom they might displace all of their pent-up hostility.

As the data from the faculty meetings reveal, during the second year and until the spring of the third year, the psychiatric nurse seldom showed initiative in directing the faculty discussions. Withdrawal from the faculty had become her *modus operandi*; it was a way of running away from the situation when it was her job to lead. This withdrawal, however, was not synonymous with lack of participation. Rather, it was a particular kind of participation. The psychiatric nurse was much more reactive to what was happening than was the psychiatrist, who tended to remain detached, probably because he had no opportunities to become involved with the faculty members as a group other than in the faculty discussions.

Apparently the psychiatric nurse's withdrawal only aggravated the faculty members' frustration. It also aroused the psychiatric nurse's feelings of guilt for abandoning her responsibility to the faculty. These guilt feelings seemed to slake her thoughts about how she might interrupt her withdrawal and get closer to the faculty.

The psychiatric nurse then resorted to seduction, which was based on the erroneous assumption that she was entirely at fault. She spent much of her effort in expiating her guilt by being a "nice gal" and by behaving like one of those diplomats who specializes in being cooperative and in making mollifying summaries of what has been said. She recognized that she was indulging in this behavior but tried to justify it on the grounds that according to her definition of the situation, the psychiatrist seemed to be seducing the faculty members into a patient-analyst relationship.

Both the psychiatric nurse and the psychiatrist fell into the trap of dictation, which as Herbert Thelen has pointed out, occurs when a leader becomes hostile and blames the group members for not measuring up to his expectations (12). This dictation was most apparent in the areas of selecting the topics for discussion, structuring the discussions, and making decisions. Some of the faculty members reacted to the psychiatrist's and the psychiatric nurse's dictatorial approach by scapegoating the psychiatric nurse and by trying to sabotage her group discussions with students.

Even though the psychiatric nurse bought the partnership with the psychiatrist at the price of concession to the other faculty members and the assumption of the servant role with them, she did not stave off the disorganization of the faculty group which occurred in the third year. As a matter of fact, one reason for the disorganization may have been the psychiatric nurse's retreat from the situation.

During this entire period of the psychiatric nurse's dependency, the psychiatrist continued to draw her in on discussions, give her recognition as a team member, and refer to her contributions in the group meetings. Never once did he confront her with her withdrawal from the faculty group. Only after his individual faculty interviews did he become aware of the degree to which the psychiatric nurse had estranged herself from the rest of the faculty.

Stage of Interdependency: Period of Collaboration

During the period when the psychiatric nurse had withdrawn from the faculty discussions, her interest and participation in the other activities of the integration project had not abated; if anything, the effort that she put into them increased. This investment led her to re-enter the faculty discussions and thus to resume her journey toward collaboration with the psychiatrist.

The event that precipitated this re-entry occurred in a faculty meeting in April of the third year, when several of the younger faculty members made a concerted effort to sabotage the unstructured conferences which the psychiatric nurse had been holding with groups of students. Because the psychiatrist had not been participating in these conferences, the psychiatric nurse realized that she could not look to him to defend them. Moreover, the conferences could not be saved through compromise. If she decided the conferences were worth fighting for, she must abandon all her tactics of dependency and rely on her own resources to save them.

Her decision was in the affirmative. She marshalled the strength that during the period of her withdrawal she had been gaining from self-knowledge and reflection and left no doubt in the faculty members' minds that she would not permit the destruction of the student conferences. For the first time in a long while the faculty members were given an opportunity to experience the psychiatric nurse on a human and personal level.

The second event that marked the psychiatric nurse's reinvolvement in the faculty meetings occurred when, in one of these meetings, she directly confronted the faculty members with her feelings about her relationship with them. Again, she did not look to the psychiatrist for succor, but saw the incident through on her own. The period of dependency was over.

In abandoning dependency, the psychiatric nurse did not retrace the road between dependency and independency, but headed in the direction of inter-dependency. She recognized that the psychiatrist's role in the work with the faculty as a group was an essential one; she must look to him for help in understanding the psychodynamic operations in the intrafaculty relation-ships, including those in her own interactions. At the same time, she was beginning to distinguish her unique role and recognize it as essential. Because of her close association with the faculty members in all their professional activities and her consequent knowledge about the ongoing issues and problems confronting them and the students, she was better equipped than the psychiatrist to draw from the faculty members their characteristic responses and distortions.

From this recognition of her place in the faculty discussions, the psychi-atric nurse proceeded to a realization of another role that she should assume in the faculty group—that of a bridge between the power group and the rest of the faculty. As an objective participant-observer who was not identified with any group, she was able to keep her finger on the pulse of the depart-ment of nursing and was therefore an appropriate representative of objec-tive reality with whom those with administrative power could test out their ideas and plans for action before presenting them to the total faculty. Thus she was in a position to intervene and to apply alternative methods when a proposed or tentatively introduced method seemed fated to miscarry. An illustration of such intervention was her initiation of conferences with the individual faculty members during the crisis concerning the new curriculum.

Secure in her role, the psychiatric nurse no longer felt the need to compete with the psychiatrist, but instead wanted to see him make the full use of his abilities. This attitude led her to an even greater awareness of the psychia-trist's potential contribution to the project, but her evaluation was based on his real abilities rather than on the imaginary powers with which she had first endowed him. She saw that he had limitations as well as strengths and realized that both must be taken into account in the further development of the integration program.

The arrangements for the conferences between the psychiatrist and the individual faculty members might be offered as a case in point. It was important that the psychiatrist should move from his position of outsider in the faculty discussions and his pinnacle of omniscient and omnipotent authority and be absorbed into the circle on a first-name basis. However, the faculty members were apparently unable to experience him as a person in the group meetings. His psychoanalytic orientation, so valuable to the project in many ways, was in this respect a limitation, because of its emphasis on one-to-one relationships. Thus, the need for conferences in which each faculty member could experience an individual relationship with him. In enthusiastically agreeing to these conferences as a way in which another team member—not herself—could make maximum use of his abilities, the psychiatric nurse arrived at real collaboration. The psychiatrist, in turn, underscored the fact that the conferences constituted a team enterprise when he made it clear that he would share with the psychiatric nurse the aspects of the conferences that were pertinent to her. The discussion between the psychiatrist and the psychiatric nurse that followed these conferences symbolized their fusion into a team.

By the end of the third year, when the psychiatric nurse and the psychiatrist had established a sound collaborative relationship, the role of leader in the faculty meetings associated with the integration project and the degree of status that was accorded to each of the team members shifted in relation to the nature of the particular problem under discussion. When the psychiatric nurse had more of the knowledge and skills required for approaching a problem than did the psychiatrist, she became the leader and was ascribed higher status by the faculty. Similarly, the psychiatrist was the leader when his special abilities were the ones that were most needed. During the last two years of the project, the faculty members were quite aware of the separate roles of the psychiatric nurse and the psychiatrist and of their role as a team. The wide gap which they once saw between the degree of authority and influence of the psychiatrist and that of the psychiatric nurse was closed.

The collaborative relationship between the psychiatric nurse and the psychiatrist, like any other relationship, did not represent a static condition, but continued to develop after teamship had been reached. The well-spring for their deepening relationship was their interest in a common problem. Understandably, the psychiatric nurse had come to the project more highly motivated than the psychiatrist. As the project progressed, however, the motivation of each increased. Each served as a catalyst for the other.

During the fourth and fifth years of the project, they had weekly conferences during which they discussed their observations and analyzed them from the standpoint of psychiatry and nursing. They discovered that in many situations in their work with faculty members and students they used a common pool of knowledge to understand the group dynamics, resistances, and reactions. They worked well together because they tended to describe interpersonal relations in terms of observable behavior and, in communicating their observations, to use the same operational yardsticks.

In these meetings there was a constant interchange between the roles of teacher and student. Each was eager to learn from the other. The psychiatrist, among many things, taught the psychiatric nurse how to recognize masked aggression and to understand some of the dynamics underlying scapegoating. He also helped her to become more sensitive to the consequences of her individual interviews with faculty members and students. On other occasions, he became the student as the psychiatric nurse oriented him to the concept of the professional nurse's role, the areas of conflict, confusion, and controversy in carrying out the nursing role, and the role of faculty in the integrative process. In crossing the borders of their own discipline, the psychiatrist and the psychiatric nurse discovered something new. This new understanding, however, did not mean loss of professional identity.

As in all significant relationships, the learning derived from this one did not end when the team disbanded—at least insofar as the psychiatric nurse is concerned. For example, at the time the collaborative work was going on, the psychiatric nurse found it difficult to understand why, at times, the psychiatrist handled his feelings of disappointment, discouragement, and frustration with the integration program by becoming angry and impatient with her, only to enter a faculty meeting and be warm, supportive, and understanding. The psychiatric nurse had unrealistically expected their teamwork to be a one-way street for pouring out troubles—her troubles. Such would be the case in psychotherapy, but not in a genuine collaborative endeavor. It did not then occur to her that the psychiatrist's ability and willingness to unload his concerns about the integration program on her was a prerequisite to his productive functioning with the faculty. Like so many other insights, this one came only with the writing of this book.

REFERENCES

1. Allen, Frederick H. "Psychiatry and Social Work in Cooperation," *American Journal of Psychiatry,* **104,** 554–557 (March, 1948).

2. Arieti, Silvano. *Interpretation of Schizophrenia.* New York: Robert Brunner, 1955, pp. 468–471.

3. Bush, Vannevar. "Professional Collaboration," *Science,* **125,** 49–54 (January, 1957).

4. Caudill, William, and Bertram Roberts. "Pitfalls in the Organization of Interdiscplinary Research," *Human Organization,* **10** (12) 15 (Winter, 1951).

5. Eaton, Joseph W. "Social Processes of Professional Teamwork," *American Sociological Review,* **16** (707) 13 (October, 1951).

6. Federn, Paul. "Psychoanalysis of Psychosis, 1. Errors and How to Avoid Them, II. Transference," *Psychiatric Quarterly,* **17** (3), 246 (1943).

7. Huxley, Aldous. "Knowledge and Understanding," *Collected Essays*. New York: Harper & Row, 1958, p. 379.

8. Kluckhohn, Clyde. "An Anthropologist Looks at Psychology," *American Psychologist*, **3**, 439–442 (October, 1948).

9. Luszki, Margaret Barron. *Interdisciplinary Team Research: Methods and Problems*. New York: New York University Press, 1958, pp. 10, 11.

10. Mann, Floyd C. "Human Relations Skills in Social Research," *Human Relations*, 341–354 (April 1951).

11. Schmahl, Jane A. "The Psychiatric Nurse and Psychotherapy," *Nursing Outlook* (July, 1962), 460–465.

12. Thelen, Herbert. *The Dynamics of Groups at Work*. Chicago: University of Chicago Press, 1954, p. 319.

13. Weber, William F. "An Educational Experience for Psychiatric Nurses in the Use of Self and the Awareness of Interpersonal Processes," unpublished paper, p. 6 (November, 1963).

PART III

CHANGE
AND
GROWTH

Chapter Fourteen

THE COLLEAGUE'S PERSPECTIVE

By Montague Ullman, M.D.

Consultant in Psychiatry and Mental Health, Skidmore College, Department of Nursing, New York City, Director of Psychiatric Services, Maimonides Hospital of Brooklyn, and Professor of Psychiatry, State University of New York, Downtown Medical Center.

The essence of my contribution to the psychiatric integration program comes through in the pages of this book. In adding a commentary to the felicitous account rendered by the author I have two points in mind. First, writing this chapter provides me with the opportunity to add my own perspective * to the events described in the preceding pages. Second, I should like to offer several suggestions for future integrative efforts based on what I believe were limitations, omissions, and errors in our own approach. The good will endure by its own merit.

From the vantage point of eight years after the start of the project, the events of the earlier years sometimes assume different proportions, even startlingly different ones. In the beginning, at least from a theoretical standpoint, the concept of psychiatric integration seemed straightforward enough. From a practical viewpoint the psychiatric nurse and I were both in complete agreement about an experiential approach to the problem. Life, being full of surprises, held some for us too. I think we were far from any accurate awareness of the true dimensions of the task we had set ourselves and of the dialectical growth process as we were to experience it later.

I would like to say a word about my own starting position as of eight years ago. It contained the paradoxical elements of sophistication and

* Although I use the collective pronouns "we" and "our" throughout, the evaluative statements are purely my own.

naiveté, the sophistication derived from many years of teaching psychiatry at a resident physician and medical student level and the naiveté from a profound ignorance of all matters pertaining to nursing and nursing education. The cross-currents and complexities of the current scene in psychiatric integration in nursing education were not known to me until I was well along in the project. In some ways this may have been an advantage. I simply assumed our approach was the most natural one and the one most generally followed.

There were a number of minor integrative goals that had to be achieved before the major task of integration could be tackled. As I worked alone during the initial months of the project, the first question to be resolved concerned my own response to finding myself an integral part of a busy program in nursing education. In other teaching situations in which I had participated, psychiatry was at the hub of things, or close to it. The relationship between what I had taught and the needs of patients was immediately visible. The role of integration in nursing education differed in at least two respects. First, there was the task of discovering the proper place for psychiatric concepts in the total scheme of things. Second, one had to learn how most effectively to bring together the psychiatric concept, the nurse teacher, and the situation. The immediate awareness of the great need for the introduction of these concepts into nursing education and practice and the readiness of the faculty to move in this direction were instrumental in resolving whatever qualms I had initially about moving into unfamiliar territory.

The second integrative effect that had to come about concerned the working relationship that developed between the psychiatric nurse and myself. Here, as already noted by the author, there was a fortunate dovetailing of theoretical orientation and a certain complementarity of style. We early and rather easily developed a freewheeling and flexible exchange of leadership role and resource person role, so that a certain fluidity of approach characterized our joint participation in many varied situations. The psychiatric nurse, by virtue of her background in nursing education and psychiatric nursing and her day-to-day contact with faculty members and students, generally made the first inroads both with faculty members and with students in eliciting and sifting the experiences around which the discussion became organized. My own contribution focused more on the task of distilling from the shared experience the relevant concepts which, if they had been clearly grasped, would have made the initial experience less problematic.

The commonality of our theoretical orientation was fortified by another fairly important factor, which has also been touched on by the author, that is, the different levels of intensity that characterized our individual relationships to the project. Because I was on the job part-time and was involved in many other arenas of activity, my relationship to the integration project was less exclusive and less consuming than that of the psychiatric nurse. Hence, I had the distinct advantage of being able to view certain events from a greater distance and, I hope, at times with more perspective.

The freedom of communication and lack of role conflict between the psychiatric nurse and myself made for a workable approach to the problems of individual students. In evaluating the students' behavior, meeting their counseling needs, and at times smoothing the transition to individual psychotherapy, we were able to coordinate our efforts.

Here, then, were the two preconditions for my own participation—the existence of a real need and the availability of a colleague who was familiar with the terrain to be traversed because of her previous experience as a psychiatric nurse and a nursing educator.

It is a difficult proposition to scan the intervening years and to evaluate change, especially when one is so close to the scene one is judging. The task becomes doubly difficult as soon as one attempts to separate the change that may have come about merely from the fact that a psychiatric team was available from the change brought about because we were able to impart to the faculty members, in our role as integrators, a sufficiently broad grasp of those strategic psychiatric concepts that would insure growth and change in themselves and in their students. Perhaps this is not merely difficult but impossible.

In practice, our impact was achieved in many different ways which related to the many different things we attempted to do. We sought to relieve intrafaculty tensions by a direct examination of the intrafaculty communication process. We tried to identify key psychiatric concepts and to explore their relevance to everyday teaching experiences. We were there to analyze and clarify specific problems arising in the day-to-day work. In sum, we gave advice and counsel, when sought, on administrative, educational, and medical problems in addition to carrying out the activities directly associated with our avowed aims and goals.

The fulcrum of our approach was, of course, the experiential techniques we employed. I think we were aware at the start, and later more explicitly so, of the problem of setting up the parameters for experiential learning while avoiding the misuse of group psychotherapeutic techniques. Except for one or two situations in which things almost got out of hand, I think that we succeeded in not traversing into group psychotherapy. The actual measure of success was closely related to the degree to which each faculty member was capable of participating spontaneously, or could be induced to participate in, the sharing of a felt reconstruction of a significant problematic event relating to her professional experience.

About half of the faculty members appeared to be ready to do this from the very beginning. By virtue of their own stable orientation to new experience they were prepared to relate realistically to what we were trying to do. This was the group that was able to see the identity of what we were doing with other forms of learning. They were the least encumbered by transferential phenomena, factional diversions, and irrelevant preoccupations with status, group acceptance, and other issues that lead into cumbersome defensiveness rather than straightforward relatedness to an issue. In a few instances this kind of orientation, although not present initially, came about at a late point, generally following a successful personal experience with the psychiatric team.

Two other reactions prevailed among the other members of the faculty. In the first of these reactions positive motivations were present but were contaminated by defensive maneuvers triggered by the circumstances of actual participation. In the case of some younger faculty members, for example, the opportunity to work with the psychiatric team was complicated by the necessity to do so under conditions, such as the faculty discussions, which exposed unresolved feelings toward authority and the use of authority. Here we witnessed on the surface much lip service to the integration program, occasional meaningful forays into participation, retreat into dissension and dissatisfaction, and renewed explorations.

It was in relation to the faculty discussions that the male-female, doctor-nurse dichotomy of the psychiatric team offered the most trouble. The psychiatric nurse, in contrast to myself, posed a threat to the instructor's own recently acquired and zealously guarded specialty status as a nurse teacher. Whereas the members of the psychiatric team tended to function in a unitary fashion rather than on a status or hierarchical basis, this group subtly tended to elicit and re-establish status lines. As is so often the case, the very things they were rebelling against were often part and parcel of their own makeup. Progress did occur with the group, although at times the course was a bit stormy. These instructors did much better in individual conferences with the psychiatric nurse or myself.

In the second group the connection with the integration program was so tangential to begin with that there was either little interest or little opportunity to articulate meaningfully with our work. This was so either because of problems of rapid turnover, as in the case of the nurse in charge of the student health office, or because their work was somewhat apart from the mainstream of the clinical experiences, as in the case of the instructor who was responsible for integrating the principles of nutrition into the nursing courses.

What has become more apparent to me in the recent period, with time lending some perspective to our efforts, is that psychiatric integration has to encompass two types of approaches in order to accommodate to two types of growth processes. There are cerebral and there are visceral approaches to change, and each approach requires its own strategies and tactics. One of the flaws in our approach, in my opinion, was to blur the difference and apply the same techniques across the board, interpreting it as resistance when one or the other group was out of kilter.

In the cerebral approach to change, the internal core of the person is changed by slow, quantitative accretions from the outside. This remains a somewhat one-sided equation until a level is reached at which a qualitative change occurs. True interaction then occurs at a new and advanced level. The faculty members who approached change in this way were the ones who responded best to a more didactic and analytical approach.

In the visceral approach there is an attempt, gross, qualitative, and un-controlled, to move from the core out to embrace and, in fact, to incorporate the new situation. A rapid, intense, and overwhelming identification is formed, which has the virtue of immediately and meaningfully linking the two parties concerned, but also has the troublesome disadvantage of doing it almost solely on the learner's terms and at the cost of the learner losing sight of the separate and objective existence of the teacher or, as in this case, the psychiatric team. The faculty members who approached change in this way responded to every issue in terms of an implicit judgment as to whether we were with them or against them, that is, total incorporation or total ejection. Whereas in dealing with the first group we had to move in constantly to make contact with the core, with this group we were constantly enmeshed in a disengaging process in an effort to define the proper limits of effective interaction.

Being the most challenging, the members of this group were also the ones with whom we made the most mistakes. They were most in need of indi-vidual attention, and this was not always forthcoming. Too often provoca-tions (really bids for this kind of attention) were allowed to build up to explosive proportions before official notice was taken. Early in the project our abortive effort to meet separately with the older and younger faculty groups was a somewhat crude and amateurish attempt to respond to the problems between the two groups. It naturally failed as there was no explicit understanding of precisely what the problem was at that time. We inter-preted the faculty schism mainly along the lines of seeing the authority-conformity conflict as the schismatic one. The remedy based on this view was to alter the external conditions, that is, to separate the faculty physically into two groups and then to deal with the two groups separately. This did nothing to touch the heart of the issue, but did give us the feeling we were doing something. The problem was more complicated than we took it to be and involved our own shortcomings as well as those of the faculty. Our approach was so geared to the expectancy of a uniform response that it did not allow for the kind of individual variation and improvisation needed to help the lone faculty member caught up in the emotional currents we had helped to unleash but had offered insufficient help in controlling.

In the year after the author left the situation I worked with the faculty alone. During this year my own time was about equally divided between clinical seminars with the junior students and group meetings with the faculty. It has not been easy to assess the effect of the absence of the psychiatric nurse on the faculty even by direct inquiry. In my own case, my window into the issues that arose and the variations of the emotional atmosphere within the faculty was temporarily blocked, and as a result I felt at some distance from their concerns and preoccupations. This tended to have the overall effect of moving the content of these discussions closer to issues involving the students than the faculty itself. It was in this situation, in particular, that the sensitivities of the psychiatric nurse could galvanize the group into action by a well-timed comment, observation, or question, and it was in this setting that her many different roles as faculty member, intermediary between the faculty and myself, and my colleague melded into an effective unity.

In my work with the students her absence proved to be less intrusive. The residual effects of their exposure to the psychiatric nurse and the general atmosphere of acceptance of the integration program that had been created within the student body over the years made for relatively free and effective engagement with the goals and purposes of the conference without the qualms, misgivings, anxieties, and hostilities that had been mobilized on earlier occasions. The students were no longer coming to be "psyched," but to learn in an area where they themselves sensed their own needs. There was no longer the explicit need to relate what we were doing to good nursing care. Much of the ground-breaking and orienting activity was by now built into the atmosphere of the department of nursing itself and was clearly reflected in the way the individual students conducted themselves at these conferences.

Through an inquiry directed to the faculty members one year after the author of this book left the situation, much that could have been inferred concerning the absence of the psychiatric nurse became explicit. Mention was made of the fact that even though she had returned for the sixth year of the project, it was difficult to evaluate her absence because her withdrawal from the program had been gradual during the fifth year, when she was preparing this book. From time to time situations arose which were difficult for the instructors to handle because of their closeness to the problem. Here their contacts with the psychiatric nurse in the past had afforded them the opportunity to "unwind" and to get a fresh point of view. One of the more recently appointed instructors commented on the personal help the psychiatric nurse provided in learning how to combine faculty and social life "without being guilty." All were agreed that her sessions with the students provided valuable learning experiences for the instructors as well. There was general appreciation of the help that had been provided in the interpretation and management of individual student behavior. There are times in the course of the school year when a high anxiety level besets the student body as a whole; in the past a skilled inquiry into the cause provided some of the answers. One particularly difficult situation involving the separation of a student from the school might have been managed somewhat less traumatically had the psychiatric nurse's counsel been available.

On a dissenting note, mention was made of the "stirring-up" activity of the psychiatric nurse and of the belief that at times she had encouraged too great a focus on the personal preoccupations and emotional embroilments of the individual students. The feeling was expressed that more of this time and energy should have been devoted to the clinical area. "Sometimes you have to know when to let students grow up by themselves."

The experiential approach to the integration process came off well in our direct sessions with the students. There were, and are, many elements in the situation which place the students in double jeopardy. The students are subjected to considerable stress associated with their particular developmental stage. In addition, they face the stresses of an exacting, demanding, and condensed program in nursing education. There is also the problematic feature of these stresses taking place in a large metropolitan area not only away from their own homes but away from their initial adaptive successes on the college campus. One of the recurrent themes when they return to campus is their immediate awareness of their own seriousness and maturity vis-à-vis their fellow students in other programs. The leavening experience of clinical exposure has made them grow up faster than, in some instances, they themselves want to. Most of them look upon this changed state of affairs with mixed satisfaction and regret.

The fact that young nursing students are in a state of unremitting stress with their wonderful intellectual and emotional openness provided a very natural and mutually rewarding opportunity for the exploration of the interpersonal aspects of their clinical experiences. Of particular interest to me was the observation that even though the main themes were recurrent and easily identified (death and the dying patient; cancer and the seriously ill patient; the acting-out patient; sexual exhibitionism; responses of patients to handicaps and deformities; difficulties in assuming the professional role with patients, other nurses, and doctors; overinvolvement with patients; and so on), the contexts in which they occurred were always novel enough to maintain a liveliness and interest for all participants in the discussions.

The student, in the transformation she undergoes in becoming a professional nurse, is successful only to the extent that she learns what a patient is. It takes some doing to move a student from her initial concept of a patient, whatever that may be (and sometimes it is as naive as that of a handsome, unattached young male convalescing from a not-too-serious illness), to a concept of what a patient really is. From an operational standpoint a patient is the more or less helpless, more or less innocent victim of an infinite number of, for the most part, malevolent occurrences, some of which evoke suffering in kind and degree that at times approaches indescribable horror. To expect a young person whose firsthand knowledge is only that of health and of an expanding universe to see and adapt to illness and constricting horizons is somewhat like asking her to peer out at the world through prisms that turn everything upside down. That this is a task in which she, as well as the instructor, can utilize the services of a psychiatrist and a psychiatric nurse should come as no surprise. Indeed, what is surprising is how well this is often carried out in the absence of such a team.

In connection with the needs of students, I might mention one area which is sometimes glossed over and which, to be handled properly, does require the teaching services of a physician, preferably a psychiatrist. I am referring to the task of orienting students to the motivational aspects of behavior. Students need help in making the connection between the behavioral end result, the underlying pathology, and the defensive operations mobilized by the illness process. Too often the natural tendency is for the response to organize itself around the overt act without a sufficient inquiry into the factors leading up to the act. Let us take somewhat similar external acts and explore the different contexts in which they occur. All are drawn from actual occurrences and ones that are by no means infrequent. All tend to elicit sharp withdrawal or hostile responses. In each instance the nursing student finds it difficult to free herself from her built-in judgmental apparatus.

A young male patient with a medical condition exposes himself and masturbates in front of a nursing student. The student, frightened, strives compulsively and desperately to lose herself in the act of making and re-making one corner of the bed. The anxiety precludes any exploration of the meaning of the behavior in terms of the way the patient is experiencing his relationship with her at the moment and hence precludes any effective management of the behavior. The patient's behavior has to be terminated but in a way that will strengthen rather than weaken the relationship. To accomplish this the student has to look at it from the point of view of what the patient is trying to do rather than on purely moralistic grounds of "good" and "bad," as titrated against the backdrop of an abstract ethical system.

A student finds a middle-aged man lying in bed masturbating as he is about to be taken to the operating room for a serious procedure. She flees the scene in obvious distress. Some awareness of what the patient is going through at this time might have crowded out the obvious hypothesis that has formed in her mind that the patient had "blown his top" to do such a thing in an exposed situation, and made room for the more humane possibility that prior to the plunge into what might be utter and unending darkness the patient may be seeking solace in one further contact with one of life's most deeply pleasurable experiences.

Or still another experience. Following a stroke, an elderly male patient tends to exhibit himself and make lewd remarks to a nursing student. She promptly and primly reminds him of his place, of the proper order of things, and of the importance of immediately restoring himself to gentlemanly grace. That this response is more comforting to her than effective with him is obvious when his next gambit takes the form of reaching for her posterior as she walks by the bedside. What the student has failed to consider, of course, is that the patient "in his right mind" would no more have condoned such behavior than she would. Moreover, if she had undergone the same sudden and catastrophic realignment of inhibitory and excitatory processes in her cerebrum, the shoe might well have been on the other foot. This does not do away with the need to manage such behavior, but the key to effective management lies in understanding the source and not in immediately mobilizing value judgments that relate only to one's own experience and have no bearing on what the patient may be experiencing at the moment.

Somewhat in the same vein is the great need the students have for help in understanding the phenomenologic aspects of illness. What are the different dimensions in which the brain-damaged patient experiences his body? The amputee his phantom phenomena? The paraplegic? The patient with mutilating and deforming illness? How is the altered self-experience translated into behavioral terms?

Many fruitful sessions were had with students around the topic of how patients, under the pressure of the illness and the symptoms they are experiencing, use language more to express the way they feel rather than as statements to be taken literally and objectively. They may talk in terms of the terrible world situation when they are really expressing their own sense of defeat at the hands of an unknown agency in the form of illness. The patient who seems inexorably dedicated to the task of having regular bowel movements and whose verbal communications hover repeatedly close to this theme is using language in this experiential sense. He cannot be dissuaded from this insistent preoccupation by any objective measures or rational explanations. This kind of verbal communication is the result of complicated defensive internal processes whereby the patient, instead of confronting himself with the realities of the illness process and thereby rendering himself potentially helpless, turns aside from a concern with the actual pathology and engages with the enemy on a battleground of his own choosing, namely, his gastrointestinal tract, whose functioning can be controlled by the proper combination of diet and medication. No such combination is effective as long as the underlying disease process continues, but the elaborate charade protects the self-system through the omnipotence it confers on the nurses and doctors in whose power it lies to find the right combination.

I can best summarize my feelings in regard to the students as one of wonderment at how much can be learned in so short a time by so young a group. This is particularly impressive when you realize that much of the character of what is learned comes under the rubric of wisdom and perception of and sensitivity to the needs and feelings of others.

I should like to direct my final comments to a brief listing of recommendations for the future, based on my own estimate of the shortcomings in our past efforts.

1. With regard to our work with the total faculty, we took what might be called a leveling rather than a sharpening approach. We sought to make gains across the board rather than focus differentially in relation to the receptivity and response potential of the individual faculty member. Certain members of the faculty might have become much better protagonists for the integration program had they been given the opportunity. They tended to get lost in the shuffle when too much time was spent courting those with the least potential in this area. In medicine, certainly, many doctors are uninterested and unresponsive to psychiatric ideas and know-how, and I suppose one might expect the same situation to prevail in nursing.

2. Our meetings with the faculty might have been enriched by greater familiarity with and knowledge of the problems and attitudes of the individual instructors. More time spent with individual faculty members would have diluted our meetings with the faculty as far as number of meetings was concerned, but might have enabled us to set our sights more realistically and effectively for each such session. In general, there should have been a freer interplay between individual and group meetings.

3. Some of the issues we chose to focus on fanned the flames of sectionalism and furthered existing schisms. It might have been better to have minimized issues relating to the status dichotomy, because many of these were natural and unavoidable in the first place.

4. Not enough of the valuable distillate of our experiences in the clinical seminars with students and the individual instructors was brought back to the faculty as a whole. In the case of the by now famous or infamous examination question referred to in Chapter 8, our efforts to gain acceptance for this question might have proceeded more smoothly had I reported to the faculty the events in the clinical conference in which the incident described in the examination question was discussed. As it was, the tide was turned in favor of the question when the instructor who participated in the conference in which the incident occurred spoke about it in the faculty group discussions.

5. The clinical conferences could have been immeasurably enhanced had the psychiatric nurse and I had greater accessibility to the clinical material under discussion. Some progress toward this end was achieved during the latter part of the five-year period of the project. The students are far from

expert reporters, so that firsthand knowledge would have provided a more reliable starting point.

6. As the program developed there was a greater awareness that a proper approach to integration was multifaceted and complicated and that it should include various service operations (for example, seeing students in psychiatric consultation and counseling instructors in the management of problem students) as well as those that might be construed as more directly integrative. In our own instance, service operations tended to be too much in the shadow and integrative activity too self-consciously in the foreground. A more judicious acknowledgment of the importance of both would have been more realistic and more appropriate.

7. The final point to which I wish to address myself has to do with the ultimate role of the psychiatric team in the ongoing collegiate undergraduate nursing program. As originally projected, psychiatric integration was seen as a process which was localized in time, and which, if successful, would leave in its wake a faculty which could further the general aims and goals of the integration program without the presence of specialized personnel. There is a question in my mind as to whether this was a proper projection. What tends to happen is that whenever psychiatric personnel and services are available, dormant needs spring to life. My own feelings are that, although the overall aims and goals would be somewhat different and the day-to-day functioning somewhat changed, a nursing program such as the one under consideration could continue to make good use of the full-time services of a psychiatric nurse (to work in integration) and a psychiatric consultant.

The need would arise from two sources, both of which are indigenous to the program. The first relates to the very difficult task previously alluded to of orienting young people to the complexities of the illness process as this unfolds in the hospital environment and to help them face the task of relating themselves to this process at a professional level. This involves the management of their own anxieties, greater knowledge of their own defensive operations, particularly in response to the seriously ill patient, the dying patient, the handicapped patient, and the like, and exposure to the kind of learning situation that can help the students conceptualize the various ramifications of the illness process as this is experienced by the patient.

The second source is related to the first and derives from the fact that this learning process has to take place in a situation where many kinds of tensions converge upon the faculty members who are responsible for the teaching experience. To begin with, the goal is not a cut-and-dried one that has to do with imparting to the student a clearly demarcated body of knowledge. It has more to do with helping the student evolve into the kind of person the professional nurse should be. This means the constant orientation of the instructor and the student to the interactional aspects of the nurse-patient relationship. Because the teaching-learning process is influenced by the relations with nursing service personnel, with medical personnel, and with other professionals both in the hospital and community settings, there are many opportunities for tensions, misunderstandings, and problematic situations to occur.

The uncertainties and unsettled issues within the nursing profession contribute to the problems and confusions that arise from time to time. The hospital milieu is not an uncomplicated social situation either for the patient or for any of the professionals who participate in it. The services of a team consisting of a psychiatrist and a psychiatric nurse would be of help in smoothing over the rough spots that are bound to appear when a faculty group, regardless of how dedicated its members may be, takes on the challenging task of transforming, within a short time, a class of eager adolescents into responsible nurses.

In short, there are built-in trouble spots in any enlightened nursing program. It is in the nature of the trouble to call for the services of such professionals as the psychiatric nurse and the psychiatrist to help in their solution. This kind of collaboration would result in greater diffusion of, and familiarity with, psychiatric principles and concepts, in addition to furthering the general goals of psychiatric integration on a day-to-day basis. The problems would be different from those faced in the initial phases of the integration program, but they would be no less real and their alleviation would certainly be no less demanding of specialized personnel.

I do not think any statement of mine would be complete without my making explicit, as the author has done, the gratitude I feel to those members of the faculty whose foresight made the experience possible and whose courage, open-mindedness, and tolerance helped us immeasurably during those periods, particularly at the beginning, when we ourselves were very much in the dark.

Chapter Fifteen

A RETROSPECTIVE APPRAISAL
OF CHANGE AND GROWTH

It was the best of times, it was the worst of times, it was the age of wisdom, it was the age of foolishness, it was the epoch of belief, it was the epoch of incredulity, it was the season of Light, it was the season of Darkness, it was the spring of hope, it was the winter of despair.

CHARLES DICKENS, *A Tale of Two Cities*

As has been pointed out, the three primary goals of the Skidmore psychiatric integration project were:

1. To foster the students' willingness and ability to become personally involved in and committed to their professional role and, through experiencing the full awareness and impact of their own feelings, to emancipate and develop their creativeness in all aspects of nursing practice.

2. To develop the students' ability to help persons with emotional and social problems through increasing their awareness and understanding of the emotional, cultural, and social factors of illness and personality growth and development.

3. To develop the students' ability to recognize, identify, examine, formulate, and intervene with guidance in the interpersonal and social problems of patients and personnel that occur in those situations in which they will work as staff nurses.

Because the psychiatric nurse project director believed that these goals could be achieved only to the degree that every faculty member was able to identify emotional and social problems that arise in nursing situations and to apply psychiatric concepts and processes in exploring these problems with students while teaching them the physical components of nursing care, the development of the instructors' skill in this area became a secondary goal of the project.

To what extent were these goals achieved during the five-year period covered in this book? The answer to this question is of utmost importance to those who are searching for ways of utilizing psychiatric knowledge for the improvement of nursing care and nursing education.

Yet the question cannot be answered by a simple yes or no. In the first place, the professional growth of the students and the faculty constituted the real measure of the project's success, and it is extremely difficult to evaluate professional change and growth. The complexity of such an appraisal is due to the fact that acquisition of knowledge is not the only criterion of growth. Professional behavior, as this refers specifically to the ability to take responsibility, to use judgment, and to exert initiative and leadership, is also being evaluated. Secondly, the project was not conducted in a vacuum, so that even when the psychiatric nurse and the psychiatrist recognized that the faculty, the students, and they themselves had grown professionally, they could not ascribe such growth solely to the effects of the integration project.

Thirdly, the time scale for evaluating professional change and growth must be in terms of years. An inherent aspect of the process of change includes waiting periods of many months during which assimilation and slow and imperceptible change have been going on. It is therefore much too soon to make a systematic assessment of the results of the Skidmore psychiatric integration project.

Because of these complexities the psychiatric team was deterred from building into its design of the project methods for evaluating its results, nor did it try to develop a valid instrument for measuring precisely what occurred. However, an attempt to appraise the results of the integration efforts was made by using the method of ongoing participant-observation of change and growth. To collect further data which might indicate such development, the psychiatric nurse also had individual interviews with all the faculty members, had a conference with the educational director of the affiliating agency where the course in psychatric nursing had been taught, and had individual interviews with selected students.

Collection of Data

INDIVIDUAL INTERVIEWS WITH THE FACULTY

At the end of the fifth year, when the psychiatric nurse's partial leave to work on this book was almost at an end, she interviewed each faculty member in the department of nursing and asked a series of questions designed to achieve the following purposes (see Appendix B).

To ascertain whether psychiatric integration had become something that belonged to the faculty—a legacy left by the psychiatric nurse and the psychiatrist.

To identify areas of the faculty's realistic dependency on the psychiatric nurse and the psychiatrist as well as the areas in which the faculty members were using initiative and were a realistic authority, and to appraise the faculty's acceptance of these two points.

To identify specific areas of endeavor or problem situations in which it was necessary for the faculty members to utilize psychiatric concepts and thereby to identify those areas of work that were specific to the psychiatric nurse's and the psychiatrist's roles.

To explore the influence of the faculty's experience or the lack of it in clinical psychiatric nursing on the acceptance or rejection of the psychiatric integration project.

To uncover attitudes toward individual psychotherapy as a medical treatment.

To clarify the faculty's perception of the role and functions of the psychiatric nurse and the psychiatrist as individuals and as a team and to uncover attitudes and feelings toward the team.

The nature and quality of the interaction between the majority of the faculty members and the psychiatric nurse in the interview situation—the degree of freedom in communication—was a partial barometer of the measure of success of the integration program. In most situations the faculty members were open, direct, and receptive during the interview experience. They were eager to share their thoughts about the progress that had been made during the fifth year, as well as to discuss some of the existing problems that had emerged during the team's partial leave. In the discussion of problem areas there was a noticeable decrease in the faculty members' tendency to place blame on others. They spoke about their reactions to the psychiatric nurse and the psychiatrist in a spontaneous and relaxed manner. The give-and-take quality of the interviews indicated that the psychiatric nurse had secured the faculty members' trust and confidence and that the differences in their respective roles were less of a barrier between them. A feeling of genuine self-satisfaction permeated many of the interviews.

One faculty member continued to be ingratiating and sedulously emphasized her own successful accomplishments. It seemed to the psychiatric nurse that she was almost parroting some of the verbalizations of the psychiatric team. As in the case of this instructor's limited and guarded participation in the faculty group discussions, it was extremely difficult to know whether her responses were the expression of what she really felt or were a means for gaining the approval of the psychiatric nurse.

In another situation a faculty member's former covert, negative, and rejecting attitudes were somewhat neutralized. She still was reluctant to recognize or to accept the fact that she might have needed some help in certain areas of her work, let alone to entertain any notion that the psychiatric team had helped her in any way.

Although some faculty members utilized the interview also to discuss personal problems and to seek help in handling them, on the whole they showed less tendency to do so than they had in previous interviews.

Conference with the Educational Director of an Affiliating Agency

As a method of evaluating the students' growth in their performance in psychiatric nursing, the year after the project director had left the Skidmore setting she had a conference with the educational director in the affiliating agency where the course in psychiatric nursing had been taught. The conference was geared to achieve the following purposes.

> To estimate the degree to which the students had resolved the authority-dependency conflict and thus were able to relate more effectively with authority figures.

> To identify the influence of the integration project on the students' initial presenting attitudes of hopelessness and helplessness about caring for psychiatric patients.

> To evaluate the students' ability to conceptualize a psychiatric nursing problem, to formulate psychiatric nursing interventions, and to appraise realistically the nursing care that had been given.

> To assess the students' willingness to become involved with psychiatric patients through personalizing the professional relationship and to appraise their ability to penetrate the meaning of disturbed behavior.

> To estimate the students' ability to identify and to formulate the dynamics operating in group interaction and their ability to identify the conjunctive and disjunctive forces as these operate in the clinical setting.

Individual Interviews with Students and Graduates of the Program

As has been noted, early in the fifth year of the project, for the purpose of collecting data for this book, the psychiatric nurse had individual interviews with fourteen students in the sophomore, junior, and senior classes and with four members of the class that had graduated in 1961 (see Chapter 12 and Appendix B). Three questions in the series were designed for the following purposes.

To identify the students' perception of the nature of student-faculty relationships in terms of the faculty's expectations of students, the quality of guidance and evaluation, and the degree to which students experience the faculty personally.

To uncover attitudes toward the specific learning experiences in the psychiatric integration program and the influence of these experiences on the students' behavioral change and growth.

To identify alterations in the students' perception of psychopathology, psychotherapy, and psychiatric patients.

The evaluation of the outcomes of the Skidmore psychiatric integration project will be discussed under the following four categories—the curriculum, the faculty, the students, and the methods of psychiatric integration that were utilized. Because the synthesis of the psychiatric nurse and the psychiatrist into a team has been analyzed in detail in the chapter on interdisciplinary teamwork (see Chapter 13), further evaluation of the psychiatric team will be limited to an appraisal of the growth in faculty-psychiatric team relationships and an assessment of the advantages and disadvantages of interdisciplinry collaboration as a method of psychiatric integration.

The Curriculum

Several important changes in the nursing curriculum occurred during the five-year period of the psychiatric integration project, some of which undoubtedly were facilitated by the project.

The thirty-hour course in interpersonal relations in nursing, which was taught by the psychiatric nurse, became a permanent part of the curriculum. Some changes were made, however; from an exclusive focus on the exploration and analysis of psychiatric concepts, its content and methods were expanded to include student presentations of clinical case material and the discussion of comprehensive nursing care. This course had to be flexible in order to avoid too much duplication of content as the faculty members began to include certain psychiatric concepts in their own teaching.

Several changes took place in the content and structure of the nursing care conferences which the instructors held in connection with their courses. These conferences were no longer focused exclusively on the discussion of particular disease entities; topics evolved from students' problems, and frequently these pertained to difficulties in understanding and handling patient behavior. Much progress was made in incorporating psychiatric concepts into clinical teaching. Anxiety, role behavior, verbal and nonverbal communication, dependency, self-concept and body image, regression, cultural differences and isolation, and fundamental human needs were some of the concepts that were woven through several aspects of the nursing curriculum in the sophomore year and through the courses in communicable disease and long-term-illness nursing, public health nursing, and team nursing in the junior year. The discussion of the psychodynamics of alcoholism and the social structure of Skid Row and their relationship to the impact of hospital-ization on homeless male patients with tuberculosis became a permanent part of the junior-year course in communicable disease and long-term-illness nursing.

A second area of content focused on recurrent problems in nurse-patient relationships. During the first clinical experience, which occurred on medical and surgical units, the students come face to face with the dying patient. All the instructors had increased their skill considerably in helping the stu-dents to deal with this problem more effectively. Other nurse-patient prob-lems that received emphasis concerned the patient who denies his illness and refuses to follow his doctor's orders or to allow a nurse to take care of him and the patient who fears loss of sexual identity, such as the male patient who needs to prove his sexual prowess by being seductive with the nurse. More attention was also directed toward the problem of interpersonal tensions and difficulties arising with the clinical personnel.

Another curriculum change effected by the integration project concerned the clinical conferences in psychiatric nursing, which functioned as a bridge between the course in psychiatric nursing in the affiliating agency and the rest of the nursing curriculum. The course in psychiatric nursing therefore was somewhat less detached from the total educational program.

The Faculty

In her appraisal of the faculty as the most important resource for psychi-atric integration, the psychiatric nurse, in the first year of the project, had given special consideration to the faculty members' knowledge of psychiatric concepts and their ability to apply these to the teaching-learning process. She also had identified the factors in intrafaculty, in faculty-psychiatric team, and in faculty-student relationships which facilitated and those which seemed to impede progress toward the goals of integration. The evaluation of faculty change and growth will be discussed therefore within the context of the four areas of knowledge and application of psychiatric content; com-munication, power, and intrafaculty relations; faculty-psychiatric team re-lationships; and faculty-student relationships.

KNOWLEDGE AND APPLICATION OF PSYCHIATRIC CONTENT

The areas which the faculty members identified as being ones in which they were realistically dependent on the psychiatric team for help included the ability to conceptualize and apply psychiatric content to the teaching-learning process. The comments of the faculty members further indicated that many of the instructors had begun to recognize and to evaluate their limitations in psychiatric knowledge and skill and to express them openly to the psychiatric nurse. The following comments were made by some older faculty members.

I think most of the faculty members have been insufficiently aware of the psychiatric implications of illness. We knew that mental health is important, but we did not have the necessary knowledge and skill to get this across to students. I have felt that our faculty was psychiatrically unsophisticated.

We need further work with both you [the psychiatric nurse] and Dr. Ullman to deepen our knowledge of psychiatric content and to increase our skill in applying it in teaching. Also, we still need more help and guidance in working as a group.

The following comments were made by some younger faculty members.

I think that one faculty member tends to give lip service to psychiatric concepts, and she seems to take whatever point of view she feels is most apt to gain her the approval of the rest of the faculty. I don't see any real change in her behavior since the beginning of the project.

I think that Miss X really appreciates the need to use psychiatric concepts, but she still seems a little apprehensive about applying them in her own classes and seminars. I think she may be afraid of psychiatry, but I think she has made a genuine effort to learn. She is much more flexible in evaluating students, and I think she uses psychiatric concepts on an intuitive level when she evaluates them.

Many faculty members had become more aware of anxiety and were more adept at recognizing how it operates in the clinical and teaching situation; some of the dynamics of illness and the dying process, including denial; the principles of personality development, particularly as these apply to student behavior; the concept of authority; and group dynamics and interactional processes, as well as some principles of communication theory.

Many faculty members grew in their ability to lead small groups of students and to explore nurse-patient relationships in action. They became quite skillful in eliciting topics for discussion, in securing the students' participation, and in uncovering their feelings about the situation. One of the most rewarding aspects of the psychiatric team's work with the faculty was the increase in the ability of all the instructors to tolerate higher levels of anxiety, as manifested by their ability to wait for the problem-solving process to evolve. The instructors were less inclined to close students off, and most of the time they were less preoccupied with arriving at pat solutions. In their interviews with the psychiatric nurse, several faculty members referred to this area of growth in themselves. An older instructor made the following comment.

> I have become enchanted with learning how to identify the process involved in evaluation and in the students' growth and learning. Also, I seem to have less need to give answers in handling problems.

A younger instructor made the following observation about her growth.

> During the psychiatric team's leave last year, I developed a greater appreciation of the importance of providing students with a flexible structure for discussing their experiences, and I learned that some floundering is usually an essential part of the learning process. Also, I became more aware that whenever I try to identify the principles or try to tie up some of the loose ends too soon, the problem we are trying to resolve always ends up by becoming more obscure.

All the instructors with whom the psychiatric team had participated in clinical conferences continued to have a good deal of difficulty in summarizing all the data they teased out of the student presentations. They also still needed much help in conceptualizing and formulating a problem; in the interviews with the psychiatric nurse most of the instructors indicated that they were unable to formulate the concepts underlying grossly disturbed behavior. In this latter area, the psychiatric team functioned as resource persons.

In regard to the range of growth in learning to formulate and apply psychiatric content, the instructors who were responsible for the supervision of students on the medical units and who, during the first year of the project, had been identified as being at the lower end of the scale in psychiatric knowledge and skill, were among the most eager and willing to learn psychiatric concepts. This growth may in part be accounted for by the nature of a medical patient's illness and hospitalization. The fact that many medical conditions can be brought under control but may not be curable insofar as cure pertains to abolishing the disease condition and that neither a patient nor a nurse can visually observe or point to the area of disturbance is bound to arouse a good deal of anxiety on the part of the patient. Then, because of the amount of time that frequently is required for anatomical healing and for establishing physiological healing and equilibrium, prolonged hospitalization often is an essential part of treating a medical condition. In these circumstances, a nurse generally is required to spend rather long periods of time with medical patients, and much of her nursing care must be geared toward recognizing and handling a patient's emotional responses to his illness and hospitalization.

The instructors who taught pediatric nursing, with the possible exception of one, demonstrated marked growth in their ability to apply psychiatric concepts to nurse-patient situations in action and to the evaluation of student behavior.

The growth among the instructors in public health nursing did not appear as marked as in the case of some other instructors, perhaps because this group originally had been at the highest level of psychiatric knowledge and skill.

Most of the instructors in surgical nursing continued to have considerable difficulty in learning to formulate and to apply psychiatric concepts to their teaching.

As far as a comparison of the growth of the older group to the younger group is concerned, four of the younger members and two of the older members demonstrated the most apparent growth in knowledge of and ability to apply psychiatric content; one younger instructor and three older instructors demonstrated the least growth.

Integration or Fragmentation. Any inclination on the part of the psychiatric team to retreat into Olympian serenity about the success in integrating psychiatric concepts was tempered by a new trend that began near the end of the fifth year of the project. A less desirable effect of the project was that at this time several instructors became involved in a serious love affair with the emotional aspects of illness and nursing care, sometimes to the point that these aspects took priority over the physical requirements of nursing care or that the physical and emotional components of nursing care were not integrated into a cohesive whole. This problem first became evident to the psychiatric nurse in her work with the students in individual conferences, in the students' responses to the examination questions prepared by the psychiatric team, and the students' written analyses of nursing-care studies.

The psychiatric nurse expressed concern about this problem on numerous occasions when the faculty met as a group. Some of the faculty, both younger and older members, responded by becoming defensive and by denying that such a problem existed, even when the psychiatrist suggested that perhaps he and the psychiatric nurse had done too good a job of psychiatric integration. Some older members raised the point that because the psychiatric team had consistently focused on the students' own emotional reactions and attitudes, perhaps the students tended to become overly concerned with themselves and less concerned with patients.

As has been emphasized, there is no such thing as too much emotional care or too much physical care; there is just good nursing care, which is, of course, the ultimate reason for psychiatric integration. However, in overzealous attempts to integrate psychiatric content, danger of fragmentation is always present. How had the faculty members facilitated the students' exclusive focus on the emotional aspects of nursing care? Had the psychiatric integration program helped to increase such fragmentation? What are some of the issues that may be involved in the fragmentation of emotional and physical nursing care?

One of the issues may have evolved from the focus and structure of both the psychiatric team's and the psychiatric nurse's clinical conferences with the individual instructor and her group of students. It was to be expected that the team's emphasis on the students' emotionally disturbing experiences would create problems of fragmentation unless this emphasis was counterbalanced by the instructor's emphasis on the physical plus the emotional aspects of nursing care. The psychiatric nurse's and the psychiatrist's emphasis would contribute to the synthesis of all aspects of nursing care only to the degree that the students' orientation to physical care had been solidly entrenched.

Another issue which was referred to by several faculty members was that perhaps the students tended to equate collegiate nursing education with an exclusive emphasis on the emotional needs of patients and to think of physical care as demeaning. If this appraisal of the students' perception of nursing care was accurate (and many of the psychiatric nurse's experiences with the students would seem to validate it), the more important issue at stake was the need for the nurse teacher, including the psychiatric nurse and the members of other disciplines who may be engaged in psychiatric integration, to be alert to any tendency on her part to increase whatever bias against physical nursing care the students might have.

Still another issue concerning the faculty members' overemphasis on the psychiatric aspects of illness and nursing care may have been related to the problem of one-upmanship (or who is at the top of the pecking order). Such preoccupation could be a defensive operation—a way for the faculty members to ingratiate themselves with the psychiatric nurse and the psychiatrist. To the extent that the faculty members were anxious about the psychiatric team's evaluation of their knowledge of and ability to apply psychiatric concepts, they most likely would try to emulate the psychiatric nurse and the psychiatrist by overemphasizing the emotional area. It is at that point that psychiatry becomes too important; and once anything has become too important, anxiety can be deduced.

In subsequent discussions of the problem of fragmentation, several younger and older instructors suggested that the feeling of power a nurse teacher can derive from the knowledge and application of psychiatric concepts might be another issue in the fragmentation of the physical and emotional components of nursing care. The following comment of a younger faculty member illustrates this point.

> Learning to observe behavior, to uncover problems, and to understand behavior is so fascinating because we have to become like detectives who are trying to solve a mystery.

Inasmuch as the psychiatric nurse's evaluation of the effects of the integration project represented an interim and open-ended appraisal of the faculty's change and growth, it is important to recognize that the problem of fragmentation of knowledge and skill, instead of signifying a final end-point that was reached, might well have constituted a transitional phase in the developmental process of learning psychiatric concepts and how to apply them. What the psychiatric team had contributed in terms of helping to bring about some resolution of the problem of the faculty's fragmentation was principally a matter of having brought the problem into the open so that all the faculty members were fully aware of it.

COMMUNICATION, POWER, AND INTRAFACULTY RELATIONS

One of the most important and apparent areas of growth in intrafaculty relations pertained to the schism between the older faculty group and the younger group. By the end of the fifth year of the project the split started to be cemented. Although, in some spots, the cement was still soft and at these points imprints of intrafaculty pressures were readily embedded, some of the places that had hardened were able to hold up under a good deal of force and agitation. Other areas were more fragile, and these readily cracked. Several of the faculty members indicated that they had initiated steps toward closing the gap between the younger and older groups. The following comments reflect some of the faculty members' attitudes about the closure of the faculty schism. Two older members' comments pointed to some resolution of the problems associated with the emphasis on conformity.

> There seems to be more tolerance among faculty. You [psychiatric nurse] have worked with us for a long time, and your acceptance has rubbed off on us. However, it is more difficult for a new faculty member to be tolerant of differences because she has not experienced the process of working this through together as we have done.

> I no longer feel there is any schism between the older and younger groups. I think faculty line up on issues now. This I can work with. I like different points of view. There are no more secret conclaves behind closed doors.

In their observations of faculty growth, three younger members stated,

> The psychiatric integration process is part of me, not only in my teaching, but in my personal life. My relationship with the faculty members in the older group has improved. I have become more accepting of difficulties, and I don't take things as personally as I used to.

> Lately it appears to me as though there has been a shift in faculty interaction. Up until now, I had not been aware of any interpersonal difficulties among the members of the older group. I have become aware, however, that they too have some interpersonal difficulties among themselves, because from time to time these now erupt into the open. But I think the gap between the two groups has been narrowed. The power among the total faculty seems to have been more evenly distributed.

> There is much more sharing now among members of the older and younger groups.

The power of the older group had waned but still was formidable. Never-theless, because many of the younger members had uncovered and tapped reservoirs of strength they never knew they had, they had grown less de-pendent on the older members for their approval. Potential leaders among the younger group had been identified. As some faculty comments reveal, the older members began to be more comfortable with the younger group and had less need to present themselves as a united front. The older mem-bers had come a considerable distance in learning to accept the value of individual differences and to give sincere recognition. As with any change, they needed sufficient time to become more comfortable with this new ap-proach. The members of both groups were more tolerant of each other's idiosyncrasies and were less inclined to take disagreements personally.

The faculty's growth in regard to the placement of greater value on differences than on conformity was dramatically demonstrated in the change of attitude toward the time of arrival at and departure from the work situ-ation. Early in the integration project the faculty members abandoned the ritual of arriving and leaving at a specific hour and checking on each other's whereabouts, and the younger instructors discarded the habit of tip-toeing in and out of work in the hope of remaining unnoticed by the older in-structors. The older and younger faculty members were no longer as defen-sive about their comings and goings, nor did they take advantage of the freedom they had struggled for and now enjoyed. On the contrary, all of them invested many hours beyond the eight-hour day.

On those sporadic occasions when a comment was made about the seem-ing unavailability of a particular instructor, that instructor was less inclined to feel guilty and submit to the old ritual of conformity in order to avoid the anxiety of possible disapproval. This was one example of the fact that the younger members were beginning to handle their former irrational attitudes toward authority figures and, concomitantly, to assume more responsibility for their own behavior rather than blame the older members for it.

The resolution of some of the problems associated with competitiveness among the faculty members and between the faculty members and the psy-chiatric nurse occurred in two areas. Pervading all levels of the faculty hierarchy was an increased ability to keep faculty and student confidences. It was a joy to observe and experience an instructor's pride when a student or a colleague revealed herself to her. Such evidence of trust and intimacy was cherished as a gift.

The other change which resulted in a noticeable reduction of competitive-ness was the increase in effective collaboration. Two members emphasized this point in the following comments.

While teaching jointly with an older instructor, I did not sit back passively and let her take the exclusive leadership. I felt I had something of value to give. In the beginning of psychiatric integration, I was uncomfortable in the clinical conferences with you [psychiatric nurse] and Monte, but now I enjoy collaborative teaching very much.

The opportunity to collaborate with an older instructor helped me to feel very comfortable with her. I think she too has grown tremendously and has become much warmer. Also, she is more direct about her feelings and attitudes. Students respond positively to this.

In one situation a younger and an older member who for a prolonged period had been bitterly critical of each other, taught collaboratively. The younger member, who was enthusiastic about the success of the experience, took positive steps in communicating her feelings to the other faculty members and in so doing diluted some of the other instructors' negative attitudes toward this older member. Both the younger and the older instructors' positions were enhanced significantly as a result of this experience.

The faculty continued to have a good deal of difficulty in utilizing the problem-solving process in reaching decisions. Many faculty members identified the continuation of a strong tendency on the part of the faculty group to avoid decisions by talking around them, to make decisions prematurely without uncovering the various conflicts and examining the consequences, and to change decisions once they were made. In discussing problems associated with decision making, some younger members commented,

We still have trouble in identifying the problem at hand. When you [*psychiatric nurse*] are present, you help us to uncover various feelings, reactions, and opinions. You point out the process and get us refocused. Sometimes I am able to do the latter, as is another faculty member. But without you, we still tend to plunge in and make premature decisions.

There doesn't seem to be much growth on the part of the faculty when it comes to making a decision about whether a student should pass or fail.

Some of the older members identified problems in decision making in the following way.

There is the ever-existing problem of faculty moving so slowly on decisions, and this makes me apprehensive about progress that must be made. We tend to talk around problems. Then there is the need for some members to hold forth and philosophize.

Perhaps there has been too much emphasis on a team approach to the detriment of individual recognition and responsibility.

Although blaming and scapegoating decreased, they tended to go into motion whenever decisions miscarried.

Some growth in regard to the faculty members' unrealistic and unclarified expectations of each other was manifested in the instructors' evaluation of students. When problems arose concerning a student's academic achievement or clinical performance, rather than wait until a problem had become serious, the instructor intervened by conferring with the student when the problem was first recognized. There also were fewer instances in which there was a discrepancy between an assigned grade, an instructor's evaluation of the student, and the quality of the student's performance. As a consequence of these changes in the instructors' evaluation of students, there were fewer breakdowns in faculty communication concerning student evaluation.

In the psychiatric nurse's interviews with the faculty members, the one area of the faculty's overdependency on the psychiatric team that was referred to by several instructors was the evaluation of student behavior. Some faculty members felt that because they had become more secure and skillful with this process, the psychiatric team should be used more selectively as resource persons. They also were concerned that some faculty members' request for the team's help might degenerate into a compulsive ritual. One younger member wondered if the continuous concentration on students was a way to avoid handling more troublesome problems and issues.

There is no question that a great deal of time in the faculty group discussions during the fifth year of the project was being devoted to exploring student behavior. This emphasis may have been caused by several circumstances—the psychiatric nurse's unavailability for on-the-spot consultation during the fifth year; the difficulty experienced by the faculty members in trusting their own judgment in evaluating behavior; some residual apprehension that a decision to fail a student might create an unpleasant situation with parents, which in turn might backfire with the college administration; and finally, attempts to learn from past mistakes in making decisions. Nevertheless, the time and effort that had been spent on student evaluation paid dividends, as was reflected in the degree of the faculty's perception and sensitivity in realistically evaluating themselves, each other, and the group as a whole.

It should be recognized, however, that the problem of unrealistic and unclarified expectations was not completely resolved. As has been pointed out, this problem frequently develops in response to the bureaucratic structure of American colleges and health institutions. In addition, because of the nature of the historical development of the nursing profession, the authority-dependency conflict as it pertains to unrealistic expectations probably will always be a central problem in nursing education.

Some faculty members felt that the fear of criticism continued to operate in faculty-group activities. One younger member stated,

> I feel that we are expected not to have problems. One never hears another faculty member talk about her failures, only her successful accomplishments. I think we still are afraid to expose our own deficiencies.

An older member commented,

> I don't think we tolerate mistakes. We still tend to attack each other. I must learn to move in and intervene when this happens.

Irrespective of some of the faculty members' continuing fear of attack from each other, the undertow of blaming and scapegoating had weakened somewhat, especially in the area of curriculum matters, an area in which all the instructors tended to feel the most secure.

As revealed in the faculty members' verbatim comments to the psychiatric nurse, some of the most significant change and growth occurred in regard to the degree of insight most of the faculty members had developed about their own and the other instructors' behavior. Unlike their behavior in group situations, the majority of the instructors were willing and able to expose their own strengths and limitations to the psychiatric nurse. The depth of the instructors' perceptions and insights indicated that in their individual relationship with the psychiatric nurse, they had traveled a long way from denying the existence of their problems.

Although the faculty members' newly developed freedom and openness in facing problems with the psychiatric nurse was a crucial step in the process of change and growth, it did not automatically follow that they had arrived at the point where they also were willing and able to personalize their professional relationships with each other by revealing their attitudes toward each other's behavior on an individual and group level.

The one truly tragic flaw in the overall picture of change and growth in intrafaculty relations was that little improvement seemed to have been made in the faculty members' ability to communicate directly with those colleagues with whom they had interpersonal difficulties or who they felt were not effectively fulfilling their professional responsibilities to the other faculty members, to the students, or to the clinical personnel. There continued to be generalized avoidance of direct confrontation of faculty members on an individual level and of setting realistic limits on inappropriate behavior. Both the younger and older members frequently referred to the lack of direct confrontation as a problem that continued to concern them. Some younger faculty members appraised the situation as follows.

> Problems relating to one faculty member were dealt with indirectly and they were discussed in small groups with everyone but the person who was involved. It seems to me that many of the problems that have arisen in intrafaculty relationships are due to our lack of directness with those persons with whom we have difficulty.

> One instructor seems to isolate herself now more than ever from the rest of faculty and from the rest of the curriculum. She seems to do whatever she wants to do without collaborating with faculty. None of us, including those in author-

ity positions, say anything to her or set any limits. We all act as if we are afraid of her.

Two older faculty members spoke much in the same vein.

There is the problem of one faculty member who tends to cut off others, and she arouses a great deal of anger when she does this. But all of us allow this to happen because we allow her to do this to us. For example, why have I allowed her to do this to me without saying anything to her?

Sometimes we find it is easier to express negative feelings toward an individual faculty member in a group than to do so in a face-to-face situation with the individual involved.

Commencing in the fourth year, both the younger and the older faculty members individually consulted with the psychiatric nurse and the psychiatrist about problems with some other faculty members. Some of these problems were serious enough to warrant immediate intervention. In spite of the psychiatric team's encouragement, support, and guidance, it was the exception when one faculty member could intervene in the disruptive behavior of another.

Considering the extended period over which the communication lines within the faculty group had been crossed, how much growth in the area of direct confrontation and limit setting was it realistic to expect in five years? On the other hand, without some beginning resolution of this problem, how much permanent change and growth in the overall picture of intrafaculty relations could legitimately be expected and realized? The achievement of intellectual awareness alone could not bring about qualitative change in the faculty members' feeling, thinking, and doing—the ingredients of genuine understanding. Nevertheless, with the development of intellectual awareness of the impact of their own and their colleagues' professional behavior, a vital step in the process of transforming profesisonal behavior had been achieved.

Despite some of the limitations in change and growth, some of the fear had been dispelled, thus revealing considerable potential strength and creativeness. It seemed as though the faculty had derived greater appreciation of the fact that to be human is to be different from others, to make mistakes, to know fear, and to feel anger, affection, despair, and hope. It seemed as if the faculty members were beginning to learn that it was all right to be human with each other.

The Image of the Psychiatric Nurse and the Psychiatrist. The psychiatric nurse's conferences with the faculty members yielded data indicating that their perception of the psychiatrist and his role had become more realistic. The faculty members recognized that they were less inclined to ascribe ascendancy in status to the psychiatrist and that they had come to appreciate his respect for individual differences, the positive force of his objectivity, and his tendency to deliberate before taking action.

Among the older members' comments were,

> He makes it clear to us that he expects us to make our own decisions and respects them when we do. We have come to expect him to throw the responsibility for decision making back to us.

> We can always count on how he will react—that he will look at the whole problem objectively. I expect this and would be disappointed if he didn't behave in this way.

The younger members' comments included the following.

> I see him as a thoughtful person who moves slowly. We understand his hesitancy. It makes us think. I have learned it is not too bad to wait.

> I don't feel I have to accept everything the psychiatrist says or that I have to agree with him without question. Before, I would have followed him blindly.

The data from the psychiatric nurse's interviews also identified that the psychiatric nurse and the psychiatrist, like the other faculty members, had as individuals shown evidence of change and growth during the integration project.

The various areas of change and growth of the psychiatric nurse that were identified by the other faculty members were (1) moving from competition to collaboration and from dependency to interdependency; (2) increased ability to communicate directly; and (3) increased concern and respect for the faculty. Included in the older faculty members' comments were the following.

> I think there was a time that you were competitive and aggressive with the rest of the faculty and that this was a period during which you were struggling to establish your place. But now, you show no envy, no competition, no aggression, and no desire to control. You have a great desire to share with all of us.

> I get the feeling that you may wait for the faculty to do now in a group what you would have done yourself a couple of years ago.

> You seem clearer about your nursing role. You are not as dependent on the psychiatrist, and you are better able to disagree with him. The first two years I think you would have submerged yourself. And two years ago, I couldn't have told this to you, either. Nor could I have been this direct with you then.

Included among the younger members' comments were the following.

> You are more direct and don't have to work up to a situation as carefully, perhaps because now you can depend on a certain amount of acceptance from us, which you didn't get in the beginning.

> You are much less dependent on the psychiatrist now. You will move in on your own.

> In reading some extracts from the book and looking back over the integration project in retrospect, I have often wondered how you ever managed to survive this situation. I have greater respect for you because of all you went through with us. You proved that you really cared about us as people.

In evaluating the change and growth of the psychiatrist in the interviews with the psychiatric nurse, the faculty members realized that he had become freer in expressing his thoughts and feelings. Among the older members' comments was the following.

> He demonstrates more animation, warmth, and vigor, but still is nonjudgmental. I think he likes us.

The younger members' comments included the following.

> He is much more relaxed. He is neither as hesitant nor as guarded in his reactions. His own feeling of freedom had to develop slowly until faculty trusted him and could accept his feelings.

Faculty and Psychiatric-Team Relationships. Having lived through the psychiatric integration process together and having shared their satisfactions and frustrations, the faculty members and the members of the psychiatric team viewed each other in a new light. By the fifth year of the project, as reflected in the faculty comments, the faculty members as a group and individually had begun to seek help from the psychiatric team with problems that pertained to students, to the utilization of psychiatric concepts, to the employment of certain teaching methods, and to difficulies in intra-faculty relationships. The value of the team's unique contributions was no longer questioned. As one of the younger faculty members said in her interview with the psychiatric nurse,

> Both of you are now accepted, looked to for help, and used, rather than merely tolerated. The psychiatric team is viewed as a vital part of the total situation. Faculty no longer ask, "Should we use them?" but rather, "When can we make time for them?"

The faculty members also identified several areas in which they experienced realistic dependency during the psychiatric team's curtailed activities in the fifth year. Their ability to acknowledge this dependency was closely allied to their acceptance of the psychiatric team as a realistic authority. In the absence of the team, the faculty had been thrown on its own resources regarding psychiatric integration and it had had the opportunity to test various psychiatric concepts and techniques that had been elucidated over the five years. From the verbatim responses obtained in the interviews, it was possible to formulate the faculty's concept of the role of the psychiatric team in an integration program. In most cases this role was communicated in terms of functions which were described as follows.

1. To act as a sounding board for the faculty members' problems and as a testing ground for their ideas and plans.
2. To provide consultation to the faculty regarding students with problematic behavior, particularly when this behavior had psychopathological dimensions.
3. To make referrals for psychotherapy.
4. To give assistance in acquiring, broadening, and deepening knowledge of psychiatric concepts and of the processes in applying these concepts to teaching students.
5. To participate as leaders and resource persons in faculty group discussions by:
   a. Summarizing reactions in an objective and nonjudgmental way.
   b. Refocusing discussions as necessary through on-the-spot recognition of a problem and analysis of the group interaction.
   c. Permitting and expecting the faculty to take the responsibility for making its own decisions.

Both the younger and the older faculty members continued to look to the psychiatric team to bring into the open within the faculty group discussions touchy issues that were disturbing to them, but which they themselves were reluctant to raise. Both of the faculty groups still were inclined to wait either for the psychiatric nurse or the psychiatrist to raise issues and to handle problems that arose among individual faculty members and to set limits on inappropriate behavior. The resolution of this area of overdependency hinged in part on whether the older and the younger faculty members would grapple with some of the realistic and unrealistic aspects of their fear of reprisal from each other.

As has been pointed out, the faculty members' candidness during their conferences with the psychiatric nurse substantiated the fact that she had succeeded in establishing a relationship with them in which they trusted her enough to evaluate her in a face-to-face situation. Various comments during these conferences revealed that efforts to foist conformity on the psychiatric nurse had long since been abandoned. The faculty members had begun to view her as a peer, while at the same time most of them acknowledged and accepted her legitimate authority as a specialist in psychiatric nursing.

One of the more obvious changes in the faculty members' behavior was their greater comfort with the psychiatrist. They had crawled out from their shells of reticence and diffidence and were beginning to question him, at times disagree with him, and even have fun with him. The most remarkable change of all was that some faculty members were less inclined to ascribe to him higher status than the psychiatric nurse. One older faculty member stated, "You and Dr. Ullman, together, are more than just 'half and half.' At one time, I looked to the psychiatrist as the authority, and now I see you both as one unit."

However, most of the faculty members still were not very clear about how to use the psychiatrist, either individually or in the group, and they relied on the psychiatric nurse to bring him into a situation as necessary. Possibly they were still lacking sufficient knowledge about psychiatric matters, and therefore insufficiently understood the psychiatrist's role, to be able to initiate contacts with him on their own and to utilize all he had to offer them.

Another reason may have been that although the psychiatric nurse and the other faculty members had resolved the status problems between them, the psychiatric team had not yet synthesized with the faculty. In such circumstances the psychiatric nurse rather than the psychiatrist may have come to represent psychiatry to the faculty members, and they would be able to use him to the degree that the psychiatric nurse was able to represent him by interpreting and clarifying his role.

Faculty-Student Relationships

From the beginning of the psychiatric integration project it was apparent to the psychiatric nurse that many of the major assets of the faculty members— those factors which fostered group cohesiveness and thereby advanced the integration process—were associated with the positive quality of faculty-student relationships. Even though concern with the students' welfare had always been a priority among the faculty members, it nevertheless was in the realm of their relationships with students that their change and growth were most clearly discernible.

As revealed by several of the students' comments one of the most significant areas of growth was in the faculty members' increased willingness and ability to move from an impersonal to a personalized professional relationship with students. Most of the faculty members had become more aware of both their positive and their negative reactions to students and to the rest of the instructors and were more comfortable in communicating directly their genuine concern for students' successes and failures. Among the student comments, the following emphasized this aspect of faculty growth.

> Our instructors let us see them as people, not just as teachers.

> The informal and relaxed atmosphere helps to reduce our tension.

> Faculty are not only interested in your clinical competence, but in you as a person.

> This is the first time in my life I ever became close to a teacher, anywhere.

In regard to change in the instructors' tendency to emphasize the negative aspects of the students' performance and to show insufficient recognition of their strengths during the day-to-day supervision of clinical experiences, some of the students commented,

> There is a tendency of the faculty to overemphasize the problems of students. We always know what's wrong with us, but we aren't very clear about what we do well.

> There were times when I was supervised that I felt cut down by the instructor instead of being helped by her.

> There is so much emphasis on tiny details that sometimes I am foggy about what is important. The faculty seem to emphasize our mistakes, and they give very little praise for what we do well.

Although there were some desultory attempts on the part of some instructors to emphasize both the positive and the negative aspects of the students' clinical performance as they occurred on the spot, from the psychiatric nurse's viewpoint, not much in the way of change in this area seemed to have occurred. Certainly this tendency of the faculty to focus on students' mistakes was not unique to the Skidmore situation, nor is it limited to education in nursing. In the literature there are frequent references to a similar problem in medical education, for example.

One of the central issues in the nurse teacher's preoccupation with the student's mistakes may be, as has been emphasized, that because the nurse teacher is the guardian of the nursing profession, she is responsible for safe and effective nursing care and she therefore must prevent anything from occurring that might endanger human welfare. Within this framework the patient rather than the student becomes the nurse teacher's focus of principal concern and the student's best interest may fall, at least temporarily, by the wayside. The degree of resolution of this problem, which can realistically be expected, probably is contingent on whether or not nursing educators develop sufficient understanding of the learning process.

The faculty members' unrealistic and unclarified expectations of students continued to be a problem throughout the project. The instructors' unrealistic expectations frequently resulted in many students feeling aggressive and hostile, as is illustrated in the following comments.

> During the sophomore year, students felt negatively about the faculty. We didn't know where we fitted in or how to act. [*Senior student.*]

> I think the faculty has too high expectations of the beginning student. We get tense and scared and feel overwhelmed. [*Sophomore student.*]

> One minute we are buddy-buddy with faculty, and we are supposed to speak openly about our reactions. In the next, we are being laced up and down in the clinical area. We are never sure where we stand. [*Junior student.*]

There was too much emphasis on grades, and unless you toed the line and lived up to the Skidmore image of a nurse, you were out. [*Recent graduate of the program.*]

A central theme of the students' comments is the instructors' unrealistic expectations of beginning students. As has been pointed out, the most reasonable explanation for these unrealistic expectations, particularly of sophomore students, related to the curriculum design in the junior year. The courses in obstetric, psychiatric, and public health nursing did not become the responsibility of the faculty until after the first five-year period of the project had come to an end.

Another crucial area of the faculty members' growth was in the quality of help and guidance they gave to students. The majority of the faculty members became more cognizant of and comfortable in accepting the relation of the student's personality to her professional behavior. They were more perceptive in recognizing the student's emotional strengths and deficiencies and were better able to identify some of the relationships between these and the student's level of academic and clinical performance. One student made the following observation.

Faculty are extremely sensitive. Their evaluations of us are uncanny. They are so clear about our strengths and limitations.

With the exception of one instructor there was overall movement in the direction of seeking students out to give them help instead of waiting for them to come to the instructor as had frequently been the case in the beginning of the project. Among the student comments that emphasized the faculty's helpful role were the following.

The support that the faculty gave me when I was having so much difficulty made me feel I could do almost anything.

Faculty don't merely tell us when we aren't doing well, but they investigate with us as to the reasons why.

The following comment of a younger faculty member emphasized the area of faculty growth.

I think we all have grown in our observation of student behavior, and some of us now are able to make up our own minds about referring students to you [*psychiatric nurse*]. Your absence has made us aware that preparation of the student for seeing you is the responsibility of the instructor. While you were here, I think all of us waited for you to call the student yourself.

In her individual conferences with students it became most apparent to the psychiatric nurse that there was a marked improvement in the instructors' interviewing skills, particularly in the area of raising critical questions and in listening. The faculty members progressively took more responsibility in working with students to clarify the problem and to collect important information. Just as the psychiatric nurse helped to "loosen up" students before they were referred to the psychiatrist, the faculty had become a bridge between the students and the psychiatric nurse.

A particularly satisfying aspect of the faculty's growth was that several members became more comfortable in allowing students to express their negative feelings about those instructors with whom they were having interpersonal problems, and they also developed some beginning skill in helping the students to come to a more realistic appraisal of the instructor under discussion. This desire for new experience was a far cry from the diatribe against the psychiatric nurse and her unstructured group discussions with sophomore students that had occurred a few years earlier. Their fear that those discussions were principally sessions in which members of the faculty were derided—chiefly themselves—had been penetrated, possibly as a result of their attendance at the conferences. The following comments of younger faculty members revealed much satisfaction with their own growth in this area.

> A group of students came to me with a problem about another instructor. I had a conference with the whole group so they could discuss the problem in the open. I was terribly apprehensive about it at first, but it went very well. The students seemed to come out with a more objective and positive view of the faculty member.

> Your [*the psychiatric nurse's*] absence stimulated me in some ways because I never would have attempted to handle problems concerning the students' relationship with another instructor.

A point not to be overlooked is that unless both of these instructors had recognized their own feelings about the faculty members in question and also had come to grips with some of their own negative reactions, they could have further complicated the situation by knowingly or otherwise taking sides with the students against the other faculty members, or by putting all their efforts into unrealistically humanizing them. The fact that both the instructors apparently had handled the situation satisfactorily suggests another dimension in their growth—a beginning resolution of their interpersonal difficulties with some faculty members.

Along with the faculty's increased skill in giving sufficient guidance to students without overprotecting them, on the part of most instructors there also was greater awareness and acceptance of their own limitations in handling students' emotional responses to their educational experiences.

PSYCHIATRIC INTEGRATION AND THE CAPACITY FOR CHANGE

The faculty's verbatim responses in evaluating change and growth revealed that the psychiatric integration program was no longer a mere superstructure or appendage to the curriculum, but instead had become an inherent part of it. Many faculty members indicated that the integrative process also had become part of themselves rather than an outer skin to be put on for selected occasions and then shed again. The psychiatric team's partial separation from the integration program during the fifth year entailed some calculated risk of the faculty becoming detached from the program. It is important, however, to recognize that the psychiatric team reduced their activities at a time when the integration program and the philosophy underlying it had been accepted generally and when the stage of synthesis had been in process for a year.

In their work with the faculty members the psychiatric nurse and the psychiatrist learned that the most important quality making for the success of a psychiatric integration program relates to the individual's capacity for change rather than to any other single personality endowment, such as intellectual ability or achievement. The team members also found that the expectations of the faculty's growth must be different for each individual member. One of their mistakes was that they had expected all the faculty members to grow with the students and with them. As might be expected, there were instances in which faculty members did not grow, but instead, reinforced and strengthened their defenses against change. These situations became more pronounced as the other faculty members operated on a more productive level.

Despite the improvement of intrafaculty relationships that had been achieved, the faculty members' participation with each other and the psychiatric team in all significant experiences continued to involve the various stages of growth identified in this book—impact, recoil, and synthesis—but they became condensed in time because of the greater freedom of communication and cohesiveness (3).

The Students

The effects of the psychiatric integration project on the students will be discussed from the following aspects: the marriage-career conflict, the authority-dependency conflict and relationships with authority figures, and the knowledge and application of psychiatric concepts and of the problem-solving process.

THE MARRIAGE-CAREER CONFLICT

Because of the numerous and complex social and psychological factors involved in the attitude of many students that marriage and a nursing career are incompatible, neither the psychiatric nurse nor the psychiatrist ever attempted to deal explicitly with the problems associated with this false dichotomy.

In her individual and group work with the students the psychiatric nurse did try indirectly to modify some of their attitudes; for example, she repeatedly stressed the importance of students having a well-rounded social life, she encouraged some students to go on to graduate school, and she shared some of her own interests and experiences outside the realm of nursing. How much, if any, change in the students' perception of the role of women and attitudes toward work occurred could not be determined.

THE AUTHORITY-DEPENDENCY CONFLICT

The students showed most growth in their attitudes toward authority and dependency. Accounting for part of this progress, possibly, was the fact that students were interacting with a group of faculty members who concurrently were struggling with their own authority-dependency conflicts and who were therefore becoming more aware of and sensitive to their own role as a legitimate authority.

By the end of the sophomore year or the early part of the junior year, the students had become primarily patient-oriented rather than task-, teacher-, or doctor-oriented. They were inclined to be more concerned with the welfare of their patients than with achieving a good grade or presenting a positive picture of themselves as students and nurses. It was rewarding to observe the students' intrepid flight from denying problems and from resisting help in recognizing them. They were better able to face problems and to seek help from the instructors. They were less afraid of becoming involved in their experiences, as was demonstrated by their giving examples which concerned their own feelings and responses and by their willingness and eagerness to explore and analyze their work with patients. They were more comfortable in acknowledging what they did not know and were motivated to search for whatever help was available to them.

The students' resolution of their authority-dependency conflict was further demonstrated by their improved communication with the faculty members. For example, some students were willing and able to initiate contact with the instructor for the purpose of openly discussing problems that had arisen in their relationships with her. These students had learned the value and skill of direct confrontation.

At the same time the students became quite perceptive in identifying the instructors with whom it was less safe for them to be open and free. As the students became more comfortable with authority, concomitantly they tended to give up some of their rigid and unrealistic expectations of the faculty. On those occasions when a student felt she could not be as free with an instructor as she might wish, she was less apt to place blame or to feel thwarted. It seemed that if the students had had positive experiences with several faculty members, most of the time they could weather the storm with those instructors who appeared more threatening to them. If they needed help in working out their interpersonal difficulties with an instructor, most of the students had become secure enough to seek such help on their own.

As might be expected, some students continued to have difficulty in establishing positive relationships with the faculty. These students had difficulty in becoming comfortable with supervision and in accepting help and guidance, let alone in seeking it on their own. There also continued to be occasional episodes of reality testing and negative acting out against authority.

The students' positive relationships with the faculty tended to carry over to their relationships with clinical personnel. When a problem concerning a patient arose, for example, the students sought those who seemed to be in the best position to help them. As time went on, the individual's rank within the hierarchy (head nurse, physician) seemed to make little difference.

In a personal communication, Gertrude Clawson, assistant director of nursing, New York State Psychiatric Institute, stated that the junior students who had had the twelve-week affiliation in psychiatric nursing during the period of the integration project were considerably more mature than their preproject predecessors in their ability to relate with authority figures. On several occasions, for example, when problems arose between themselves and the clinical personnel of the affiliating agency, they requested a meeting with those who were concerned, during which they were able to discuss the problems in a nonjudgmental way. In spite of the fact that the students were in an entirely new environment, and moreover in a psychiatric setting, which was bound to be somewhat threatening, instead of regressing even temporarily in their ability to relate effectively, they continued to communicate on a high level with those in authority positions.

Closely related to the students' increased freedom with authority figures was their emerging perception of themselves as a rational authority. Correspondingly, many students tended to develop a strong sense of leadership and were fairly consistent in exercising initiative.

The final but by no means least important evidence of the students' emancipation from their authority-dependency conflict was their ability to appraise more realistically the strengths and limitations of the faculty. As some of the previously cited comments reveal, many students were able, with what sometimes seemed uncanny perception, to pinpoint a faculty member's positive points as well as to find her Achilles' heel.

Conversely, there were still students who needed to deny that a faculty member had some limitations, but these students were by far in the minority. The majority of students had grown to the place where they could recognize and accept that their teachers, like themselves, had human weaknesses.

KNOWLEDGE AND APPLICATION OF PSYCHIATRIC CONTENT

Growth in the students' understanding of psychiatric content, particularly the concepts of anxiety, frustration-aggression, conflict, and denial was demonstrated in part by their increased ability to observe their own behavior: to recognize the presence of anxiety in themselves and to identify their characteristic modes of adaptation to it. Their progress in learning to tolerate the anxiety engendered by their experiences was exemplified partly by their greater freedom in revealing their feelings of anger, sadness, sexuality, sympathy, and tenderness in response to a situation, and they arrived at the point of development where they viewed their own attitudes and responses as one of the most important sources of data in problem solving. Among their comments in appraising this area of their growth was the following.

> As students in the psychiatric integration program, we went through different stages of problem solving together. This process has become an integral part of my life. I use it all the time and find myself asking, "What am I feeling?" When one does this at least she becomes aware that a problem exists.

The students were able to use psychiatric content to identify and understand clinical problems. Every student was able to recognize a patient's anxiety in her first or second contact with him. In the early stage of learning psychiatric concepts, a student's observations were limited to a patient's manifest behavior. In later steps of the learning process, she was able to observe problems in thinking and perceiving as indicated by such processes as dissociation and denial and to incorporate these observations into the data about a patient's behavior. For example, in her work with a patient who, by going counter to medical and nursing prescriptions, was conspiring with fate not to recover from his illness, the student was able to recognize the manifestations of denial of illness. Although many of the students also had learned to appraise the level of anxiety (mild, moderate, severe, or panic) that was operating, errors in such an appraisal did occur, usually in the direction of underestimating the anxiety level.

The students' understanding of communication theory was exemplified not only by their more highly developed powers of observation but also by their ability to elicit patients' feelings, to raise pertinent questions, and to conceptualize some of the themes in interpersonal transactions. They were able to use the principles of communication on an operational level as was partially demonstrated in their effective relationships with authority figures, with whom they had established a higher order of explicit communication. In their analysis of patient behavior, the students had progressed from stereotyping behavior with such abstractions as *attention getting, complaining, demanding, depressed, hopeless, seductive,* and *uncooperative,* to describing a patient's verbal and nonverbal behavior, to exposing their own feelings in response to it, to conceptualizing some of the principles under-lying it, and to clarifying its meaning. On the other hand, the students continued to have considerable difficulty in applying their knowledge of personality growth and development except in their work with children.

The students' deeper grasp of role theory was evidenced by their increased ability to formulate the principles of their professional role and to make these operational, as for example, by setting appropriate limits with a patient who tries to set up a relationship that is antagonistic to the student's goals as a nurse.

They also had matured in their ability to give patient case presentations and were comfortable in exposing their relationships with patients to the total group. They analyzed and summarized the pertinent data. When miscar-riages occurred in their relationships with patients, they frequently were able retrospectively to conceptualize the process involved and to evaluate their nursing care. As was to be expected, it took them longer to transfer these formulations into the nursing situation, and they usually could do this only with help from the instructor.

When students functioned as observers of the group process, they re-ported their observations, which included their own subjective responses to the group interaction. As they progressed in the program they were able to identify, analyze, and summarize such elements of group dynamics as shifts in participation, role taking, and feeling tones and nuances, and to identify the steps in the problem-solving process. Some students were able to identify various conjunctive and disjunctive forces that operated in the clinical setting. Consequently, when disjunctive forces seemed to over-shadow the cohesive forces, the students were less apt to become blocked or to withdraw into passivity.

As might have been expected, the one overall area in nursing practice that continued to arouse a great deal of anxiety was the care of a dying patient. A few students gradually were able to relinquish some of their unrealistic hope and expectation that somehow they could cure the dying patient through nursing care, but these students were in the minority. Although the students continued periodically to resort to withdrawal from the dying patient, or to bury their feelings of sadness and their sense of loss in self-recrimination or in censuring clinical personnel for not having accom-plished the impossible, these feelings and attitudes came into the open sooner and, for the most part, after discussion of the dynamics involved, the students were able to handle the situation effectively.

In regard to the students' growth in psychiatric nursing performance, during the years when the psychiatric team had clinical conferences with the junior students, the initial period during which the students were unable to interact with patients was considerably shortened. In the project director's weekly clinical conferences in psychiatric nursing, she observed that the students' feelings of hopelessness about the psychiatric patient and about their own helplessness to alter his course came into the open earlier and that, although these feelings were intense, they were more quickly resolved. Accordingly, students became involved with patients sooner and were less preoccupied with themselves.

Clawson has also pointed out that during the period of the psychiatric integration project the students were able to work in greater depth with patients, they were eager to try out various approaches, and they became skillful in evaluating these approaches. It appeared that the students had started to close the gap that existed in their perception of normal and psychopathologic behavior and that perhaps they were beginning to view all behavior on a continuum.

It is important to point out, however, that in the clinical conferences and while serving as a psychiatric nursing consultant in medical and surgical situations, the psychiatric nurse observed that many students, even after having completed the course in psychiatric nursing, frequently were still unable to recognize the overt manifestations of psychopathology in patients on medical and surgical units. Upon further investigation of some of these examples of fragmented knowledge and experience, the psychiatric nurse learned that the students had come to identify psychiatric patients not so much in terms of behavior but rather with placement in a psychiatric setting, especially in terms of the routines that such settings have established for handling and controlling patients. Such a clear-cut example of selective inattention would seem to indicate the presence of a good deal of residual anxiety in relation to psychiatric patients. This finding underscored the necessity for keeping in mind that the integration of psychiatric concepts into professional nursing practice is not synonymous with the practice of psychiatric nursing.

By the junior year in their courses in psychiatric nursing, public health nursing, and team nursing, the students had made a good deal of progress in withstanding the anxiety that accompanies a problem-solving approach. Although they frequently bewailed the loss of credulities and on such occasions tended to lapse into a search for pat answers, they had begun to accept the principle that answers to the question of how to handle a patient's problems effectively evolve out of the analysis of the nurse-patient interaction. Included among the students' comments in reference to the emphasis on problem solving was the following comment of a senior student.

> We are taught to think—to use our past experiences in terms of the present and to problem-solve. I can go on a clinical unit where I have never been before and still work effectively. I think this is because there is such emphasis on principles. Then you can figure out the concrete. I learned a process, not just the facts.

As for the ability to apply the steps in the learning process in bringing about change and in solving clinical problems, as has been pointed out, the students were able to collect the pertinent data concerning emotional and social problems, to describe what was observed, to analyze these data, to formulate meanings and relationships including connections between past and present events, and to validate these meanings and relationships with other persons (the patient, a family member, the physician, the instructor, or the psychiatric nurse). Concerning the ability to intervene in patients' problems, for the most part, the students' competence was limited to initiating interventions in superficial problems. Generally, the students were unable to intervene in problems which involved a good deal of anxiety, conflict, dependency, regression, severe psychosomatic disorders, and personality disorganization. When on those rare occasions a student was skilled in negotiating such interventions, she usually did so on an intuitive level, and as a consequence, she was unable to formulate the principles underlying her interventions.

The psychiatric nurse did not concur with the commonly professed belief that the generic baccalaureate program in nursing either does or should prepare students to initiate nursing interventions in people's problems. She believed that it is the function of the collegiate program to impart the knowledge that is necessary to understand the meaning of behavior and to teach the processes that are involved in approaching and handling people's problems, but that it is as a graduate rather than as a student that the nurse moves into competency in intervention. Moreover, as has been pointed out, the psychiatric nurse did not believe that the graduate of a generic baccalaureate degree program in nursing should be prepared to initiate and implement nursing interventions which require her consciously to set up situations in which a patient's problems come into the open and are handled. Rather, this function is the responsibility of the clinical specialist in psychiatric nursing prepared in a master's degree program.

As has been pointed out in relation to the faculty's budding preoccupation with the psychiatric aspects of illness and nursing care, the students' tendency to fragment physical and emotional nursing care continued during the five years of the project. However, a qualitative change occurred in the character of the problem. Instead of avoiding the anxiety of interpersonal involvement with patients, the students, sometime in the junior year, were able to establish and become professionally involved in nurse-patient relationships.

Despite the psychiatric nurse's efforts to bring about some resolution of the students' bias against physical nursing care (by focusing on both the physical and emotional components in her course on psychodynamics and in the clinical conferences and by demonstrating the synthesis of nursing care in medical and surgical situations), the students' bias was still observable after they had completed the clinical program.

Methods of Psychiatric Integration

To assist others who conduct projects of this kind in the selection of the methods that they might use, an attempt has been made to appraise the effectiveness of each of the various methods employed in the Skidmore project and, in addition, to evaluate interdisciplinary teamwork as a method of psychiatric integration.

The three learning experiences for the faculty—the participation of the psychiatric team in the individual instructor's clinical conferences with her group of students, the individual conferences that each faculty member had with each member of the psychiatric team, and the weekly faculty group discussions with the psychiatric team—each had its strong points and its weak points.

CLINICAL CONFERENCES WITH THE INDIVIDUAL INSTRUCTOR AND STUDENTS

The clinical conferences which the instructors had with their students were in many ways superior to the faculty group discussions for the purpose of learning and teaching psychiatric concepts. In the clinical conferences with students, the sharply circumscribed nature of the subject matter, the focus on the instructor, and the psychiatric team's expectations of her opened the way for the instructor to seek help from the psychiatric nurse. Within this framework the clinical expertise of the psychiatric nurse became evident and could be more readily accepted. Neither the instructor nor the psychiatric nurse was required to take on the added burden of having to deal with the rest of the faculty members' approval, disapproval, lethargy, frustration, resentment, or competitiveness, and it was less necessary for the instructor to maintain a wall of resistance in the effort to keep from losing face with her professional colleagues.

The conferences also provided the psychiatric nurse with a greater opportunity to develop a personal relationship with each instructor than that provided by the faculty discussions, and she was less concerned with the instructor's approval or disapproval. Her role conflict was resolved when she became useful to the instructors, so that she did not find it necessary to relinquish her role or to engage in a power struggle with the psychiatrist.

One of the greatest advantages of the clinical conferences was that not only did they serve as a steppingstone in developing the instructor's ability to collaborate effectively with others but this goal was achieved within an interdisciplinary context.

This method also had some shortcomings. As has been pointed out, most of the instructors quite naturally approached the experience of working with the psychiatric team in the clinical conferences with students with greater apprehension than was evident in their approach to the faculty discussions. Although some of this apprehension undoubtedly was a carry-over from the instructors' negative attitudes toward the psychiatric team members during those sessions, some of this apprehension was also related to the fact that the instructor essentially was trapped as far as hiding her limitations in knowledge and skill from the psychiatric team was concerned.

Another disadvantage of this method was that the students could have interpreted the psychiatric team's presence in the conferences as signifying that their instructor was not knowledgeable and skillful enough to deal with the material herself; in the case of the Skidmore project, however, this issue never became a problem.

Another disadvantage related to the fragmentation of physical and emotional nursing care. Even though the psychiatric team's emphasis on understanding and handling patient behavior had always been within the context of a patient's medical condition, the presence of "behavioral experts" may have reinforced the faculty's and the students' inclination to play down the physical aspects of nursing care. One of the psychiatric team's mistakes was to assume that the instructors were putting equal stress on physical nursing care and that therefore the students' appreciation of the importance of meeting physical needs was firmly rooted. Such was not the case in all situations.

In the effort to intervene in the fragmentation of physical and emotional nursing care, the psychiatric team had considered the possibility of broadening the focus of the clinical conferences so as to include a detailed exploration and discussion of all the aspects of nursing care. Such a focus would have required extending the time of the clinical conferences from one hour to at least one and one-half or two hours. Because of the already crowded curriculum it was not possible to implement this modification.

INDIVIDUAL CONFERENCES

One of the chief advantages of the individual conferences that each member of the psychiatric team had with each faculty member was that these conferences provided a framework in which both members of the psychiatric team and the faculty members could personalize their relationship with each other. Another advantage was that the conferences made it possible to explore the problems of overlapping memberships in the groups of older and younger faculty members, to identify the controversial issues where the lines of conformity were sharply drawn, and to correct some of the faculty members' distorted notions about the integration program and the psychiatric team. In these interviews it was also possible for the faculty member to uncover and discuss problems which in her opinion were too threatening for group discussion.

The psychiatric nurse and the psychiatrist learned that the more two-way contacts they had with the faculty, the greater chance there was of establishing a higher order of communication between and among the faculty members, the students, and the psychiatric team. The individual conferences frequently opened the way for introducing changes that otherwise might have been more difficult, if not impossible, to implement.

The principal disadvantage in this method of psychiatric integration was that the time required in frequent individual conferences was considerable. However, because those experiences that were not shared automatically led to some misunderstanding between the faculty members and the psychiatric nurse and the psychiatrist, the team came to the realization that individual contacts are essential if maximum freedom of the faculty and the psychiatric team was to be achieved.

The Faculty Group Discussions

Because of the experimental nature of a psychiatric integration project, it is incumbent upon the person who directs such a project not only to utilize methods that hold some promise of achieving the goals of integration but also to try new methods as a way of broadening the professional field of endeavor. In the case of the Skidmore integration project, the small size of the faculty in the department of nursing provided the psychiatric nurse project director with an invaluable opportunity to experiment with group methods of bringing about change in the professional behavior of the faculty members.

The major contribution of the faculty group discussions was that they functioned as an instrument in facilitating the professional change and growth of the faculty members by setting up a higher order of communication—the secondary goal of the integration project. They helped to change some of the faculty members' professional standards and values, such as those that pertained to the expectations and evaluation of students. They helped to change the atmosphere of the faculty group by uncovering and healing over the schism between the two authority structures.

Another asset of the discussions was that they functioned as a medium through which the younger faculty members came to recognize their unique strengths and to learn how to more effectively handle their relationships with the older members. Among the younger members' comments about this value of the faculty discussions was the following.

> Even though I used to churn a mile a minute before going into the faculty discussions and, depending on what was happening, sometimes churned all through them, the meetings helped to free me professionally with the faculty and the students. I even find they helped me in my personal life. Because the

older faculty members already had authority and status within the group, they may have felt less need to have had the spotlight put on our relationships with each other. It was the younger group members who needed help in learning to recognize their own strengths and in learning how to handle their attitudes toward authority.

By focusing on intrafaculty relationships, it was almost as if you [*psychiatric nurse*] and Dr. Ullman became a voice for the younger members, who felt less powerful. With this kind of support, they came to recognize their own strengths and to feel more secure so that they no longer felt they had to crumble under or rebel against authority.

In discussing the advantages of the faculty group discussions, several faculty members emphasized that the psychiatric nurse's and the psychiatrist's acceptance and respect was a requisite for a successful learning experience. Among the comments of the older members the following was included.

The faculty group meetings were very helpful to me. We did a great deal of groping and exploring at first, but we were encouraged by you [*the psychiatric nurse*] and Dr. Ullman, and we needed your help. Although a certain amount of leadership came from the team, we were never pushed by them.

When someone did voice her anger, she was not rejected by the group. There were times when I expressed fears without being made to feel I was a coward for being afraid. It was a relief when tentative solutions to a problem had been worried through by the group. One reward of the meetings was the spirit of respect, trust, and comradeship that gradually built up in the group.

A younger faculty member made the following comment.

Of course there were occasions when I felt that our individual personalities were under scrutiny, and sometimes this made me very uneasy; there were times I got angry. But neither you [*the psychiatric nurse*] nor Dr. Ullman gave me the feeling that you thought I was stupid, or that you ridiculed me for my deficiencies. You both communicated respect, and I felt you accepted us even when we goofed. I think it was your and Dr. Ullman's acceptance of us, plus your expectation that we could and would change, that was the crux of the success of focusing on faculty relationships. Such an approach would be dynamite and be doomed to failure before it started if the psychiatric nurse or the psychiatrist communicated disrespect.

Despite the advantages of focusing on intrafaculty problems at the time of their occurrence, as far as the Skidmore project was concerned, the timing of this emphasis may have been unfortunate. A basic principle of any change process is that the process must begin at the point where the satisfactions derived from change are apt to outweigh the frustrations. Because the faculty schism was so apparent that it overshadowed the faculty members' problems as instructors, the psychiatric nurse and the psychiatrist may have been in too much of a hurry to try to resolve the faculty cleavage. They did not sufficiently consider or appreciate the fact that faculty schism is a social phenomenon inherent in the organizational structure of the American college and university. Perhaps the psychiatric nurse's and the psychiatrist's principal mistake was that in their work with the faculty they began at the highest level of psychiatric integration before the faculty members' confidence in them had been built up. The point at which the faculty members were being helped with their problems as nurse teachers—the fourth and fifth years of the project—might have been the starting point rather than the end-point of the group discussions.

As for the emphasis on the resolution of the difficulties in intrafaculty relations, perhaps this focus should have been perceived as a desired end rather than a beginning. As the data from the faculty discussions reveal, intrafaculty difficulties emerged also during the discussions of the faculty members' problems associated with their taking the role of teacher. It is within this context that intrafaculty relationships might have been discussed without adding further to the existing anxiety.

The central issue that continues to intrude itself, however, is that despite the numerous opportunities that existed for the faculty members and the psychiatric nurse to work together on problems and issues that arose in regard to teaching and to identify how these related to the need for psychiatric knowledge and skill, during the early years of the project the faculty members were fearful of exposing themselves and discussing their concerns as nurse teachers. Instead, the faculty was embroiled in the crossfire between the younger and older members.

Another alternative would have been to postpone all group work with the faculty, regardless of the focus, until each faculty member had had sufficient opportunity to experience the psychiatric nurse and the psychiatrist in an individual relationship and to be helped by them in the area of their teaching responsibilities. However, much of the difficulty in helping the faculty communicate more effectively stemmed from the influence that the faculty group had on the individual faculty member's attitudes. To appraise realistically the advantages of the group discussions for the Skidmore project, it should be recognized that as long as the values of the faculty as a group remained the same, the individual faculty members in the group continued to hold on to them tenaciously (1). It is highly questionable, therefore, whether the higher order of explicit communication that was established among the faculty members would have been achieved through methods other than the faculty group discussions with the psychiatric team.

In contrast to the psychiatric team's individual conferences with each faculty member, one of the principal disadvantages of the group discussions was that in the attempt to obtain the cooperation of both authority groups, it was extremely easy to bypass the leadership of either group or to become identified with one of them, thereby alienating the other group and widening the breach between the two. Another shortcoming was that unlike the situation of the psychiatric team's work with the individual instructor in her clinical conferences with her students, the instructor and the psychiatric nurse had to handle the rest of faculty members' and the psychiatrist's approval, disapproval, anxiety, frustration, hostility, and competitiveness. The constant interplay of statuses heightened the possibility that the faculty members and the psychiatric nurse would lose face in front of each other and the psychiatrist.

Another limitation was inherent in the experiential nature of the method, namely, the danger of crossing the border between experiential teaching and group psychotherapy. This possibility never materialized in the Skidmore project. A requisite for a successful group problem-solving experience is that any person who utilizes this method must be aware of and continually alert to the limits of an experiential teaching approach as contrasted with a formal psychotherapeutic approach. The following limits of the experiential group method are therefore made explicit (3).

1. The prevailing issues that are explored among the faculty members should be limited to those arising in connection with professional nursing practice, teaching, and colleague relationships.

2. Within this focus individual personalities should be under scrutiny only insofar as the attitudes and behavior intrude in the professional experiences of the nurse teacher. Concern should be centered exclusively on the present situation; the individual genetic and motivational factors should never be considered.

3. The desired increment in professional behavior should be one that can reasonably be assumed to be possible in persons who are striving toward greater professional competence. No such assumption can be made in a formal psychotherapeutic situation until unconscious sources of resistance have been eliminated.

Because the worth of any endeavor has to be measured against its cost, as a final point in assessing the value of the faculty group discussions, a central issue is whether in the long haul, the results of the faculty group discussions with respect to the degree of professional change and growth that were realized were worth the trauma to the psychiatric nurse and the rest of the faculty members. Would the psychiatric nurse use the method again in another situation?

In answering both questions the psychiatric nurse recognizes that the experiences of the Skidmore faculty never could be fully replicated. She also is cognizant that her own professional change and growth would enable her to perceive in new light whatever problems might arise in the future and to cope with them more effectively. Despite the anxiety, frustration, and hostility that were generated by the discussions, as far as the psychiatric nurse is concerned, she definitely would utilize this method again, provided the needs of a faculty indicated its use and if the circumstances were such to make its use feasible.

ACTIVITIES WITH THE STUDENTS

Because of the large number of activities in which the members of the psychiatric team worked with the students and because of the interlocking nature of many of these activities, it has been impossible to isolate what each one contributed to the students' change and growth. Among the students' comments on the general value of the psychiatric team's work with them, the following were included.

> Nursing itself can be learned anywhere. The psychiatric integration program broadened me as a person. It changed me and the way I think about things.

> The emphasis on the psychiatric aspects of nursing is the strongest and most valuable part of the Skidmore program.

Methods of Teaching Psychiatric Content. The value of the course in psychodynamics taught by the psychiatric nurse was demonstrated by the fact that it became a permanent part of the nursing curriculum.

In regard to the clinical conferences, in which the psychiatric team members served as resource personnel, among the comments made by the students was the following (see Chapter 11).

> That one particular clinical conference with you [*the psychiatric nurse*] and Dr. Ullman, in which we were discussing the problem of our poor class morale, was a turning point in my whole life. For the first time I understood what you both were trying to get across to us. When Dr. Ullman illustrated our problem with his diagram, it was as though my own problem had been drawn out on the blackboard. It was as if I could see my name, in lights.

The principal strength of the psychiatric team's participation in the clinical conferences with the sophomore and junior students was that, because the focus was on their work with other than psychiatric patients and behavior was discussed as existing on a continuum, the conferences helped to close the gap between the students' perception of normal and abnormal behavior. Another advantage was that the conferences provided the one opportunity for working with all the students on clinical problems in a group setting. A concomitant advantage, which was due solely to the nature of the curriculum, was that the clinical conferences during the junior year helped to build a bridge between the courses that were taught at the affiliating agencies and the rest of the curriculum and also to establish continuity of psychiatric integration in all the courses for which the Skidmore faculty assumed total responsibility.

The psychiatric nurse's work with selected patients on medical and surgical clinical units in collaboration with the students, the instructors, and the clinical personnel provided one of the most effective methods of psychiatric integration. The instructors and students increased their skill in identifying and formulating patients' problems, in recognizing situations when psychiatric nursing consultation seemed indicated, in utilizing the psychiatric nurse's knowledge and skills, and in collaborating with her. By taking care of patients herself, the psychiatric nurse demonstrated the synthesis of physical and emotional nursing care and thereby began to counteract the faculty's and the students' tendency to fragment total nursing care.

Although change and growth of the nursing service personnel was not a central aim of the project, the effect of these psychiatric nursing consultations on the hospital nursing staff should not be minimized or dismissed. Many positive relationships were established with staff, to the degree that some members regularly requested the psychiatric nurse to work with certain patients. Several unsolicited comments from nursing personnel indicated that they were beginning to recognize the value of psychiatric nursing consultation.

> We have enough patients with emotional problems to keep you busy all day, everyday.

> I'm beginning to think that maybe we should have a psychiatric nurse on the hospital staff that we can call upon to help us with difficult patients, just like the students have you to help them.

> When are you coming back again? I wish you could spend more time with us.

The nursing personnel started to come to grips with their need for help in developing their ability to apply psychiatric concepts to their nursing care of medical and surgical patients.

One of the disadvantages of this method of integration was that the student was not always readily available to participate directly with the psychiatric nurse in her work with a patient. From time to time, there was also some difficulty in clarifying with a head nurse the objectives of psychiatric nursing consultation and in evaluating with her the impact of the experience on nursing personnel.

As a method of integration, psychiatric nursing consultation opened up a myriad of possibilities for the future. For example, the psychiatric team began to explore the possibility of working with the instructors in the clinical setting with the purpose of further developing the instructors' skills in the supervisory process. Also there was the point that the psychiatric nurse's work may have contributed to laying the groundwork for the practice of liaison psychiatric nursing in the particular general hospital.

Methods in Helping Students to Change and Grow. In appraising the results of the unstructured student group conferences with the psychiatric nurse, some of the sophomore students at the end of the experience evaluated it as follows.

In these discussions I have found out more about the dynamic behavior of a group than I ever learned before. I feel that something very new and wonderful has been pointed out to me which I had never thought of before—that people in a group are very reluctant to talk about themselves. I think that this experience would be hard to improve upon. The difficulties we had were a normal part of the whole process of our learning to work as a group; this process is in itself a phenomenon that I am glad I have experienced.

In the beginning, I didn't understand the meaning or the reason for having these discussions, but toward the end of the experience, I was beginning to see their value. At the beginning I didn't see what could be discussed: I didn't think that people would have troubles concerning work they loved. This was my picture of things. Since then I've seen that no matter how much you love or enjoy something there will always be problems. As for improving this experience, somehow we needed to get this feeling of trust in each other and of closeness communicated before these discussions could be any help. This closeness has to come from the students. Only when they realize and see this fact can we start on a forward path. I realize this growth depends upon the students in the group.

I feel that these discussions have begun to show me many things, some of which are: how to look at group relations objectively and how to attempt to analyze these relations; how to come to some definite conclusions concerning the group's interaction and the role of each participant; and how to recognize that growth in group and individual personal relations is a long-range project requiring *hard work* and all of one's mental capacities. I have come to understand that the hindering factors are stages through which we must pass to achieve a mature level from which to "take off" for further growth.

Junior students who were having their experience in psychiatric nursing made the following comments.

In the small group discussions that we had with you [*the psychiatric nurse*] last year, I began to get clear on how much more effective we can be once we get out our feelings about what happens to us. I used to feel such relief. This experience made our whole class very close to each other.

I feel that the conferences helped me to better understand psychiatric patients.

All the students' reactions indicated that the unstructured student group conferences had helped them in at least two ways. First, by giving them the opportunity to work through some of their problems with authority figures, this experience helped them to become more comfortable with their instructors. Second, in the process of acquiring an appreciation of the importance of understanding the meaning of behavior and of learning how to handle it, the students became more receptive to psychiatric nursing.

Although the series of unstructured student group conferences was an excellent method for achieving the goals of psychiatric nursing, it is incumbent on any person who plans to utilize this method to recognize that successful outcomes besides being dependent on the leader's knowledge and skill are also dependent on the following three requisites.

1. The person who leads these conferences must be aware of her own anxiety. Her anxiety tolerance level must also be high enough for her to withstand faculty disapproval.

2. There must be agreement with both the faculty members and the students regarding the degree of confidence that is to be maintained and how confidential material is to be dealt with.

3. There must be recognition that the obstacles that are encountered in working with the students are an inherent part of the evolutionary process of group development.

The impact of the psychiatric nurse's and the psychiatrist's individual conferences with students was described in the following student comments.

> My conference with you [*the psychiatric nurse*] helped me to understand myself.

> It is important to have someone to relate to without being afraid of punishment. I felt I needed objectivity, and talking to you [*the psychiatric nurse*] helped me tremendously.

> The talks I had with you [*the psychiatric nurse*] and Dr. Ullman were most helpful to me during college.

Beginning in 1962–1963, a psychiatrist and a psychiatric social worker were employed by the college on a part-time basis. They were available for guidance and psychiatric consultation to students in all departments on the Skidmore campus. The psychiatric team members' experiences with those students who had problems that had interfered with their productivity and their guidance activities were a powerful motivating force in the action taken on the campus.

USE OF INTERDISCIPLINARY TEAMWORK

The welding of the psychiatric nurse and the psychiatrist into an effective collaborative team was a slow and arduous process and one punctuated with anxiety, challenge, conflict, and satisfaction. In the quest for new and better ways to deal with a broad spectrum of interpersonal problems, it is the wise psychiatric nurse educator who remains alert to the various advantages and disadvantages of interdisciplinary collaboration both to the project with which she is connected and to her as a member of the team.

From the point of view of the project as a whole, the main advantages of an interdisciplinary approach over an unidisciplinary one are the following.

1. More kinds of problems can be studied. In the Skidmore project, because of the psychiatrist's knowledge of diagnosis, treatment, and the psychodynamics of human behavior and the psychiatric nurse's knowledge of the psychodynamics and sociological principles of behavior, nursing care, and nursing education, they were able to undertake activities that neither could have handled alone.

2. Problems can be studied in greater breadth and depth when they are explored from more than one point of view. Moreover, the outcome of combining two points of view is greater than the sum of the separate points of view. The previous experience of both members of the Skidmore team with respect to teaching and focusing on interactional processes had been limited to work with patients and students. In their collaboration, their activities were expanded to include the faculty and its individual members.

3. The faculty and the students have the advantage of two specialists, each with unique knowledge and skills. They also have the opportunity to observe the physician-nurse relationship in action in other than a clinical situation and to see how the physician and the nurse utilize each other in an educational situation, how they deal with the problems of communication, and how they handle the differences that arise between them.

From the point of view of the team member, the advantages are the following.

1. The provision of a testing ground for different frames of reference enables the team member to expand his vision as he sees problems in a wider perspective.

2. In explaining the reasons for his conclusions about a problem to a member of another discipline, the team member has to clarify his own concepts and ideas. In the Skidmore project, the psychiatric nurse uncovered many of her blind spots about nursing, medicine, and teaching.

3. In the process of explaining his point of view, the team member develops a higher order of explicit communication.

4. Teamwork offers a challenge and an opportunity for the development of greater flexibility, security, and maturity since, as Redlich and Brody have emphasized, these characteristics are required to a considerably higher degree in interdisciplinary group work than when problem solving is carried out in isolation or in collaboration with colleagues of a homogeneous background (2).

From the overall point of view, the disadvantages are the following.

1. Teamwork is expensive. (This is a disadvantage of all teamwork, unidisciplinary as well as interdisciplinary.)
2. The team approach is time-consuming because of the time needed for the team members to communicate with each other. (Again, this applies to all teamwork, but it is particularly applicable to interdisciplinary teamwork because of the team members' differences in viewpoint and terminology.)

From the point of view of the team member, the disadvantages include the following.

1. Some autonomy and individual freedom must be relinquished. It is not as easy for a team member to take off on various excursions and tangents as it would be if he were working alone. (This is applicable to all teamwork.)
2. There is a greater pressure to arrive at answers and demonstrate positive results. (This is applicable to all teamwork.)
3. Learning about another's discipline is often accompanied by frustration.
4. Interpersonal pitfalls are greater than when one works alone or with a homogeneous group, and personal defenses against anxiety are not as effective in a group.

In this summary of the advantages and disadvantages of interdisciplinary collaboration, the bias on the side of the advantages is undoubtedly very much in evidence. This is natural, because it is based on the psychiatric nurse's experience in interdisciplinary collaboration. Had she had a different partner with whom to collaborate, quite an opposite picture might have emerged.

Summary

Insofar as could be determined without any instrument for objective measurement, the primary and secondary goals of the psychiatric integration project were achieved and each of the activities with the faculty and the students contributed to this achievement. If the project director were asked to rank the methods according to their productiveness, she would select, as most useful, two activities with the faculty—the faculty group discussions and the work with individual instructors in clinical conferences with their student groups—and three activities with students—the unstructured group discussions, the course in psychodynamics, and the psychiatric nursing consultations with selected patients on medical and surgical units.

REFERENCES

1. Lewin, Kurt K. *Resolving Social Conflicts*. New York: Harper and Row, 1948, pp. 49, 50.

2. Redlich, Frederick C., and Eugene C. Brody. "Emotional Problems of Interdisciplinary Research in Psychiatry," *Psychiatry: Journal for the Study of Interpersonal Processes*, 233–239 (August, 1955).

3. Schmahl, Jane A., and Montague Ullman. "The Three Phases of Psychiatric Integration in Nursing Education," *Integration of Psychiatric Nursing Concepts in Baccalaureate Basic Programs*. New York: National League for Nursing, 1963, pp. 4–13.

Chapter Sixteen

CONCLUSIONS: NEED
FOR FURTHER CHANGE

If the way which, as I have shown, leads hither seems very difficult, it can nevertheless be found. It must indeed be difficult since it is so seldom discovered; for if salvation lay ready to hand and could be discovered without great labour, how could it be possible that it should be neglected almost by everybody? But all noble things are as difficult as they are rare.

BARUCH SPINOZA.

The significance of the Skidmore psychiatric integration project is not limited to the educational program in which it was conducted. The remainder of the discussion will be devoted to a consideration of what the author believes to be some of the implications of her main findings for master's education in nursing, psychiatric integration in baccalaureate education, and nursing practice.

In the formulation of these conclusions, recognition was given to the built-in limitations of the Skidmore faculty as a representative sample of nursing faculties in baccalaureate programs across the country—the small size of the faculty; the fact that the graduate preparation of all but one nurse faculty member was obtained in two institutions, both of whose programs focused on the functional aspects of the nurse leader's role rather than on the development of clinical expertise and neither of which had a generic baccalaureate program in nursing. Nor was the possibility overlooked that by mere coincidence a group of faculty members who had difficulty in applying psychiatric content had converged in one particular setting. In other words, it was necessary to curb the kind of premature generalizations that lose sight of what is peculiar to the situation under study and to attend to only what this situation shares with other baccalaureate programs in nursing.

The author took into account the reports of the other psychiatric integration projects, Jean Campbell's report on a study of master's education in nursing (3), and the report of a study on teacher preparation in the United States (4), as well as her own experiences with faculty members and students in other baccalaureate and master's degree programs and her personal communications with persons who have directed or are directing psychiatric integration projects. These various studies and experiences have indicated that a number of the problems and issues that were encountered by the psychiatric team who worked in the Skidmore project occur in varying forms and degrees in other college and university settings.

The Challenge to Master's Education

Before consideration is given to some of the possible implications of psychiatric integration in baccalaureate education for the preparation of nurse teachers, it seems important to consider two questions. Is it realistic and in the nursing profession's best interest to expect all nurse teachers in baccalaureate and master's degree programs to be able to utilize psychiatric content in nursing practice and in the teaching-learning process? What about those nurse teachers who have highly developed skills in other areas such as administration or research, or superior knowledge in other fields important to nursing education, such as the physical or biological sciences?

The answers to these questions most likely depend upon whether the nursing profession as a whole, nursing educators in general, and a particular faculty subscribe to or eschew two assumptions: (1) that professional nurses can and must carry a greater share of the direct nursing care of patients, and (2) that in addition to the functions delegated to the nurse by the physician (which because of this delegation might be classified as dependent functions), professional nursing has independent *nursing* functions.

Acceptance of the first assumption requires nursing educators to be aware of changes of the ecology of illness. Because many of the physical illnesses have been conquered, the balance sheet of illness in this country is heavily weighted on the side of chronic illness, the illnesses of old age, and the yet incurable diseases, the very nature of which requires the nurse to recognize and to reduce stress and fear. Acceptance of the second assumption also leads to educational emphasis on the behavioral sciences, on which the independent functions of nursing are primarily based, in contrast to the dependent functions, which are to a considerable extent based on the medical, physical, and biological sciences (1).

In the Skidmore program, the curriculum revisions and the psychiatric integration project were based on these two assumptions, as is this book. Therefore, the conclusions and recommendations presented here are based on the belief that the purpose of baccalaureate education in nursing is not to prepare nurses to give *more* nursing care but rather, to give a *different kind* of nursing care.

This concept of baccalaureate nursing education requires that the nurse teacher be a clinical specialist who is skilled in recognizing and identifying overt and covert nursing problems, analyzing them in terms of scientific and nursing principles, and formulating and initiating interventions that are founded on such principles. From this it follows that master's education in nursing has no other recourse but first, to prepare all future nurse teachers to achieve mastery in the practice of their chosen clinical specialty, and second, to achieve a high level of competence in teaching professional nursing care to students.

In emphasizing the need for this kind of advanced preparation, the author is not suggesting that the task of master's education is to turn graduate students into jacks of all trades and masters of none. Nor is she implying that one of the goals of master's education should be to transform all future nurse teachers into psychiatric nurses; it cannot be expected that every nurse teacher will be able to initiate and implement interventions on psychopathologic behavior which require her consciously to set up situations in which a patient's problems come into the open and then are channeled. This level of intervention continues to be the function of the nurse who has been prepared in a master's program in psychiatric nursing.

If the author's findings in the Skidmore study of psychiatric integration are correct, the majority of the faculty members were inadequately prepared to function either as a clinical specialist or as a teacher. As has been emphasized, whatever knowledge of the learning process and of social science content they had acquired was apparently "known" only on the verbal level. One might postulate, of course, that the Skidmore faculty consisted essentially of a group of nurse teachers who, by chance, happened not to be comfortable in dealing with the subjective responses of patients and students and in utilizing the problem-solving process, or who, for personal reasons, during their master's programs resisted all attempts to educate them to utilize this knowledge. However, the extent to which their knowledge was increased and the degree to which their skill in translating verbalized formulations into nursing practice and teaching was developed during the project, constitutes valid testimony that they possessed the necessary potential to have acquired this knowledge and to have developed these skills in their graduate programs. It therefore seems likely that their deficient preparation did not stem solely from personal resistance (of which there was a great deal in response to the psychiatric integration program) or from limited intellectual capacity, but that, instead, it could be charged to inadequate preparation.

The author further believes that master's education in nursing has been woefully inadequate in preparing the future nurse teacher with respect to the other essential clusters of knowledge and skill: to utilize what man has discovered about the learning process; about the growth and development of physical and intellectual competencies; about the cognitive processes involved in speculating about unobserved events from empirical data, in tracing the implications of these events and in judging and conceptualizing the whole piece by the pattern that has been identified; and about the methods and techniques of communicating to others what one has learned. Similarly, judging from the outcomes, master's education in nursing has not been particularly successful in helping the student to develop her potential for *feeling* professional experience in its totality so fully that she is well on her way to knowing any particular corner of it. In the author's opinion, these deficiencies are not likely to be overcome until some consensus is reached concerning the characteristics of master's education in nursing—its students, its curriculums, and its faculties—vis-à-vis its purposes.

THE GRADUATE STUDENTS

As has been pointed out in Campbell's report, the first decision that must be faced about master's programs in nursing is whether they are to serve as a "fifth year of undergraduate study, postgraduate study, a first period of graduate study, or *the* [only] period of graduate study." As far as clinical nursing content is concerned the decision at present is a dictated one because of the educational foundations of many graduate students.

As was noted by Margaret Bridgman over a decade ago (2) and more recently by Campbell, the upper-division major in baccalaureate programs should be the base on which specialization in nursing on the master's degree level is built. However, a large number of candidates for the master's degree have come from the pool of diploma program graduates who earned a baccalaureate degree specifically designed for registered nurse students and which, in many instances, has not adhered to the requirements of most generic baccalaureate programs in nursing (5, 6).

As a consequence of the deficiencies of candidates for the master's degree, one of the principal functions of master's education in nursing has, to date, consisted of filling in the gaps in preparation that is neither adequate nor appropriate for truly professional nursing and then attempting to build a superstructure on this pieced-together foundation. The first part of this task is by no means easy or always possible; it requires the nurse teacher on a graduate faculty to stir a sediment of stereotyped ideas and to break through crystallized perceptions, codified values, and ritualized approaches to problem solving that have been inculcated upon graduate students in their undergraduate preparation. The second part of the task is therefore usually abandoned. In essence it appears that, insofar as nursing content is concerned, most master's programs in nursing have functioned as a fifth year of undergraduate study.

THE CURRENT CURRICULUMS

There appears to be little agreement among graduate faculties on a definition of nursing as a subject for advanced study. Historically, the focus of specialization has been a functional one—the preparation for positions as administrators, supervisors, teachers, and consultants, who usually functioned in nursing service settings and diploma programs in nursing. The curriculum pattern was adapted from the pattern of preparation of teachers and administrators for the elementary and secondary school levels. Campbell's findings have revealed that the functional focus in master's education in nursing persists to a considerable degree. Of the thirty-five institutions in her study, the focus of seventeen was identified as clinical, of twelve as functional, and of four as both clinical and functional, whereas two had varied concentrations for specialization (3).

Because the nursing profession must take more responsibility for providing direct nursing care to patients and because the fulfillment of this responsibility is dependent on the development of clinical and teaching expertise, the following recommendation is made regarding the focus of specialization in nursing.

Nurse-teacher preparation requires a double focus: the study of a delimited area of clinical nursing which is based on upper-division courses of the undergraduate major, and the study of the teaching-learning process.

The Clinical Focus. As a result of the tendency to neglect the clinical aspect of master's degree education and the deficient preparation of many master's degree students, nursing education has been handicapped in the identification of advanced content in nursing. Even when these handicaps are overcome, the development of advanced content will be obstructed by the lack of consensus about what areas of knowledge are foundational requisites for clinical expertise. As has been pointed out, it is this author's belief that knowledge derived from graduate-level instruction in the social sciences is essential if systematic and theoretically sound analysis is to replace the present intuitive and anecdotal state of nursing practice and education. Such a belief presumes consensus about a core of social science content that is common to all master's curriculums in nursing.

That such a consensus is far from being arrived at is attested to by Campbell's study. Of the fifty-six clinical nursing faculty members in graduate programs who were asked to identify the specific subject areas in the undergraduate nursing curriculum that are crucially relevant to graduate study, only nine, all of whom taught psychiatric nursing (of whom there were twelve in all), specified growth and development. Of the respondents who specified the social and behavioral sciences as being crucial, the instructors in psychiatric nursing were at the top of the range; next were the instructors in maternal-child nursing, then the instructors in medical-surgical nursing, with the instructors in public health nursing being at the lower end of the range. Of the eighty-nine respondents who were asked to identify the aspects of the undergraduate major in nursing that are crucial for graduate study, seven respondents—six instructors in psychiatric nursing (out of twenty-two) and one instructor in medical nursing (out of twenty-nine)—specified the ability to use knowledge of psychiatric nursing (3).

No single subject area was identified as essential for the master's curriculum by at least 50 per cent of the eighty-six respondents in Campbell's study. The only respondents who specified growth and development as essential for the advanced core were some of the instructors in maternal-child nursing, and they represented only 38 per cent of their group. The only respondents who specified the discipline of psychiatry were some instructors in psychiatric nursing, who represented only 36 per cent of their group. The pattern of respondents who specified the social and behavioral sciences as an essential aspect of the graduate core of study was identical with that pertaining to the essentiality of this area in the undergraduate program: the instructors in psychiatric nursing ranked first in percentage of affirmative answers and the instructors in public health nursing ranked last (3).

In view of the absence of a generally accepted theory of professional nursing practice and of sufficient consensus about the subject areas that should provide the core of master's education in nursing, the recommendations are the following.

1. In the attempt to build a theory of professional nursing practice, nursing research should begin to focus on studying the methods the professional nurse uses to facilitate change in the patient's responses to illness, medical treatment, hospitalization, and nursing care and to facilitate change in his willingness and skill in the use of positive health practices, and also to study the kind of patients in whom such change is brought about.

2. The results of this research should be used in the development of a core of social science and nursing knowledge for all master's degree curriculums in nursing.

The Functional Focus. The discrepancy between the nurse teacher's acquisition of knowledge of clinical nursing and her ability to apply it in her work with students reflects limitations in knowledge about what kind of educational practices have what effects on what kind of students (8). It reflects the absence of a generally accepted theory of human growth and development from which the nursing faculty can state certain hypotheses about the relationship between educational goals and teaching methods.

The gap between knowledge and application also reflects a major bias of nursing educators, namely, the assumption that "talking about" psychiatric content and the principles of the learning process is synonymous with applying them in action and that to wax dithyrambic about feelings is equivalent to the life experience of feeling. This assumption is built solidly into the learning experiences, the methods of teaching, and the language used in graduate nursing education. As a consequence, the nurse teacher in a graduate program is apt to be unable to develop learning experiences and to utilize teaching methods and operational language that would assist future nurse teachers to develop the cognitive skills of abstraction and conceptualization and would enable them to connect these skills with the use of the self in professional relationships.

Because the preparation of nurses for teaching now consists largely of courses in methodology rather than an analysis of how to consciously relate the ends and means of educational practices, the following recommendations were made.

1. Nursing education should begin to focus on studying the effects of teaching methods on students by identifying which methods facilitate what kinds of professional change in what kinds of students.

2. The methodology of teaching, instead of being presented in separate courses as a distinct body of knowledge (which assumes that predictive generalizations which are valid in every teaching-learning situation have been identified), should be presented within the context of a practicum of teaching.

A field practicum in teaching of approximately eight weeks, preferably concurrent with other courses, should be required of all future nurse teachers. During this experience the competence of graduate students would be evaluated under conditions set up by the university. There would be continuous observation of students by experienced, cooperating nurse teachers in basic programs in nursing. The experience would include several weeks of full-time responsibility for conducting classes in their respective area under the guidance of the cooperating nurse teacher.

3. A master teacher, whose qualifications include much practical experience, should be appointed to the graduate faculty to function as an instructor in clinical teaching. This faculty member, in consultation with the instructors in each clinical nursing specialty, would have the responsibility to place students where the finest quality of nursing instruction is available. In seminars with small groups of students, the instructor in clinical teaching would function with the graduate student in a master teacher—apprentice relationship by amplifying and extending what the cooperating teacher is teaching.*

* This recommendation is based in part on recommendations by James Bryant Conant (4).

THE FACULTY

One way in which nursing education is attempting to develop a graduate nursing education of consequence is by dealing with the problem of inadequately prepared nurse teachers in master's programs. Graduate education in nursing is moving in the direction of requiring the doctorate as the minimum degree for teaching in graduate programs, thereby bringing itself in line with graduate education as a whole. At least two problems emerge in this connection, however.

The first problem pertains to the insufficient number of recruits and inadequate facilities for doctoral programs. According to Campbell's study of the 360 faculty members who were involved in graduate instruction (which included non-nurses holding doctorates from other disciplines), 75, or approximately 21 per cent, held a doctoral degree, 283, or approximately 78 per cent, held a master's degree, and of the remaining two individuals, one held a certificate from graduate school and the other a baccalaureate degree (3).

The second problem pertains to the spiraling effect of the past and present deficiencies of baccalaureate degree programs in nursing. In view of Campbell's findings that, insofar as nursing is concerned, most master's programs have functioned as a fifth year of undergraduate preparation, to what extent are the sins of master's programs being visited on doctoral programs?

It will be some time before there is a sufficient supply of adequately prepared nurses to teach in master's programs. Therefore the immediate question is: Pending the improvement of master's programs in nursing, how are the inadequately prepared graduate faculty members to be helped to become the kind of teachers they are capable of becoming?

As a way of trying to close the hiatus in the teaching of psychiatric content, two recommendations are made concerning the continuing education of graduate faculty members.

1. Any university that offers a graduate program in nursing should arrange for those of its faculty members who either have not had psychiatric nursing experience or whose experience has been inadequate, to make up this deficiency either in its own psychiatric nursing department or in another university which has psychiatric nursing faculty members who are competent to provide and supervise a graduate-level educational experience. This experience should consist of the graduate faculty member working with psychiatric patients in individual relationships and in groups. The selection of the experience should take into account the clinical specialty of the graduate faculty member; for example, the nurse who teaches in a graduate program in pediatric nursing would work with emotionally disturbed and mentally retarded children.

To facilitate the transfer of psychiatric nursing knowledge thus obtained, the psychiatric nursing experiences should be augmented by seminars planned and conducted jointly by the psychiatric nurse teacher and a faculty member in the area of the learner instructor's clinical specialty. Such a provision assumes that the university offering the experience also offers advanced preparation in the clinical specialty of the learner instructor.

2. To provide nurse faculties in graduate programs with an opportunity for a group attack on professional problems of mutual concern, including the improvement of their members' effectiveness in utilizing psychiatric and behavioral science content, universities conducting graduate programs in nursing should institute ongoing in-service education programs similar to those that have been utilized in some of the psychiatric integration programs in baccalaureate-degree nursing programs.

Because in-service education in nursing has to date been restricted largely to nursing service settings and diploma programs in nursing, and because of the resistance that is bound to be engendered when a graduate faculty member is faced with the disturbing reality that her graduate preparation no longer is adequate to meet the rapidly changing health needs of society, unbiased consideration of the advantages and disadvantages of these two proposals is not easy. Such consideration requires graduate faculties to be willing and able to look at the way things are as well as at the way they might wish them to be. As has been pointed out in reference to psychiatric integration projects in baccalaureate programs (see p. 4), continuing education for graduate faculties would not serve as a substitute for appropriate doctoral preparation of nurse teachers, but, rather, would be a way of handling the present situation. Whether or not graduate faculties would need the impetus of a formal integration project probably would depend on the degree of motivation on the part of the faculty members and their capacity for and the degree of resistance to change. Another factor, which pertains to both of the recommendations, is the availability of sufficient funds to implement them.

The second problem that emerges in relation to improving the quality of teacher preparation in master's programs is the lack of the graduate faculty's direct teaching contact with students in a generic baccalaureate program. For example, of the 127 faculty members in Campbell's study who were not directors of programs, 62 taught graduate students only and 45 taught graduate students and registered nurse baccalaureate students. Campbell has stated (3),

> Only 20 individuals indicated a specific teaching involvement with basic baccalaureate students. Of the 20, 11 also taught registered nurse baccalaureate students. . . . In 5 of the study programs, a basic program was not offered at the time of the interview, therefore, direct opportunity for validation was

never available. In 17 other programs, no graduate faculty member interviewed, with the exception of four directors, had a teaching load involving basic students. In six other institutions, only one faculty member in each indicated such teaching responsibility.

In regard to the significance of the insulation of graduate from generic baccaulaureate education for the quality of graduate teaching, Campbell has stated (3),

> Advanced study at the graduate level presumably rests upon an undergraduate major. It would seem logical, therefore, for much of the involvement at the baccalaureate level to be with the standard establishing group—the basic student group.

She further has stated,

> The extensive involvement of graduate faculty with the registered nurse student and the exclusion of the generic student raises many questions. . . . How delayed or distorted may the development of content in nursing be if those developing it do not have continuing recourse to the reality of the nursing subject as it develops and changes? How adequate is the preparation of future nurse teachers when faculty providing the instruction in the role area have little contact with learners in the curriculum which prepares for professional practice and in which these future teachers will teach?

The time has come for weighing the advantages against the disadvantages of masters programs in nursing conducted by educational units in nursing which do not offer a generic baccalaureate program. In the author's opinion, the disadvantages of such master's programs seem to outweigh the advantages.

Psychiatric Integration in Baccalaureate Education

One of the principal findings of the Skidmore project was the tendency of the faculty members and students to fragment the physical and emotional-social components of illness and nursing care. This finding has particular relevance for the structure of the nurse teacher's role in baccalaureate degree programs.

On the one hand, it might be assumed that the deepening of some grooves of professional practice is apparently inevitable in any profession or occupation and that this emphasis of the part must involve some deterioration of the whole. On the other hand, the problem of fragmentation of nursing care points up the underlying issue that the teacher of baccalaureate-level nursing is caught within the administrative line of the hierarchal structure of both the university and health agencies, insofar as they do not encourage her to function as a clinical practitioner in the sense of giving nursing care to patients.

Even though the baccalaureate nursing teacher works with patients through her students, this role is not synonymous with the continuing development of her own clinical expertise by the giving of direct care to patients. The nurse teacher's contacts with patients are segmented and for the most part limited to the level on which the baccalaureate student is able to function at a given time. It might well follow, therefore, that little by little, without becoming aware of what is happening, the nurse teacher loses her perspective of the total picture of nursing needs and thereby cannot synthesize all aspects of nursing care.

In regard to the problem of role structure of the baccalaureate nursing teacher, the following recommendation is made.

Research should focus on the identification of ways in which the two aspects of the role of the nurse teacher in a baccalaureate degree program— a teacher of students and a nurse who provides direct nursing care for patients—can be reconciled.

The belief that there is need for psychiatric integration programs in master's education leads to the sticky issue of whether the psychiatric nurse who works primarily in integration should be regarded as a temporary or a permanent member of the staff of a baccalaureate degree program in nursing. With the improvement of baccalaureate and masters degree programs in nursing, it is to be expected that there will follow a new generation of nursing educators who in their own undergraduate and graduate programs have attained reasonable knowledge of psychiatric content and skill in applying the content to the care of patients as well as to the teaching of students. Does this mean that the psychiatric nurse teacher will be freed from the obligation of leadership in psychiatric integration and will be able to concentrate on her other responsibilities to continue to teach psychiatric nursing on the undergraduate level, prepare psychiatric nurse specialists in master's degree programs, work with psychiatric patients, and do research?

Because of rapid changes and progress in the field of psychiatry, there will probably always be need for a psychiatric nurse to assist the undergraduate faculty in the teaching of total nursing care to all patients. But as the preparation of nurse teachers improves, the psychiatric nurse will have to modify her goals and *modus operandi*. For the purpose of establishing and maintaining continuity between the course in psychiatric nursing and the rest of the curriculum, the following recommendation is made.

In the case of a baccalaureate program whose faculty is well prepared in psychiatric concepts, rather than bring in an outside expert in psychiatric nursing to function on a part-time basis as a consultant and resource person to the faculty, the psychiatric nurse faculty member who is charged with the overall responsibility for the course in psychiatric nursing should take these roles. It would be her function to stimulate further the faculty's interest in social behavior, interpersonal relations, and research germane to their area of work.

QUALIFICATIONS FOR WORKING IN PSYCHIATRIC INTEGRATION

Considering the broad gulf that yawns between the quality of current baccalaureate and master's degree programs in nursing and the cultural lag that exists between the recognition of the need to improve master's education for nurses and the implementatiion of such changes, it is likely that psychiatric integration programs as they are known today will continue to play a vital part in baccalaureate nursing education for some time to come. In both her present role in psychiatric integration and her future role, which would include responsibility for the course in psychiatric nursing, the psychiatric nurse functions as a change agent in relation to faculty, students, and clinical personnel. Like any other approach to change, psychiatric integration, whether it is within the context of current problems raised by inadequate nurse teacher preparation or future improvements, is not a fountain at which all psychiatric nurse educators can or should bathe. However, the psychiatric nurse who is willing to invest herself in psychiatric integration either in the present or the future may want to consider how she might better prepare herself to deal with the complexities that are woven into the fabric of the integration and consultation process. In discussing the qualifications for working in psychiatric integration and consultation programs, the following three areas will be discussed: (1) education and experience, (2) degree of motivation, and (3) personal characteristics.

Education and Experience. To be able to achieve a successful and satisfying experience in integrating psychiatric content, the psychiatric nurse on the faculty of a baccalaureate degree program must be an expert clinician in the nursing care of psychiatric patients. She should have completed an advanced program in psychiatric nursing and hold the master's degree. She also should have had sufficient experience in psychiatric nursing beyond her clinical learning experiences in educational programs to have developed clinical expertise with patients. This task is not simple to accomplish, especially in view of the social structure of nursing which encourages nurses to give up direct contact with patients. With a high degree of motivation and resourcefulness, however, the psychiatric nurse can continue to develop her clinical skills, not as an administrator, not as a supervisor or teacher of students, but as a nurse of patients.* Not only must the psychiatric nurse

---

* Throughout the author's experience on two collegiate faculties, she spent approximately eight hours a week in working with psychiatric patients in a variety of clinical settings. Margaret C. Haley, dean, School of Nursing, Seton Hall University, and Agnes Gelinas, former chairman, Department of Nursing, Skidmore College, agreed to this arrangement at the time she was appointed to their faculties, and they supported her throughout the endeavor.

be an expert with the psychiatric patients, but since much of her work is apt to be in the area of liaison psychiatric nursing in which she functions as a clinical nursing consultant to the faculty, students, and clinical personnel in the general hospital, she also must have some general knowledge of medical and surgical conditions.

The very nature of psychiatric integration also requires that the psychiatric nurse be a master teacher. There already are multiple complexities built into the integrative process without the psychiatric nurse being required to synthesize what she has learned in her graduate program in psychiatric nursing with learning how to teach. Ideally, then, the psychiatric nurse should have had some experience in curriculum development and teaching psychiatric nursing, preferably in a generic baccalaureate degree program.

Degree of Motivation. During the author's work with graduate students from another university who were having supervised field practice in psychiatric integration and in conferences with other psychiatric nurses who were planning to work in integration programs or had just begun to do so, she became cognizant of the aura of magic with which many of these nurses surrounded the entire endeavor of psychiatric integration. This charismatic view was manifested by the ascription of unrealistic power and prestige to the role of project director. In several situations, it could well have seduced the future or neophyte project director into hoping and expecting that some of this magic, in terms of power and prestige, would rub off on herself.

In such circumstances, the concept of psychiatric integration is divorced from the reality problems implicit in the process of change. Instead of coping with these problems on a level of self-involvement, the psychiatric nurse with a distorted view of her power is more likely to put her major emphasis on sustaining the myth of magic.

To be genuinely motivated to work with the faculty in teaching total nursing care, perhaps the psychiatric nurse needs to have experienced some sense of frustration in achieving her goals in teaching psychiatric nursing because of the insufficient preparation of students. Before the psychiatric nurse is willing to collaborate with the faculty and members of other disciplines, she also may have needed to have experienced a lack of challenge in working alone. Perhaps before she can reach out in true partnership to others, she first must have had sufficient experience and achieved enough security to be able to face the limitations of her own professional discipline.

In a pioneer and collaborative endeavor, such as psychiatric integration, in which one's individual autonomy and freedom necessarily are reduced, the psychiatric nurse's professional goals must be synthesized with the goals of the faculty and student groups. In the face of such demands, it is perfectly legitimate for the psychiatric nurse to consider what plums are available. The personal motivating factors such as salary, prestige, and papers published are important.

Personal Characteristics. As has been demonstrated throughout this book, the psychiatric nurse is first, last, and always a human being, after which she then is a nurse, a psychiatric nurse, a teacher, an "integrator," a consultant, and a resource person. Whether she works with psychiatric patients or in psychiatric integration, she studies human life. Thus the first characteristic for working in integration and consultation programs is the willingness to become involved. Involvement requires the psychiatric nurse to be in contact with and to understand her own feelings and to relate to the human core of those with whom she works, which involves the experiencing and revelation of her own feelings.

Professional involvement leads directly into the second characteristic: eagerness to learn from others—collaborative partners, other faculty members, students, clinical personnel, and patients. The desire to learn includes the ability to appreciate differences. The psychiatric nurse must be able to function productively without having the answers. She must be able to recognize and accept her limitations and those of her discipline, as well as those of the faculty members, the students, and the other persons with whom she might collaborate.

A third characteristic is the capacity to change. In psychiatric integration and consultation, the psychiatric nurse must be challenged by the need to look at problems from different points of view and by the possibility of adapting her insights and skills to all areas of nursing education and practice. The psychiatric nurse must therefore be willing to give up some autonomy and freedom and relinquish some long-cherished ideas and concepts without experiencing a loss of herself personally or professionally.

The fourth characteristic is the psychiatric nurse's ability to tolerate high levels of anxiety, frustration, and loneliness. She must be able to wait for the faculty's acceptance even though she thinks she knows the answers to a problem. She must be tough enough to withstand battering by her professional colleagues when they feel threatened. Yet she also must be sensitive and soft enough to keep in tune with their needs, hopes, and aspirations.

These personal characteristics have particular significance for the preparation of psychiatric nurses. An essential question that must be reckoned with is how nursing education can produce the kind of psychiatric nurse that will mature not only in a technical but also in an emotional sense. It is more likely that a psychiatric nurse can better withstand the uncertainty and frustration of exploring the uncharted territories of psychiatric integration and consultation if she has achieved a reasonable degree of personal fulfillment outside the realm of her professional life. There are probably those psychiatric nurses to whom life has been kind insofar as they have been able to develop an enduring pattern of meaningful interpersonal relationships which can sustain them throughout the pushes and pulls of psychiatric integration. Then there are other psychiatric nurses who because they have experienced more serious developmental misfortunes may need to work through some of their problems of unresolved attitudes toward authority, drive for power and status, need for approval, and fear of disapproval, through the process of psychotherapy. It is not possible to say with certainty, but the process of professional change might well be facilitated if the psychiatric nurse has undergone a personal therapeutic inventory.

The Improvement of Patient Care

Somewhere along the way the nursing profession will have to disentangle the Gordian knot of how the generic baccaulaureate student can utilize her knowledge and skill as a graduate. In other words, will the nursing care provided for patients be any better now as compared with the period prior to the integration of psychiatric content in nursing education? In discussing this problem, Laura L. Simms has raised several provocative questions (9).

> How is the clinical expertise of graduates to reach patients? Through *supervision* of staff who work directly with patients? Through *consultation* with the nursing team? Through a *liaison* who coordinates services of many departments? Through a *nurse practitioner* who is charged with the ultimate responsibility for all aspects of a comprehensive type of nursing care for a selected group of patients?

These questions point to the fact that like the medical profession, the nursing profession faces the problem of how to bridge the ravine that separates the learning of psychiatric theory as a baccalaureate student and being helped to apply this knowledge as a graduate. But a much deeper problem is how the graduate is to adapt the practice of patient-centered care to the bureaucratic structure of the hospital, which, because efficiency is its major goal, has an elaborate division of labor with a lengthening line of administrative command.

As has been emphasized, the primary consequence of this bureaucratic interference for the nursing profession is that instead of giving nursing care to patients, nurses are managing the hospital. Because nurses have delegated bodily care to ancillary workers, patients are frequently cared for by persons who are least equipped to do so. It is no wonder that baccalaureate faculty and students and professional nursing service personnel may be inclined to look upon physical nursing care as unchallenging and degrading.

It is in the hospital or health agency where nursing education and nursing service must join together. If, however, nurses continue to be wholly committed to the shibboleths of "administration," "supervision," "teaching," and "consultation" rather than to patient care, there would seem to be little justification for the existence of a nursing profession, let alone the concerted effort of nursing educators to incorporate psychiatric content into baccalaureate curriculums.

Despite the overall picture of the nursing profession's flight from the patient's bedside, several attempts are being made to add another dimension—the provision of direct nursing care. To cite only a few examples, Frances Reiter has theoretically formulated and has implemented an operational structure by which the professional nurse can completely break with the traditional pattern of running the hospital and instead be able to carry out direct nursing care functions by adapting them to the existing pattern of hospital organization (7). Faye G. Abdellah, et al., have formulated the problems of patient-centered care and have identified some of the central issues that are involved in the nursing service personnel's movement from the functions of hospital management to patient-centered care (1). Simms has colorfully described an experiment in which a graduate of the Skidmore program worked directly with a group of selected patients from before admission to the hospital through discharge (9).

The work of Reiter, Abdellah, et al., and Simms, provides several guidelines for some possible ways of moving from managerial to clinical nursing functions. Among these guidelines are included the following.

1. The administration of nursing functions and the provision of direct nursing care could be set up under two separate nursing service organizational structures.

2. The professional nurses who would be responsible for providing direct nursing care would operate within the *clinical line* of the nursing service organizational structure. These nurses would not be assigned to a time shift or to a work location—their names would not appear on the time or assignment sheet. Consequently, they would be free to work wherever and whenever they might deem necessary for achieving the goals of nursing care. Regarding the lines of authority and communication, these nurses would be directly responsible to the nurse in charge of the particular department (medicine, surgery, psychiatry, and so on) rather than to the head nurse of a particular nursing unit.

3. The professional nurses who would be responsible for the administration of nursing and clinical units (among whom might be staff nurses, head nurses, and supervisors) would operate with the *administrative* line of the nursing service organizational structure. These nurses would be responsible for carrying out whatever managerial functions require nursing knowledge —for example, supervising other nurses and ancillary workers, managing the physical environment of the nursing unit, and coordinating on the unit the pharmaceutical, nutritional, transportation, and other services which do not require professional personnel to have direct contact with patients. In contrast to those nurses who would provide direct professional nursing care, these nurses would be assigned to a specific time shift and work location—their names would appear on time and assignment sheets.

The picture of clinical nursing practice that emerges from the work of these and other nurse pioneers, instead of portraying tiresome chimeras, depicts a reality for the future of the nursing profession. Perhaps this picture will be an answer to the value of psychiatric integration projects in the present.

REFERENCES

1. Abdellah, Faye G., Irene L. Beland, Almeda Martin, and Ruth V. Matheney. *Patient-Centered Approaches to Nursing.* New York: The Macmillan Company, 1960.

2. Bridgman, Margaret. *Collegiate Education for Nursing.* New York: Russell Sage Foundation, 1953.

3. Campbell, Jean. *Masters Education in Nursing.* New York: National League for Nursing, 1964, 23, 37, 38, 42, 53, 54, 59, 78, 80.

4. Conant, James Bryant. *The Education of American Teachers.* New York: McGraw-Hill Book Company, Inc., 1963.

5. Dineen, Mary A. "A Nursing Major Without Nursing," *Nursing Outlook* (April, 1965).

6. Macdonald, Gwendoline. "Baccàlaureate Education for Graduate Diploma and Associate Degree Programs," *Nursing Outlook,* 52–56 (June, 1964).

7. Reiter, Frances. "The Improvement of Nursing Practice," *Improvement of Nursing Practice.* New York: American Nurses Association, 1961, pp. 3–11.

8. Sanford, Nevitt. "Higher Education as a Social Problem," in Nevitt Sanford (ed.), *The American College.* New York: John Wiley and Sons, Inc., 1962, pp. 10–30.

9. Simms, Laura L. "The Clinical Nursing Specialists: An Experiment," *Nursing Outlook,* 26–28 (August, 1965).

APPENDIXES

THE CURRICULUM PATTERNS

1957–1962

First Year. (The academic year is spent at the Skidmore College campus in Saratoga Springs.)

Academic Year		Credits
English 101, 102		6
Biology 103–104	Anatomy and Physiology	6
Biology 106	Microbiology	3
Chemistry 105–106		6
Psychology 201b		3
Sociology 101		3
Home economics 110		3
Physical Education		0

Second Year. (The academic year and an eight-week summer session are spent at the department of nursing in New York City.)

Academic Year		Credits
Nursing 101	Foundations in Nursing	12
Nursing 201–202–203	Growth and Development	3
Nursing 204	Medical, Surgical, Pediatric Nursing	9
Nursing 205	Medical, Surgical, Pediatric Nursing	8
Summer Session		
Nursing 206	Medical, Surgical, Pediatric Nursing	9

Third Year. (The academic year and an eight-week summer session are spent at the department of nursing in New York City.)

Academic Year		Credits
Nursing 301a, b, c	Communicable Disease and Long-Term Illness	3
Nursing 302a, b, c	Team Management	7
Nursing 303a, b, c	Neuro-Psychiatric Nursing	10
Nursing 305a, b, c	Obstetric Nursing	8

Summer Session
    Nursing 315   Public Health and Public
                                          Health Nursing   11

Fourth Year. (The academic year is spent at the Skidmore College campus in Sara-
        toga Springs.)

Academic Year   Credits
    Nursing 318   Professional Nursing   3
    Electives and
        Liberal Arts   27
    Physical Education   0

                                1963–1966

First Year. (The academic year is spent at the College in Saratoga Springs and an
        eight-week summer session at the department of nursing in New York
        City.)

Academic Year   Credits
    Biology 103–104   Anatomy and Physiology   6
    Biology 105   Microbiology   3
    Psychology 201b   3
    Liberal Arts Elective   3
    Sociology 101   3
    Chemistry 105–106   General Chemistry   6
    English 101, 102   Freshman Composition   6
    Physical Education   0

Summer Session

    Nursing 101S   Foundations in Nursing   6
    Nursing 103S   Pharmacology   1
    Nursing 105S   Nutrition   1

Second Year. (The academic year is spent at the department of nursing in New
        York City.)

Academic Year   Credits
    Nursing 105   Pharmacology   1
    Nursing 201a, b   Human Growth and Development   3
    Nursing 202   Epidemiology and Biostatistics   1
    Nursing 203a, b   Medical-Surgical Nursing 1   14
    Nursing 205a, b   Nursing of Mothers, Infants
                                and Children   11

Third Year. (The academic year and an eight-week summer session are spent at the department of nursing in New York City.)

Academic Year		Credits
Nursing 303a, b	Psychiatric Nursing	7
Nursing 305a, b	Medical-Surgical Nursing II	15
Nursing 307a, b	Public Health and Public Health Nursing	8

Summer Session		
Nursing 309S	Social Science	3
Nursing 317S	Independent Study in Nursing	3

Fourth Year. (The academic year is spent at the College in Saratoga Springs.)

Academic Year		Credits
Liberal Arts Electives		27
Nursing 317	Professional Nursing	3

INTERVIEW QUESTIONS

I. Faculty Attitudes and Experiences

Early in the fifth year of the project, the following questions were used by the psychiatric nurse in individual interviews with each of the faculty members. In addition to these data, socio-biographical information also was obtained.

1. Do you feel that the faculty members' religious beliefs influence the teaching-learning process? If so, how?
   Do you feel there is any relationship between the faculty members' religious beliefs, their attitudes toward psychiatry, and their responses to the psychiatric integration project?
2. What is your perception of the way the faculty view cultural and racial differences? Do you feel their view influences the selection of faculty members or the teaching-learning process? If so, how?
3. Do you feel that the personal aspect of a faculty member being single is reflected in any way in her nursing or teaching role or in the way she carries out her functions? If so, how?
4. Do you feel your experience or the lack of it in *public health nursing* has affected your teaching, your relationships with the faculty, or your responses to the psychiatric integration project? If so, how?
5. Do you feel your experience or the lack of it in *psychiatric nursing* has affected your teaching, your relationships with the faculty, or your responses to the psychiatric integration project? If so, how?
6. What is your perception of your own professional experience; how do you feel about the length of time you have been teaching? Does your experience add up to just "more experience," more tolerance, or more frustration?

II. Student Attitudes

Early in the fifth year of the project, the following questions were used by the psychiatric nurse in individual interviews with fourteen students in the sophomore, junior, and senior classes and with four members of the class that graduated in 1961. Selection of the students and graduates was based on two criteria: religious preference and status of relationships with men. The Protestant, Jewish, and Roman Catholic faiths as well as students who were married, engaged, "going steady," and "unattached" were equally represented.

1. Do you feel that the faculty members' religious beliefs influence the teaching-learning process? If so, how?
   What is your perception of the way the students view religious differences?
2. What is your perception of the way the faculty on campus and in the department of nursing view cultural and racial differences? Do you feel this view influences the selection of faculty members or students? If so, how?
   What is your perception of the way the students view cultural and racial differences?
3. What are your views about marriage vis-à-vis a career in nursing?
   How do you feel about the personal aspect of a faculty member in the department of nursing being single?
4. How would you describe the nature of the faculty-student relationships in the department of nursing?
   What do you perceive as the primary strengths and limitations in these relationships?
   How do you feel about the degree and quality of faculty guidance of students?
5. If you had to do it all over again, would you choose the Skidmore program in nursing? Give the reasons for your answer.
6. What are your future professional goals?
7. How do you feel about psychotherapy and how did you feel about it before coming into the clinical program in nursing?
   Have you ever considered psychotherapy for yourself?
8. What are your reactions to the psychiatric integration program?

III. Faculty Opinions about the Project

The following questions were used by the psychiatric nurse in her interviews with all of the faculty members at the beginning of the sixth year of the project. Approximately one and one-half to two hours were spent with each faculty member.

1. What are your general feelings about the psychiatric team being less available this past year? Did you work at psychiatric integration on your own?

2. Were there situations in which you or the rest of the faculty members took leadership but might not have done so if the psychiatric team had been available?

3. Did any concrete situations arise in which you or the rest of the faculty members wished that the psychiatric team were available?

4. Did the psychiatric team's decreased availability stimulate, inhibit, or have no effect on your own and the rest of the faculty members' activity in psychiatric integration?

5. What have you noticed emerging in relationships among the faculty during the psychiatric team's absence? How did the faculty meetings go without the psychiatric nurse? Do you feel that the faculty members have more, less, or the same degree of tolerance for each other's positive and negative contributions?

6. At this point in the project, how do you perceive the psychiatrist? The psychiatric nurse? The psychiatric nurse and the psychiatrist as a team?

7. Do you feel your knowledge and experience or lack of it in psychiatric nursing has influenced your response to the integration program? If so, how?

8. In view of the fact that the project is concerned with the integration of psychiatric concepts, which can be achieved through the faculty members' experiences with each other and the students as well as through their personal relationships, have you ever felt the need to have some psychotherapy? If so, what did you do about it?
   How do you feel about psychotherapy for students?
   Do you feel that any of the principles and processes of psychotherapy have any implications for the teaching-learning process?

9. From your review of some of the materials which quote some of the faculty's and students' responses to the psychiatric integration process, how do you feel about the particular focus of the book that is being prepared about the Skidmore project?

Appendix C

EXAMINATION QUESTIONS PREPARED BY THE PSYCHIATRIC TEAM FOR GENERAL EXAMINATIONS

I. Responses to One Question

The following question that was developed by the psychiatric team for general examinations was given to sophomore students during the years 1959, 1960, 1961, and 1962. Subsequent to the first use of the question, only items 4 and 5 were graded by the psychiatric nurse.

QUESTION

Patient Situation. Robert S., a twenty-eight-year-old single man, was admitted with the diagnosis of spontaneous pneumothorax. His four-week hospitalization was relatively uneventful. He was on complete bed rest until four days prior to discharge, when he was allowed up.

You are assigned to care for this patient. He is able to take his own bath; you give him back care and make his bed. While you are making his bed, the patient stands a short distance away, watching you work. As you look up, you observe that the patient has had an erection and is openly masturbating.

1. What are your initial and spontaneous reactions to the patient's behavior?

I would be completely shocked! Not so much at the fact what is being done as the situation of *where* it's being done—completely in the open and in plain sight of those around. I would be disgusted at the fact that the patient was doing this in front of me. One can understand this patient's situation of being hospitalized for four weeks and not having any chance to let some of his emotions out, but he should have learned in 28 years that this was not the time nor place. My embarrassment would be overwhelming.

My first reaction would be surprise that most likely would be mixed with fright about what to do, but not fear of physical attack. I think the actual situation would leave me devoid of any power to reason or without insight into what provoked his behavior. I would say now that his behavior was a way of his regaining his power—not the power of an erection—but the power to stand alone and be out of bed. This is his first chance to exhibit that he is able to stand on his own. I would also feel embarrassed that I had caught him in the act of masturbating.

My very first thought would be that of disgust. Then I would think, "Now calm yourself. You must pretend you haven't seen this. Don't let him know you know. Get the bed finished as soon as possible and leave the room until you can collect yourself. This guy must really have a problem." If the patient has realized that I have seen him, I would try not to let him know this has upset me. I imagine my reactions in their order of occurrence would be: shocked and I would stare a second longer; jerky movements such as turning my head back to making the bed as soon as I came to the realization of what I saw. I would hurry to finish making the bed without a word, all the time thinking what should be done. I would be very scared the whole time wondering what is going to happen. Is this man a sex maniac and is he going to attack me or what?

I imagine I would probably ignore the fact that I had seen it and retreat as quickly as possible out of the room after saying something like "you can get back into bed now," or "your bed is finished." In other words, I would probably deny the situation. Actually it is much too hard to anticipate what I would do, as I've never been faced with the situation.

2. What physical manifestations specific to you would be apt to accompany your reactions?

I would turn as red as my hair! My hands would get cold and clammy as they usually do when I'm in a tight situation. If I was talking at the time, I would surely stumble over my words. I can control my facial expressions, but that blush would give my feelings away.

I would sweat from nervous tension at seeing him do it. I don't think I would say anything, although, undoubtedly my movements would be halted in mid-air for a moment, before I could grasp what was going on. Then I would hastily look for something that needed to be done to divert my attention and to try to nullify the fact that I saw him doing this.

My physical manifestations probably would include a feeling of sudden intolerable warmth, clamminess of the hands, and perhaps a sensation of nausea. My eyes would probably open wide, as they inevitably do in every startling situation. My hands might be unsteady at first, although I might try my best to remain calm.

3. On impulse, how would you automatically handle the situation?

I would throw him a pillow to fluff up or hand him his towels to straighten on the bedside—anything to get him busy doing something. In actuality I would look for something at the immediate moment that would keep him preoccupied for a while and then when he finished with that task I would try to keep him busy with something else or ask him to help me with some of my chores or strike up a conversation with another patient that would involve him and which I could leave them together, alone.

I would undoubtedly ignore his actions, finish up as quickly as possible and get out of the room—probably preferring not to return.

On impulse, I'd probably continue on with my work and not pay any attention to it, since it is normal. In either case, I might start a conversation to get his attention on something else and to not transmit my uneasiness to him. In actuality, I'd probably act more calm than I was, and appear as though I saw this often (which I haven't) because after my first reaction I would be able to understand this is normal behavior and act more calmly.

I have two responses and either one would be on impulse. 1) My being shocked and disgusted almost to the point of being angry could force a "stop that" out of me. 2) My being embarrassed to the point of shyness could cause me to turn my back and finish making the bed and let the whole thing go unnoticed.

On impulse, I believe that I should tell the man that this kind of behavior should not be indulged in while others are present and would he please cease. If he ignored this I would leave the room and get a staff nurse to handle the situation. This is what I would do if I had enough reason left (after being shocked) and felt I was in enough control of my emotions to speak with him.

4. On further reflection and analysis, evaluate the above. In what respect was your handling of the situation appropriate and in what ways was it inappropriate? Why?

Neither of my reactions were appropriate. Being angry and telling him to stop would just cause attention to what he was doing. The fact that I noticed him and showed some emotions, even though of anger, may cause him more excitement. Ignoring the situation doesn't help matters since the patient will continue masturbating as long as he desires. It doesn't say much for the nurse either who will run from the situation just because it is unpleasant to her.

My whole avoidance of the situation (denial) would be completely inappropriate as it would communicate firstly to the patient that I was uneasy and did not approve of his action. It would say "you are bad" and "I don't want anything to do with your actions." Most certainly it would communicate a lack of understanding on my part.

My complete withdrawal and denial of the action (the patient must have noticed my awareness of the situation) would make any attempt to draw feelings out of patient impossible because by my previous actions I had communicated various disapproval. I doubt therefore if the patient would openly express his feelings. My own silence (would communicate more than words) and denial that this ever occurred, certainly would not allow the patient to express his feelings. My golly, if he was bothered enough to masturbate openly, then he should have some form of personal expression—talking with the understanding nurse, but my action merely cut off his expression to the nurse and undoubtedly made him feel extremely guilty of his own method of expression—masturbation.

I think I was a little embarrassed and inwardly ill at ease because I've not had this come up. I felt this way even though I realized it was normal. I think getting his mind on something else would be the best thing I could do, as I did in this situation. By not making an issue of the act, whether or not he knew that I had seen it, he will not be embarrassed or feel uncomfortable. Since it is a natural and reasonable situation, letting it pass and encouraging another train of thought seems best.

5. If you found yourself in a similar situation again, what would you see as an effective way of handling the patient's behavior?

I think I would use the diversion method if in a similar situation. Perhaps ask him to hand me the pillow or push the chair aside so I could get through. Anything to get his mind away from his emotions. If everything fails, I would tell him to stop, but not with emotion of anger as I did before. Also, giving him a chance to talk later on may help him with any inner feelings he may have.

I don't believe I do see an effective way of handling the predicament unless we were to have a discussion on this subject. Maybe this situation could be handled using a few pooled ideas, but I frankly, on the knowledge I now have, would be at a complete loss the first time this kind of thing happened to me. However, I seriously believe that the most effective way of dealing with this is to leave the room, at least for someone of my age as compared to him.

6. How do you feel about this nurse-patient situation as an examination question?

My first reaction was thinking "How ridiculous!," and one of resentment in having to put down my feelings on paper about this subject. As I began writing, most of these feelings disappeared. I do think, however, this subject would be better brought up in a group discussion and not so pinpointed to individual reactions as on this exam. The strain of the exam itself is difficult enough without a topic like this added to it.

I think it was a good idea to ask us what our reactions would be because I'm sure many of us have had experiences with boys who have an erection on the dance floor, for instance. However, I think that few of us are qualified to handle this situation tactfully for the first time.

I think it's rather impossible to answer this question because it is too hard to imagine myself in that position. What I would actually do I cannot say. It depends on where it occurred, who else was there, if it was the first meeting with the patient and so on. This is a better question for open discussion.

I think it is a good question. First of all, congratulations for telling us that only questions 4 and 5 are to be graded. By so doing, questions 1, 2, and 3 guided me to spontaneous actions and made it easier for me to get them down on paper without feeling guilty at saying something which might be wrong. Question 4 helped me to evaluate myself and question 5 helped me to rebuild my ego. The situation itself was good as an exam question as it was dramatic and something I feel many of us have strong feelings about. But by analyzing such a situation one can look at herself more objectively without being under the pressure of the social situation itself. I think it allowed a lot of room for much self-probing—and it also provided an opportunity to analyze the "rules of communication."

I feel that it is a good exam question, for this situation is reality. It could happen at any time to any one of us. You usually don't think of something like this until it actually happens or unless you see it on paper before you. I know I never really considered this fact until now. It's sort of a shock to see this situation sitting before you on an exam, but it is true and it does happen; I guess that's the reason why it presented a shock at first.

II. Other Questions Prepared by the Psychiatric Team for General Examinations

QUESTION A

Patient Situation. A married white woman of thirty-three years, married to a Filipino, was admitted to the Hospital. She complained of palpitation, nervousness, hot flushes, and shortness of breath. She stated that she had been well until three months ago, when, while at church, she had an attack in which she felt a tingling sensation all over and thought "she was going out of her mind." She had a sensation of heat and flushing of the upper chest, over the face and neck, and had an "all gone feeling inside." Extreme weakness and palpitation of the heart followed. She reported that her physician told her she had high blood pressure and kidney disease. She said "my kidneys are shot," and stated that her doctor gave her medicine, which however did not help her. Instead "nervousness and irritability" increased and, together with palpitation, were especially marked at the time of the menstrual period. She found it necessary to keep herself busy all the time in her household tasks in an effort to allay her nervousness and she developed certain compulsive tendencies, such as not being sure that she had accomplished a task satisfactorily and as a consequence doing it over and over again.

She stated that her previous health has been good but on close questioning admitted that she was not quite up to par just before this illness began three months ago. For about two years she had felt mentally depressed, had restricted her social life, had been increasingly irritable with the children and had been frigid in her sexual life. The menstrual history had been normal. She had had sighing respirations, which is what she meant when she said that she suffered from "shortness of breath." At times she had band-line headaches and occasionally felt as though her head was "clogged up." She was very sensitive and cried easily. Her weight had not changed. She was married at the age of nineteen to a Filipino which caused great consternation in this Irish family. She has two children, eleven and thirteen years old; both are well. Three years ago she had a spontaneous abortion at three months.

Her father, sixty, and mother, sixty-one, are both living. Both were born in Ireland. The mother has hypertension which was discovered about two years ago. The patient is the oldest of eight children, all of whom are married and in good health. The patient left the sixth grade of school to work in a large bakery where she held her position a long time and was regarded as a good worker.

On admission the blood pressure was 216/140 and there was a pronounced vasomotor flush over the front of the chest mounting up the neck and face. After admission this flushing was less marked and the blood pressure varied between 160 and 200 systolic and 100 to 120 diastolic. Eyeground examination showed rather pronounced angiospasm but no retinitis and this tended to diminish during the hospital stay so that there remained only moderate attenuation of the arterioles. This was interpreted as the preorganic phase of hypertension. All of the laboratory findings were negative.

The general physical examination disclosed no evidence of disease aside from the vasomotor flush, elevation of blood pressure and the overactive heart; the latter, however, seemed perfectly normal.

1. What kind of a life situation does the patient seem to be in? (Check one)
   _____ a. expanding and developing
   _____ b. at a plateau
   _____ c. downhill
   State in one sentence the reason for your choice.
2. Which of the patient's symptoms do you think are primarily of emotional origin?
   Which of the patient's symptoms do you think have both physiological and psychological elements?
3. What are some of the social and cultural stresses that have led up to the picture this patient presents?
4. How does the patient seem to function as a woman?
5. What does the patient's choice of language ("my kidneys are shot," "my head is clogged up," "going out of her mind," "all gone feeling inside") reveal about the patient?
6. What are the implications for the total nursing care of a patient who presents these emotional problems?

QUESTION B

1. Choose a patient with whom you have worked who showed any one of the following four reactions: anxiety, depression, withdrawal, or aggression.
Describe the behavior which led you to form this judgment.
Describe and evaluate your own feelings and responses to a specific situation in which this behavior was demonstrated.
What did you do in the situation?
2. Choose another patient who showed a different one of the above reactions than you chose in the first situation.
Describe a specific situation in which this manifestation of the patient's behavior had an effect on the other people on the clinical unit.
Describe the responses and reactions of others (nursing personnel, doctors, aides, other patients, members of the patient's family, etc.) to this behavior.

QUESTION C

Patient Situation. A single, white, twenty-year-old male was admitted to the hospital with the diagnosis of diabetes mellitus. He stated that he had an upper respiratory infection and noted 4+ spillage of sugar in his urine. He also developed a laceration of the right heel.

The patient was diagnosed as having diabetes four years ago. During the period prior to this hospitalization he was careless about his diet. He skipped meals and then ate sandwiches for dinner. He was working eight hours a day doing odd jobs, while at the same time attending numerous classes in prose-narrative writing at two different schools. He has ambitions of being a famous writer. He was sleeping between four and six hours a night. During this period, he adjusted his own insulin intake. In the hospital, his diabetes was difficult to control. He described himself as "a brittle diabetic" because "the amount of sugar I spill is affected by the slightest bit of anxiety."

The patient was brought up in the Orthodox Jewish religion. While in the hospital he declared himself to be an atheist and for a time was a member of an "off-beat" group in San Francisco. His father was born in Germany and his mother was born in this country. Both are now residing in California. His father was poor but worked himself up to a high income bracket and has his own business. The patient describes his family as "nouveau riche." The father wanted the patient to be a physician. The patient attended medical school for 1½ years in California, after which he dropped out and "came to New York to become a writer." He states his father is unsympathetic about his aspirations to be a writer and impatient with his way of life. He feels his mother encourages him.

1. Focus on the cultural, social and interpersonal concepts involved in "nouveau riche," Orthodox Judaism, emphasis on intellectual pursuits, and expand these as to the way they may relate to the patient's present mode of life.

The following is an extract from one of several short stories written by the patient in the hospital. He described it as "an exercise in imitating the style of Ernest Hemingway."

The Desert
I

"In the middle of the city is the desert."

We were playing cards, talking. Three men; we were smoking, and in our hands we held aces, kings, jacks; knights too.

"Did you say *in* the city? Right in the middle?"

"That's what I said: There was city to the north, city to the west, to the east and also to the south. From the squares and from the streets the winds blew."

"And it was desert?"

"Desert! It was rock and dust, with a clump of wormwood here and there; just so; and not water; and, sometimes, vultures."

"And lizards?"

"And lizards."

"And no lights at night?"

"No stars."

We look at each other. A card was thrown on the table. Another was thrown, another, and another. The fat one won.

"Well, was it very big?"

"Yes and no. Some thought so. Some did not. There were bones of animals scattered about. Skulls with horns."

"A real desert!"

"I've seen even the ruins of houses there."

"Human houses?"

"Human houses. With light bulbs and rooms and paint and self-glass."

"Self-glass?"

"Mirrors."

"Oh!"

"And how did you get there?"

"In a taxi. I took my luggage with me."

2. The patient gives this extract to you to read. In a few sentences give your reactions to it in terms of mood and central themes.
3. Suppose the patient asks you what you thought of this extract, tell exactly how you think you would handle the situation.
4. What do you learn about the patient from this extract? What are some of the generalized meanings?

INDEX

ABOUT THE AUTHOR

JANE A. SCHMAHL was born in Chicago, Illinois and had her undergraduate preparation at the Frances Payne Bolton School of Nursing, Western Reserve University. She received her baccalaureate and master's degree at Teachers College, Columbia University. She also is a graduate of the William Alanson White Institute of Psychiatry, Psychoanalysis, and Psychology, where she received the certificate for teachers in the psychology of interpersonal relations.

Her nursing experience has included work in public health and industrial nursing, medical nursing, and psychiatric nursing. Her career in teaching has been pursued at Seton Hall University, School of Nursing and Skidmore College, Department of Nursing, where, as the director of the psychiatric-mental health nursing integration project, she collected the data for this book. She was a member of the national planning committee of the National League for Nursing Basic Psychiatric Nursing Education Project, and she has been the chairman of the Interdivisional Council on Psychiatric and Mental Health Nursing of the New Jersey and Southern New York Leagues for Nursing.

Miss Schmahl is now on the faculty of the William Alanson White Institute, where she teaches psychiatric nursing and is a full-time doctoral student in the department of sociology at Rutgers—the State University of New Jersey, where she is working for the degree of doctor of philosophy.

Experiment in Change, which is Miss Schmahl's first book, presents a unique synthesis of the principles of nursing education and of learning, psychoanalytic, and sociological theory derived from her study of the process of professional change and growth.